# Reliability and Validity of Data Sources for Outcomes Research & Disease and Health Management Programs

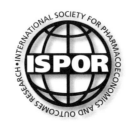

# Reliability and Validity of Data Sources for Outcomes Research & Disease and Health Management Programs

**Editor-in-Chief**
Dominick Esposito, PhD

**Assistant Editor**
Kristen Migliaccio-Walle, BS

**Managing Editor**
Elizabeth Molsen, RN

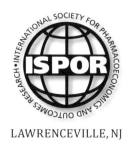

LAWRENCEVILLE, NJ

**Reliability and Validity of Data Sources for Outcomes Research
& Disease and Health Management Programs**

Published by
International Society for Pharmacoeconomics and Outcomes Research (ISPOR)
505 Lawrence Square Blvd. South
Lawrenceville, NJ 08648 USA
Tel: 1-609-586-4981 | Toll Free: 1-800-992-0643
Fax: 1-609-586-4982
Email: info@ispor.org | Website: www.ispor.org

© 2013 International Society for Pharmacoeconomics and Outcomes Research
All rights reserved.

No part of this publication may be reproduced, stored in a retrieval system, distributed, or transmitted in any form or by any means, such as photocopying, recording, electronic, mechanical, scanning, or otherwise, without the prior written permission of the publisher, except in the case of brief quotations embodied in critical reviews and certain other noncommercial uses permitted by copyright law. For permission requests, e-mail publications@ispor.org.

Every effort has been made in preparing this book to provide accurate and up-to-date information that is in accord with accepted standards and practice at the time of publication. Nevertheless, the authors, editors, and publisher can make no warranties that the information contained herein is totally free from error.

The mention of specific companies or certain manufacturers' products does not imply that they are endorsed or recommended by the International Society for Pharmacoeconomics and Outcomes Research or the authors. Citations to specific studies are included for informational purposes only, and should not be seen as an endorsement of study design, results, reference products, or any other information contained in the article cited.

No responsibility or legal liability are assumed by ISPOR, the editors, and the authors for any injury and/or damage to persons or property as a matter of products liability, negligence, or otherwise, or from any use or operation of any methods, products, instructions, or ideas contained in the material herein.

ISPOR and the ISPOR logo are trademarks of the International Society for Pharmacoeconomics and Outcomes Research.

Ordering information is available by calling ISPOR at 609-586-4981, or visit the ISPOR website at www.ispor.org.

Library of Congress Control Number 2012947209
ISBN 978-0-9743289-3-5

Printed in the United States of America.

# Contents

Section Editors . . . . . . . . . . . . . . . . . . . . . . . . . . . . . . . . . . . . . . . . . . . . . . . . . . . . vii
Contributors . . . . . . . . . . . . . . . . . . . . . . . . . . . . . . . . . . . . . . . . . . . . . . . . . . . . . . ix
Reviewers . . . . . . . . . . . . . . . . . . . . . . . . . . . . . . . . . . . . . . . . . . . . . . . . . . . . . . . xiii
Acknowledgements . . . . . . . . . . . . . . . . . . . . . . . . . . . . . . . . . . . . . . . . . . . . . . xv
About ISPOR . . . . . . . . . . . . . . . . . . . . . . . . . . . . . . . . . . . . . . . . . . . . . . . . . . . xvi
Introduction . . . . . . . . . . . . . . . . . . . . . . . . . . . . . . . . . . . . . . . . . . . . . . . . . . . . . . 1

## PART 1
## Claims Databases

**CHAPTER 1**  Administrative Claims Databases to Evaluate Health and Disease Management Programs . . . . . . . . . . . . . . . . . . . . . . . . 13

Renée J.G. Arnold, PharmD, RPh; and Iftekhar Kalsekar, PhD

**CHAPTER 2**  Characteristics of Claims Databases . . . . . . . . . . . . . . . . . . . . . . . 15

Iftekhar Kalsekar, PhD; Lisa Mucha, PhD;
and Sanjeev Balu, PhD, MBA, BPharm

**CHAPTER 3**  Scope of Claims Databases . . . . . . . . . . . . . . . . . . . . . . . . . . . . . . . . 28

Tao Fan, PhD, MS; Iftekhar Kalsekar, PhD; Sanjeev Balu, PhD, MBA, BPharm; Hans Petersen, MS; Bijal M. Shah, BPharm, PhD; and Mireya Diaz, PhD

**CHAPTER 4**  Using Claims to Guide Decision Making . . . . . . . . . . . . . . . . . . . . . 45

Heidi C. Waters, MS, MBA

**CHAPTER 5**  Retrospective Drug Utilization Review for Generating, Evaluating, and Benchmarking Health and Disease Management Data . . . . . 53

Mireya Diaz, PhD; and Bijal M. Shah, BPharm, PhD

## PART 2
## Electronic Health Records

**CHAPTER 6**  Introduction to Electronic Health Records . . . . . . . . . . . . . . . . . . 73

Ryung Suh, MD, MPP, MBA, MPH; Andrew B. Einhorn, MS;
Richard Hartman, PhD; Edward Kim, MD, MBA;
Jaspal Ahluwalia, MD, MPH; Carla Zema, PhD;
Sam Ho, MD; and Steven R. Simon, MD, MPH

*Contents*

CHAPTER 7  Uses of Electronic Health Records for Health
and Disease Management .................................. 84

    Andrew B. Einhorn, MS; Carla Zema, PhD; Steven R. Simon, MD, MPH;
Ryung Suh, MD, MPP, MBA, MPH; and Sam Ho, MD

CHAPTER 8  Strengths and Weaknesses of Using Electronic Health Records
for Health and Disease Management .......................... 98

    Carla Zema, PhD; Steven R. Simon, MD, MPH; Sam Ho, MD;
Edward Kim, MD, MBA; Jaspal Ahluwalia, MD, MPH; Andrew B.
Einhorn, MS; Farrokh Alemi, PhD; and Brent Gibson, MD, MPH, FACPM

CHAPTER 9  Electronic Health Record Implementation Challenges
at the Practice Level .................................... 107

    Rachel Shapiro, MPP

CHAPTER 10  Real-Time Applications of Electronic Health Record Data ..... 115

    Farrokh Alemi, PhD; Brent Gibson, MD, MPH, FACPM;
and Carla Zema, PhD

CHAPTER 11  Policy Maker Perspectives on Electronic Health Records ...... 122

    Ryung Suh, MD, MPP, MBA, MPH; Jason Ormsby, PhD, MBA, MHSA;
Sarah Johnson Katz, MS; and Brent Gibson, MD, MPH, FACPM

# PART 3
## Patient-Reported Outcomes

CHAPTER 12  Introduction to Patient-Reported Outcomes ................. 133

    Robin S. Turpin, PhD; and Heidi C. Waters, MS, MBA

CHAPTER 13  Patient-Reported Outcomes Instrument Design
and Development ....................................... 141

    Gergana Zlateva, PhD; Anandi V. Law, BPharm, PhD, FAACP, FAPhA;
and Elizabeth Molsen, RN

CHAPTER 14  Psychometric Methods for Patient-Reported
Outcomes Assessment .................................. 151

    I-Chan Huang, PhD, MSc; and Jane Speight, MSc, CPsychol, PhD,
AFBPsS

CHAPTER 15  Health-Related Quality of Life/Functional Status
and Health and Disease Management ...................... 172

    Anandi V. Law, BPharm, PhD, FAACP, FAPhA; I-Chan Huang, PhD, MSc;
and Jayashri Sankaranarayanan, MPharm, PhD

CHAPTER 16   Work Outcomes in Health and Disease Management .......... 188

Jayashri Sankaranarayanan, MPharm, PhD; Sue Jennings, MAEd, MPH, PhD; and Teresa Hartman, MLS

CHAPTER 17   Patient Satisfaction and Health and Disease Management ..... 206

Anandi V. Law, BPharm, PhD, FAACP, FAPhA; and Mark Bounthavong, PharmD

# PART 4
# Alternative, Population-Based Data Sources

CHAPTER 18   Introduction to Alternative, Population-Based Data Sources .. 223

Christopher R. Frei, PharmD, MSc

CHAPTER 19   Medical Expenditure Panel Survey Data from the Agency for Healthcare Research and Quality ............. 225

Jayashri Sankaranarayanan, MPharm, PhD; Mariam K. Hassan, BPharm, PhD; and Teresa Hartman, MLS

CHAPTER 20   Survey Data Sources from the National Center for Health Statistics ....................................... 239

Jayashri Sankaranarayanan, MPharm, PhD; Mariam K. Hassan, BPharm, PhD; Yaozhu J. Chen, MPA; and Teresa Hartman, MLS

CHAPTER 21   Healthcare Cost and Utilization Project (HCUP) .............. 255

Frank R. Ernst, RPh, PharmD, MS

CHAPTER 22   Medicare Databases ........................................ 281

Renée J.G. Arnold, PharmD, RPh; and Tammy G. Curtice, PharmD, MS, MBA

CHAPTER 23   Veterans Health Administration ............................ 290

Mariam K. Hassan, BPharm, PhD; and Dennis W. Raisch, RPh, PhD

CHAPTER 24   The Role of Patient Registries ............................... 298

Jayashri Sankaranarayanan, MPharm, PhD; Teresa Hartman, MLS; and William Crown, PhD

CHAPTER 25   Randomized Controlled Trial Data ........................... 315

Mariam K. Hassan, BPharm, PhD; and Jayashri Sankaranarayanan, MPharm, PhD

*Contents*

CHAPTER 26  Genetics Databases . . . . . . . . . . . . . . . . . . . . . . . . . . . . . . . . . . . . . 323

              Christopher R. Frei, PharmD, MSc; Russell T. Attridge, PharmD, MSc; and Bradi L. Frei, PharmD, MSc

# PART 5
## Statistical Approaches and Methods

CHAPTER 27  Introduction . . . . . . . . . . . . . . . . . . . . . . . . . . . . . . . . . . . . . . . . . . . 335

              Joel Hay, PhD

CHAPTER 28  Primary Data Types and How They Are Analyzed Statistically: *Demonstration Projects* . . . . . . . . . . . . . . . . . . . . . . . . . . . . . . . . . . . . 340

              Pedro Plans-Rubió, MD, PhD, MSc

CHAPTER 29  Primary Data Types and How They Are Analyzed Statistically: *Randomized Controlled Trials* . . . . . . . . . . . . . . . . . . . . . . . . . . . . . . 343

              Ashish Parekh, MS

CHAPTER 30  Primary Data Types and How They Are Analyzed Statistically: *Natural Experiments* . . . . . . . . . . . . . . . . . . . . . . . . . . . . . . . . . . . . . . 347

              Hans Petersen, MS

CHAPTER 31  Primary Data Types and How They Are Analyzed Statistically: *Prospective Designs* . . . . . . . . . . . . . . . . . . . . . . . . . . . . . . . . . . . . . . 350

              Pedro Plans-Rubió, MD, PhD, MSc

CHAPTER 32  Primary Data Types and How They Are Analyzed Statistically: *Retrospective Designs* . . . . . . . . . . . . . . . . . . . . . . . . . . . . . . . . . . . . 355

              Ashish Parekh, MS

CHAPTER 33  Statistical Methods for Randomized Controlled Trials: *Hypothesis Testing* . . . . . . . . . . . . . . . . . . . . . . . . . . . . . . . . . . . . . . . 360

              Pedro Plans-Rubió, MD, PhD, MSc; and Nalin Payakachat, BPharm, MSc, PhD

CHAPTER 34  Statistical Methods for Randomized Controlled Trials: *Discrete Outcomes* . . . . . . . . . . . . . . . . . . . . . . . . . . . . . . . . . . . . . . . 365

              Rahul Jain, PhD; and Joel Hay, PhD

CHAPTER 35  Statistical Methods for Randomized Controlled Trials: *Continuous Outcomes* . . . . . . . . . . . . . . . . . . . . . . . . . . . . . . . . . . . . 374

              Pedro Plans-Rubió, MD, PhD, MSc

| CHAPTER 36 | Statistical Methods for Randomized Controlled Trials: *Survival Analysis* .................................................. 381 |
|---|---|
| | Chenghui Li, PhD; and Qayyim Said, PhD |

| CHAPTER 37 | Statistical Methods for Randomized Controlled Trials: *Confounders* ...................................................... 388 |
|---|---|
| | Hans Petersen, MS |

| CHAPTER 38 | Statistical Methods for Randomized Controlled Trials: *Missing Data in Outcomes Research Studies* ................... 393 |
|---|---|
| | Roger Luo, PhD |

| CHAPTER 39 | Statistical Methods for Randomized Controlled Trials: *Sample Selection Bias Issues* ............................... 398 |
|---|---|
| | Joanna Campbell, PhD |

| CHAPTER 40 | Statistical Methods for Randomized Controlled Trials: *Propensity Scores* ............................................ 405 |
|---|---|
| | Hans Petersen, MS; and Joel Hay, PhD |

| CHAPTER 41 | Statistical Methods for Randomized Controlled Trials: *Instrumental Variables Methods* ........................... 409 |
|---|---|
| | Eberechukwu Onukwugha, PhD; and Emily S. Reese, MPH |

| CHAPTER 42 | Statistical Methods for Randomized Controlled Trials: *Heckman Selection Models* .................................. 415 |
|---|---|
| | Eberechukwu Onukwugha, PhD |

| CHAPTER 43 | Statistical Methods for Randomized Controlled Trials: *Bootstrap Method* ............................................ 419 |
|---|---|
| | Nalin Payakachat, BPharm, MSc, PhD |

| CHAPTER 44 | Statistical Methods for Randomized Controlled Trials: *Model Validation* ............................................ 423 |
|---|---|
| | Nalin Payakachat, BPharm, MSc, PhD |

| CHAPTER 45 | Statistical Methods for Randomized Controlled Trials: *Nonparametric Statistical Methods* ....................... 427 |
|---|---|
| | Joel Hay, PhD |

Acronym Reference List .................................................. 433

Index .................................................................. 441

# Section Editors

## Part 1: Claims Databases

**Renée J.G. Arnold, PharmD, RPh**, Principal, IMS Health, New York, New York, USA; Adjunct Associate Professor, Department of Preventive Medicine, Mount Sinai School of Medicine, New York, New York, USA; Adjunct Full Professor, Division of Social and Administrative Sciences, Arnold and Marie Schwartz College of Pharmacy, Long Island University, Brooklyn, New York, USA

**Iftekhar Kalsekar, PhD**, Director, Health Services, US Medical, Bristol-Myers Squibb, Plainsboro, New Jersey, USA

## Part 2: Electronic Health Records

**Ryung Suh, MD, MPP, MBA, MPH**, Associate Professor, Georgetown University, Washington, DC, USA

**Carla Zema, PhD**, Assistant Professor, Saint Vincent College, Latrobe, Pennsylvania, USA

## Part 3: Patient-Reported Outcomes

**Robin S. Turpin, PhD**, Senior Director and Global Lead, Health Economics and Outcomes Research, Baxter Healthcare, Deerfield, Illinois, USA

**Lisa Mucha, PhD**, Associate Director, Global Market Access, Primary Care Business Unit, Pfizer Inc., Collegeville, Pennsylvania, USA

**Anandi V. Law, BPharm, PhD, FAACP, FAPhA**, Professor and Chair, Pharmacy Practice and Administration, College of Pharmacy, Western University of Health Sciences, Pomona, California, USA

## Part 4: Alternative, Population-Based Data Sources

**Christopher R. Frei, PharmD, MSc**, Associate Professor, College of Pharmacy, University of Texas at Austin, Texas, USA; Adjunct Faculty, School of Medicine, University of Texas Health Science Center at San Antonio, Texas, USA

## Part 5: Statistical Approaches and Methods

**Joel Hay, PhD**, Professor, Pharmaceutical Economics and Policy, University of Southern California, Los Angeles, California, USA

# Contributors

**Jaspal Ahluwalia, MD, MPH**, Chief, Overseas Clinician Training, U.S. Army Medical Research Institute of Infectious Diseases, Fort Detrick, MD, USA

**Farrokh Alemi, PhD**, Professor, Georgetown University, Washington, DC, USA

**Renée J.G. Arnold, PharmD, RPh**, Principal, IMS Health, New York, NY, USA; Adjunct Associate Professor, Department of Preventive Medicine, Mount Sinai School of Medicine, New York, NY, USA; Adjunct Full Professor, Division of Social and Administrative Sciences, Arnold and Marie Schwartz College of Pharmacy, Long Island University, Brooklyn, NY, USA

**Russell T. Attridge, PharmD, MSc**, Assistant Professor, University of the Incarnate Word, Feik School of Pharmacy, San Antonio, TX, USA

**Sanjeev Balu, PhD, MBA, BPharm**, Director, U.S. Payer & Real World Evidence, AstraZeneca Pharmaceuticals, Wilmington, DE, USA

**Mark Bounthavong, PharmD**, Pharmacoeconomics Clinical Specialist, Veterans Affairs San Diego Health Care System and UCSD Skaggs School of Pharmacy and Pharmaceutical Sciences, San Diego, CA, USA

**Joanna Campbell, PhD**, Senior Manager, Health Economics and Outcomes Research, i3Innovus, Medford, MA, USA

**Yaozhu J. Chen, MPA**, Director, IMS Health, Alexandria, VA, USA

**William Crown, PhD**, Chief Scientific Officer, Optum Labs, Cambridge, MA, USA; Affiliate Faculty, Mongon Institute for Health Policy, Harvard University, Cambridge, MA, USA

**Tammy G. Curtice, PharmD, MS, MBA**, Regional Health Economics & Outcomes Research, Shire Development, LLC., Wayne, PA, USA

**Mireya Diaz, PhD**, Associate Scientist, Vattikuti Urology Institute, Henry Ford Hospital, Detroit, MI, USA

**Andrew B. Einhorn, MS**, Adjunct Instructor, Georgetown University, Washington, DC, USA

**Frank R. Ernst, RPh, PharmD, MS**, Principal, Premier Research Services, Premier Healthcare Alliance, Charlotte, NC, USA

**Tao Fan, PhD, MS**, Director, Global Health Outcomes, Merck & Co., Inc., Whitehouse Station, NJ, USA

**Bradi L. Frei, PharmD, MSc**, Associate Professor, University of the Incarnate Word, Feik School of Pharmacy, San Antonio, TX, USA; Clinical Pharmacist, Cancer Therapy & Research Center, University of Texas Health Science Center at San Antonio, San Antonio, TX, USA

**Christopher R. Frei, PharmD, MSc**, Associate Professor, University of Texas at

Austin, College of Pharmacy, Austin, TX, USA; Adjunct Faculty Member, University of Texas Health Science Center at San Antonio, School of Medicine, San Antonio, TX, USA

**Brent Gibson, MD, MPH, FACPM**, Vice President of Operations, National Commission on Correctional Health Care, Chicago, IL, USA

**Teresa Hartman, MLS**, Head of Education and Associate Professor, McGoogan Library of Medicine, University of Nebraska Medical Center, Omaha, NE, USA

**Richard Hartman, PhD**, Director, Policy and Forecasting, Veterans Health Administration, Washington, DC, USA

**Mariam K. Hassan, BPharm, PhD**, Director, Health Economics and Outcomes Research, Sunovion Pharmaceuticals, Inc., Marlborough, MA, USA

**Joel Hay, PhD**, Professor, Pharmaceutical Economics & Policy, University of Southern California, Los Angeles, CA, USA

**Sam Ho, MD**, Chief Clinical Officer, UnitedHealthcare, Cypress, CA, USA

**I-Chan Huang, PhD, MSc**, Associate Professor, Department of Health Outcomes and Policy, Department of Pediatrics and Institute for Child Health Policy, University of Florida, College of Medicine, Gainesville, FL, USA

**Rahul Jain, PhD**, Research Manager, HealthCore, Inc., Andover, MA, USA

**Sue Jennings, MAEd, MPH, PhD**, Consultant, Outcomes Measurement and Methodology Committee, DMAA: The Care Continuum Alliance, West Hills, CA USA

**Sarah Johnson Katz, MS**, Director of Development, Christ House, Washington, DC, USA

**Iftekhar Kalsekar, PhD**, Director, Health Services, U.S. Medical, Bristol-Myers Squibb, Plainsboro, NJ, USA

**Edward Kim, MD, MBA**, Clinical Indication Leader, Neurodegeneration Global Development, Novartis Pharmaceuticals Corporation, East Hanover, NJ, USA

**Anandi V. Law, BPharm, PhD, FAACP, FAPhA**, Professor and Chair, Pharmacy Practice and Administration, Western University of Health Sciences, College of Pharmacy, Pomona, CA, USA

**Chenghui Li, PhD**, Associate Professor, Division of Pharmaceutical Evaluation and Policy, University of Arkansas for Medical Sciences, College of Pharmacy, Little Rock, AR, USA

**Roger Luo, PhD**, Director, Advanced Analytics – Health Economics and Outcomes Research, IMS Health, Plymouth Meeting, PA, USA

**Elizabeth Molsen, RN**, Director, Scientific & Health Policy Initiatives, ISPOR, Lawrenceville, New Jersey, USA

**Lisa Mucha, PhD**, Associate Director, Global Market Access, Primary Care Business Unit, Pfizer, Inc., Collegeville, PA, USA

**Eberechukwu Onukwugha, PhD**, Assistant Professor, Department of Pharmaceutical Health Services Research, University of Maryland, School of Pharmacy, Baltimore, MD, USA

**Jason Ormsby, PhD, MBA, MHSA**, Senior Vice President and Chair of Health Quality and Information Technology Group, Atlas Research, Washington, DC, USA

*Contributors*

**Ashish Parekh, MS**, Candidate, Doctor of Pharmacy, Sullivan University, College of Pharmacy, Louisville, KY, USA

**Nalin Payakachat, BPharm, MSc, PhD**, Assistant Professor, Department of Pharmacy Practice, University of Arkansas for Medical Sciences, College of Pharmacy, Little Rock, Arkansas, USA

**Hans Petersen, MS**, Senior Research Associate, Lovelace Respiratory Research Institute, Albuquerque, NM, USA

**Pedro Plans-Rubió, MD, PhD, MSc**, Public Health Official, Health Registries, Public Health Agency, Health Department of Catalonia, Barcelona, Spain

**Dennis W. Raisch, RPh, PhD**, Professor and Chair, Pharmacoeconomics, Epidemiology, Pharmaceutical Policy and Outcomes Research, University of New Mexico, College of Pharmacy and Clinical Pharmacy Specialist, Veterans Affairs Cooperative Studies Program, Albuquerque, NM, USA

**Emily S. Reese, MPH**, Graduate Research Assistant, Department of Pharmaceutical Health Services Research, University of Maryland, School of Pharmacy, Baltimore, MD, USA

**Qayyim Said, PhD**, Assistant Professor, University of Arkansas for Medical Sciences, College of Pharmacy, Little Rock, AR, USA

**Jayashri Sankaranarayanan, MPharm, PhD**, Assistant Professor, Department of Pharmacy Practice, University of Nebraska Medical Center, College of Pharmacy, Omaha, NE, USA

**Bijal M. Shah, BPharm, PhD**, Associate Professor, Social Behavioral and Administrative Sciences, Touro University, College of Pharmacy, Vallejo, CA, USA

**Rachel Shapiro, MPP**, Researcher, Mathematica Policy Research, Inc., Princeton, NJ, USA

**Steven R. Simon, MD, MPH**, Associate Professor, Department of Medicine, Harvard Medical School, Boston, MA, USA; BWPO Physician, General Medicine and Primary Care, Brigham And Women's Hospital, Boston, MA, USA

**Jane Speight, MSc, CPsychol, PhD, AFBPsS**, Director, AHP Research, Ltd., Hornchurch, England, UK; Foundation Director, The Australian Centre for Behavioural Research in Diabetes and Director, Diabetes Australia Victoria, Melbourne, Australia; Chair, Behavioural and Social Research in Diabetes, Australia Centre for Mental Health and Wellbeing Research, Deakin University, School of Psychology, Burwood, Australia

**Ryung Suh, MD, MPP, MBA, MPH**, Associate Professor, Georgetown University, Washington, DC, USA

**Robin S. Turpin, PhD**, Senior Director and Global Lead, Health Economics and Outcomes Research, Baxter Healthcare, Deerfield, IL, USA

**Heidi C. Waters, MS, MBA**, Associate Director, Outcomes Management, Otsuka America Pharmaceutical, Inc., Princeton, NJ, USA

**Carla Zema, PhD**, Assistant Professor, Saint Vincent College, Latrobe, PA, USA

**Gergana Zlateva, PhD**, Senior Director and Group Leader, Global Market Access, Primary Care Business Unit, Pfizer, Inc., New York, NY, USA

# Reviewers

The authors and editors gratefully acknowledge the time, insight and expertise of the following ISPOR members who submitted chapter reviews:

| | |
|---|---|
| Patricia Alegre | Mary Gawlicki |
| Susan F. Anton | Amede Gogovor |
| Jorge Arellano | Amy Guo |
| Renee Arnold | William Hollingworth |
| Muhammad Aslam | Margaret Hux |
| Manu Bansal | Shrividya Iyer |
| Richard L. Barron | Carlos E. Izquierdo |
| Samir Bhattacharyya | Mark Jewell |
| Deepak Bhere | K. Ian Johnson |
| Sandy Blake | Sherif Kamal |
| Annemarie Braakman-Jansen | Carmen Kirkness |
| Johanita R. Burger | Maria Koltowska-Häggström |
| Tom Burke | Smita Kothari |
| John Byrd | Kathryn Lasch |
| Robyn Carson | William Lenderking |
| Liana D. Castel | Su-Ying Liang |
| Chih-Hung Chang | Marion Lindemann |
| Lee-Yee Chong | Yvonne Lis |
| Jason Cole | Miaomiao Liu |
| Karin Coyne | Xianchen Liu |
| Tuan Dinh | Andrew Lloyd |
| Cynthia Doucet | Barbara Marino |
| Gottfried Endel | Susan Mathias |
| Steven R. Erickson | Clare McGrath |
| Dominick Esposito | Lori D. McLeod |
| Emuella Flood | Richard W. Millard |

*Reviewers*

Kimberly L. Miller
Lesley Miller
Georgia Mitsi
Andrea Mraz
Rose E. Mullen
Anagha Nadkarni
April N. Naegeli
David Nerenz
Chima Ohuabunwo
Lukaso L. Onokoko
Jinhee Park
Nalin Payakachat
Gerson Peltz
Michael R. Pollock
Ghandi Pranav
Nazia Rashid
YongJoo Rhee
Annette Schmeding

Paul Scuffham
Kojiro Shimozuma
Iyer Shrividya
Meaghan St. Charles
Tara Symonds
Ebenezer Tetteh
Anthony Waka Udezi
Elizabeth Jisha Unni
Jill Van Den Boss
Vasudha Vats
F. Randy Vogenberg
Tarun Wadhwa
Michael Wang
Jeffrey T. White
Diane Wild
Gayle Wittenberg
Joanna Wu
Donald D. Yin

# Acknowledgements

The editor-in-chief would like to thank his wife and best friend, Andrea Mraz Esposito, for her support during the editing process and all his colleagues who were supportive of him taking on this endeavor.

The managing editor would like to thank Nadia Naaman, Randa Eldessouki, Rebecca Corey, and Marilyn Dix Smith for their support during this five year process, Maria Swift for her first-rate organizational assistance and contribution to finalizing the book, Eden McConnell for excellent proofreading suggestions, Steve Priori for his help with the publication, Susie Henkel for her graphic design wizardry on the striking cover design and promotional pieces, Bethann Carbone and the ExpressIt Media team for making the book a reality, and Kristin Migliaccio-Walle for coming through with superb editing when we really needed it.

Most of all, I would like to thank Dominick Esposito, Editor-in-Chief, for his tireless effort, exceptional writing and editorial skills, and unflagging sense of humor. All of the contributors and editors involved in this book owe him an enormous debt of gratitude. Without him, this book would not have been completed.

On a personal note, I want to thank my parents and grandmother for their love and support throughout my career and education and Adrian for his love, support and patience during the publication of 5 task force reports and 2 books.

# About ISPOR

Founded in 1995, the International Society for Pharmacoeconomics and Outcomes Research (ISPOR) is a nonprofit, international, educational, and scientific organization that facilitates the translation of outcomes research into useful information for health care decisions at all levels. ISPOR communicates health care information through several channels: its 3 journals, *Value in Health*, *Value in Health Regional Issues*, and *ISPOR CONNECTIONS*; annual meetings, congresses, and biennial regional conferences, as well as ISPOR's educational program that includes distance learning, short courses, and continuing education.

In addition, ISPOR provides tools for health care decision makers, educators, payers, researchers, students and patients. ISPOR has published more than 50 ISPOR Good Practices for Outcomes Research Reports, consensus guidelines on key outcomes research methods. The Society has also produced the ISPOR Research Digest, a searchable database of nearly 30,000 abstracts and presentations from ISPOR meetings; the ISPOR Global Health Care Systems Road Map; the International Digest of Databases; and web-based questionnaires on assessing evidence in observational, modeling and other types of research studies. All of these are available to the public on the ISPOR website (www.ispor.org).

ISPOR has over 7,000 active members from more than 100 countries around the world. In addition, ISPOR's 64 Regional Chapters expand ISPOR's reach to over 13,000 members.

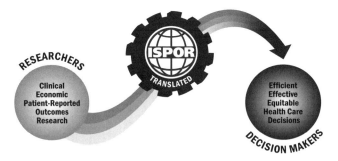

ISPOR promotes outcomes research
and its use in evidence-based health care decisions

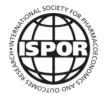

# Introduction

# Introduction

Chronic disease is a leading cause of death and disability and estimated to cost $1.3 trillion per year in treatment and lost productivity in the United States alone.[1-2] In response to the increasing prevalence of chronic illnesses and ever-rising health care costs, health and disease management (HDM) initiatives came to prominence in the 1990s as mechanisms to restructure health care. In an effort to standardize the term *disease management*, the American Heart Association generated a series of principles and recommendations which are best summarized as the use of evidence-based medical management for improving the quality of multidisciplinary care and patient outcomes.[3] Likewise, the Care Continuum Alliance (formerly, the Disease Management Association of America) defines disease management as "a system of coordinated health care interventions and communications for populations with conditions in which patient self-care efforts are significant."[4]

HDM programs promote patient-centered, integrated care with the goals of improving overall quality of care and reducing health care costs through the enhancement of patient wellness. These programs receive funding from a variety of sources, including the US federal government and individual state governments, large employers, and insurers. Although the concept of HDM is widely embraced, the nature and scope of programs vary broadly from small initiatives focused on a limited set of patients from a single payer group to widespread programs which include almost all chronically ill people across multiple payer groups. The smaller initiatives are typically directed by health care providers (either physicians, nurses, or other providers) and, sometimes, small-scale payers, and delivered within a primary care setting. Larger initiatives tend to address specific care processes or clinical outcomes and are usually offered by commercial for-profit vendors. These larger programs also commonly incorporate information systems for patient education and self-management that are marketed as a cost-containment strategy to employers and health insurers.

In their inception, HDM programs were small initiatives delivered in primary care settings; many of which still operate throughout the United States.[5-7] Such early programs focused on single conditions or diseases intended for improving patient education and medication adherence. As the idea of HDM became more widespread and the desire for health care cost containment took hold, HDM programs began to evolve into broader, population-based initiatives aimed at managing chronic conditions.[8] These programs further evolved to extend the scope to include the multifaceted care needs of people with comorbidities and multiple conditions.

## Motivation for this Book

The past decade has brought with it increasing scrutiny and requirements for accountability in the health care sector. As the demand for evidence to demonstrate the value of interventions that purport to improve health care outcomes and quality continues to emanate from stakeholders, the need for rigorous, independent evaluations of health care interventions will persist. Nevertheless, even small-scale HDM initiatives can be costly to implement thus the payers (large employers, insurers, federal and state government agencies) have a financial interest in generating evidence on the effectiveness of these programs and the comparative effectiveness of alternative approaches. Likewise, as the US federal government and private entities continue to invest in the infrastructure to conduct comparative effectiveness research in health care, the need and demand for valid and reliable data is greater than ever.

The primary mission of this volume is to provide a centralized source of information collating a variety of data sources and research methods used in HDM programs and their evaluations. It is a culmination of the efforts of many individuals motivated by the need for a comprehensive guide to improve the evidence base for HDM studies through rigorous research methods. Each section of this book addresses either critical data sources for HDM, key factors in the design of evaluation or data collection instruments, or both. In what follows, we provide a brief synopsis of the evidence base for HDM. Although this short discussion might become outdated as data become increasing available and stakeholders test new models of care for improving patient outcomes and reducing health care costs, the book itself can continue to be a resource to those stakeholders. Those who seek to understand how to demonstrate the reliability and validity of their data sources and the research methodologies used in conjunction with them will find the essential elements to do so in this volume.

## Evaluation of Health and Disease Management Initiatives

At the time of the writing of this book, evidence for the effectiveness of HDM initiatives is mixed. Although there are many peer-reviewed manuscripts that provide supporting claims that these initiatives improve specific patient outcomes, evidence of reduced health care costs is inconclusive or limited.[9-17] What is known about the impact of interventions to manage chronic disease(s) tends to be based on small studies that frequently focus on high-risk patients.[18-21] At best, the results from these studies have limited generalizability and should be interpreted with caution. Although transitional care models are supported by evidence from randomized controlled trials (RCTs),[22-26] telephonic HDM programs are generally not supported by such evidence.[27-31]

Large HDM initiatives sponsored by the federal government have not been successful at demonstrating the expected reductions in health care costs in the Medicare population. In the decade from 1999 to 2009, the Centers for Medicare and Medicaid Services (CMS) sponsored 7 disease management demonstrations involving about 300,000 beneficiaries across 35 programs, including provider-based, third-party, and hybrid models. Reducing costs sufficient to cover program fees proved particularly challenging. Final evaluations on 20 programs found 3 demonstrating evidence of quality improvement at or near budget neutrality when program fees are considered. Interim reporting on the remaining 15 programs covering at least 21 months of follow-up suggests that 4 are close to covering their fees.[12,32] For example, in one demonstration of 15 programs of coordinated care, only 3 interventions reduced overall health care costs and only 2 of those 3 were cost saving, primarily heart failure, coronary artery disease, and diabetes.[11,33]

In the world of clinical research, randomized controlled trials are the "gold standard" by which interventions are judged effective or ineffective. However, as previously noted, few large RCTs of HDM programs exist and much of the evidence for the effectiveness of these initiatives are in the form of secondary data analyses that compare outcomes of a treatment group to a nonexperimental comparison population. In addition, a systematic review of HDM initiatives in asthma, a common chronic illness, concluded that there were few rigorous evaluations of interventions and insufficient evidence to recommend any one program.[34]

## The Importance of Reliable and Valid Data

Establishing a counterfactual is a key analytic challenge for evaluations of HDM initiatives. Although random assignment of members of the eligible patient population to treatment and control groups is the preferred research design from the perspective of a clinical scientist, such a methodology frequently is not feasible or appropriate for HDM programs for reasons such as cost, ethical considerations, generalizability, and practical difficulties of ensuring accurate experimental design. As a consequence, HDM program participants are typically self-selected and have some underlying motivation or desire to participate in the program that is not captured or measurable. The bias that results from this self-selection has the consequence of potentially overstating the effectiveness of these programs.[35-36]

In the absence of an unbiased counterfactual, researchers should consider alternative comparison strategies to ensure findings of intervention effect(s) are only explained by the intervention and not other factors. However, as these strategies move further away from the RCT design, there are more threats to the validity of findings. Although evaluators can use statistical techniques such as regression discontinuity analysis or instrumental variable analysis to balance the treatment and comparison groups on observable characteristics after the fact, it is better to plan such analyses prospectively before a given intervention is implemented or evaluated. Moreover, in order to trust the veracity of claims made by operators of HDM initiatives, payers must first have faith that the data used to evaluate those claims are reliable and valid. Without such assurances, proof of program effectiveness is likely to be, in actuality, a biased assessment of the relative benefits and clinical outcomes of HDM interventions.

## Part 1. Claims Databases

The first section of this book provides a description of administrative health insurance claims databases and how they may be used for HDM. Although these data are primarily maintained for billing and other administrative purposes, they include a wealth of information on the utilization of a variety of health care services. Researchers use health care claims data regularly to examine the effectiveness of health care interventions in both prospective and retrospective studies.

This primer on administrative claims databases describes the basic characteristics of these datasets, identifies common sources of claims data used for research purposes, and summarizes key research design issues to consider when using these data. The section also describes some primary uses of claims data including informing HDM decision making through the identification of prevalent chronic medical conditions, gaps in quality of care, and variations in medical practice within a study population of interest. The last chapter of this section describes a process for comparing outcomes from a claims dataset (benchmarking) with the example of medication-use (or retrospective drug) review, one of many applications for health care claims data.

## Part 2. Electronic Health Records

The passage of the Health Information Technology for Economic and Clinical Health Act (HITECH) as part of the American Recovery and Reinvestment Act of 2009 represented a significant investment in health information technology (HIT) by the United States federal government.[37] A considerable portion of the funds allocated under HITECH support the widespread adoption of electronic health records (EHR) technology by health care providers. Because EHRs are likely to become much more prevalent, the second section of this book focuses on their use in evaluations of HDM programs.

The section begins with a description of EHRs and the evolution of paper medical records to electronic ones. In what follows, the roles of EHRs in HDM are reviewed, including specific uses of EHR data in research and health surveillance, and the strengths and weaknesses of using electronic data sources for HDM. As this section describes, the benefits include the standardized data, accurate diagnostic and procedural coding, technology-driven health applications, resulting enhanced opportunities for research analysis, and the detection of rare sentinel events. In addition, the same chapter delves into the EHR limitations, including difficulties accessing data stored on disparate systems and interoperability issues across disparate EHR systems.

To provide additional perspectives on the use of EHRs for research purposes, this section also includes chapters that examine EHR data from the provider and policy maker perspectives as well as examples of real-time applications of EHR data. Specifically, implementation challenges at the practice level are examined and barriers to adoption such as cost are reviewed. From the policy maker perspective, a number of national and international initiatives are discussed along with the role of policy makers in establishing EHR systems. Lastly, this section explores innovative approaches to EHR data management, such as the real-time monitoring of trends in disease and illness within a population, automated epidemiological systems, and enhanced reimbursement tracking.

## Part 3. Patient-Reported Outcomes

The measurement of patient-reported outcomes (PROs) or any report from patients about how they function in relation to a health condition or its therapy is an important component of HDM programs and their evaluation.[38] Because PROs can encompass a wide array of outcomes, including physical functioning, pain, psychological well-being, treatment adherence, and satisfaction, there are many issues to consider before incorporating them into HDM initiatives or including them as key outcomes in research studies. As such, the third section of this book defines PROs and their uses in HDM.

The section begins with 3 chapters on patient-reported outcome design. To start, the potential biases resulting from low or differential response rates to PRO instruments, challenges due to recall or social desirability, the issues of trust and confidentiality, and the influence of incentives on PRO data quality are presented. The second chapter describes PRO instrument design and validation with a focus on administration methods, linguistic validation, and approaches to standardization. The PRO design portion of the section is rounded out by a summary of psychometric methods and the issues which researchers should address when developing a new instrument.

The last 3 chapters of this section provide various applications of the use of PROs in health and disease management through descriptions of their utility to HDM programs and other stakeholders. First, well-known, validated health-related quality of life and functional status instruments are described, highlighting differences across them. Next, the use of PROs to measure work outcomes, absenteeism, presenteeism, and productivity is discussed. Lastly, the role of patient satisfaction measures in HDM is summarized and the relationship between satisfaction and health-related quality of life is highlighted.

## Part 4. Alternative, Population-Based Data Sources

The fourth section of the book presents alternative, population-based data sources not otherwise discussed in the preceding chapters and describes the potential uses of each one for HDM. These sources range from large public payer data and national surveys to more focused clinical registries. For example, the section begins with a description of data sources available from 2 of the largest payers in the United States—the Centers for Medicare & Medicaid (CMS) and the Veterans Health Administration. The section also describes nationally representative survey data which contain data from a variety of health care settings and are held by the Agency for Healthcare Research and Quality and Centers for Disease Control and Prevention (CDC).

*Introduction*

In addition to these data sources, this section includes a description of patient registries, focusing on those established to monitor product safety and measure comparative effectiveness of health care interventions. In addition to providing examples of existing registries, included is guidance for registry development and HDM applications of patient registry data. The final 2 chapters in this section describe the use of clinical trial data and genetic information from databases used to study the effectiveness of prescription medications through individualized medicine. The RCT chapter discusses the need for additional new outcome measures and debates the strengths and limitations of data obtained through RCT as compared to observational data. The genetics chapter highlights databases from the SNP Health Association Resource (SHARe), a major epidemiological genetics initiative by the US National Institutes of Health, and discusses current perspectives and future challenges for genetics databases that may be used for HDM.

## Part 5. Statistical Approaches and Methods

In the clinical research universe, RCTs are the gold standard by which interventions are judged safe and effective. However, as previously noted, very few large RCTs have been conducted of HDM programs and much of the evidence for the effectiveness of these initiatives is in the form of secondary data analyses that compare outcomes of a treatment group to a nonexperimental comparison population. As such, researchers and policy makers must be aware of the challenges in using and interpreting nonexperimental or observational data. Moreover, it is imperative that they be knowledgeable of potential solutions to improving the reliability and validity of conclusions drawn from these data.

The last section of this book provides a primer to understanding these issues by introducing study design options and statistical methods or approaches which address the limitations of secondary data analyses. The first part of this section describes various evaluation design methods such as natural experiments, prospective designs, and retrospective designs, and identifies their strengths and weaknesses. After this discussion, the section describes the statistical methods for evaluating outcomes of RCTs, including methods for examining discrete or continuous outcomes and time-to-event (survival) models. This part of the section also describes methodologies for dealing with missing data as well as hypothesis testing and confidence intervals.

The remainder of this section is devoted to the statistical estimation of outcomes in nonexperimental research studies. Given that such study designs are subject to a wide variety of threats to internal validity, they require more complex statistical analysis than those employed for RCTs. While no chapter in this section is intended to cover any of the statistical methods in detail, it will give readers interested in HDM evaluation an introduction to basic concepts. In particular, this section details methods for selection bias correction, including propensity score estimation and multivariable regression.

## References

1. Kung HC, Hoyert DL, Xu JQ, Murphy SL. Deaths: final data for 2005. National Vital Statistics Reports 2008;56(10). http://www.cdc.gov/nchs/data/nvsr/nvsr56/nvsr56_10.pdf. Published April 24, 2008. Accessed April 25, 2013.
2. DeVol R, Bedroussian A. *An Unhealthy America: The Economic Burden of Chronic Disease*. Santa Monica, CA: Milken Institute; 2007.
3. Krumholz HM, Currie PM, Riegel B, et al. A taxonomy for disease management. *Circulation*. 2006;114:1432-1445.
4. Care Continuum Alliance. http://www.carecontinuumalliance.org/dm_definition.asp. Accessed March 12, 2011.
5. Lorig KR, Ritter P, Stewart AL, et al. Chronic disease self-management program: 2-year health status and health care utilization outcomes. *Med Care*. 2001;39(11):1217-1223.
6. Malone R, Shilliday B, Ives TJ, Pignone M. Development and evolution of a primary care-based diabetes disease management program. *Clin Diabetes* 2007;25:31-35.
7. California HealthCare Foundation. Challenging the Status Quo in Chronic Disease Care: Seven Case Studies. http://www.chcf.org/publications/2006/09/challenging-the-status-quo-in-chronic-disease-care-seven-case-studies. Published September 2006. Accessed May 1, 2011.
8. Nolte E, McKee M, eds. *Caring for People With Chronic Conditions: A Health System Perspective*. Maidenhead, UK: Open University Press; 2008.
9. Powell Davies G, Williams AM, Larsen K, Perkins D, Roland M, Harris M. Coordinating primary health care: an analysis of the outcomes of a systematic review. *Med J Aust*. 2008;188(8 Suppl):S65–S68.
10. Mattke S, Seid M, Ma S. (2007). Evidence for the effect of disease management: is $1 billion a year a good investment? *Am J Manag Care*. 2007;13:670–676.
11. Peikes D, Chen A, Schore J, Brown R. Effects of care coordination on hospitalization, quality of care, and health care expenditures among Medicare beneficiaries: 15 randomized trials. *JAMA*. 2009;301(6):603-618.
12. Esposito D, Brown R, Chen A, Schore J, Shapiro R. Impacts of a disease management program for dually eligible beneficiaries. *Health Care Financ Rev*. 2008;30(1):27-45.
13. Peytremann-Bridevaux I, Staeger P, Bridevaux P, Ghali WA, Burnand B. Effectiveness of chronic obstructive pulmonary disease-management programs: systematic review and meta-analysis. *Am J Med*. 2008;121(5):433-443.
14. Thiebaud P, Demand M, Wolf SA, Alipuria LL, Ye Q, Gutierrez PR. Impact of disease management on utilization and adherence with drugs and tests: the case of diabetes treatment in the Florida: a Healthy State (FAHS) program. *Diabetes Care*. 2008;31(9):1717-1722.
15. Coberley C, Morrow G, McGinnis M, et al. Increased adherence to cardiac standards of care during participation in cardiac disease management programs. *Dis Manag*. 2008;11(2):111-118.
16. Morisky DE, Kominski GF, Afifi AA, Kotlerman JB. The effects of a disease management program on self-reported health behaviors and health outcomes: evidence from the "Florida: a healthy state (FAHS)" Medicaid program. *Health Educ Behav*. 2009;36(3):505-517.
17. Brennan T, Spettell C, Villagra V, et al. Disease management to promote blood pressure control among African Americans. *Popul Health Manag*. 2010;13(2):65-72.
18. Bodenheimer T, Wagner E, Grumbach K. Improving primary care for patients with chronic illness: the chronic care model, part 2. *JAMA*. 2002;288(15):1909–1914.
19. Weintraub A, Gregory D, Patel AR, et al. A multicenter randomized controlled evaluation of automated home monitoring and telephonic disease management in patients recently hospitalized for congestive heart failure: the SPANCHF II trial. *J Card Fail*. 2010;16(4):285-292.
20. Anderson DR, Christison-Lagay J, Villagra V, Liu H, Dziura J. Managing the space between visits: a randomized trial of disease management for diabetes in a community health center. *J Gen Intern Med*. 2010;25(10):1116-1122.
21. Carter EL, Nunlee-Bland G, Callender C. A patient-centric, provider-assisted diabetes telehealth self-management intervention for urban minorities. *Perspect Health Inf Manag*. 2011;8:1b.

*Introduction*

22. Coleman EA, Parry C, Chalmers S, and Min SJ. The care transitions intervention: results of a randomized controlled trial. *Arch Intern Med.* 2006;166(17):1822-1828.
23. Parry C, Min SJ, Chugh A, Chalmers S, Coleman EA. Further application of the care transitions intervention: results of a randomized controlled trial conducted in a fee-for-service setting. *Home Health Care Serv Q.* 2009;28(2-3):84-99.
24. Naylor MD, Brooten DA, Campbell RL, Maislin G, McCauley KM, Schwartz JS. Transitional care of older adults hospitalized with heart failure: a randomized, controlled trial. *J Am Geriatr Soc.* 2004;52(5):675-684.
25. Naylor MD, Brooten D, Campbell R, et al. Comprehensive discharge planning and home follow-up of hospitalized elders: a randomized clinical trial. *JAMA.* 1999;281(7):613-620.
26. Lorig KR, Sobel DS, Stewart AL, et al. Evidence suggesting that a chronic disease self-management program can improve health status while reducing utilization and costs: a randomized trial. *Med Care.* 1999;37(1):5-14.
27. Motheral BR. Telephone-based disease management: why it does not save money. *Am J Manag Care.* 2011;17(1):e10-e6.
28. Konstam V, Gregory D, Chen J, et al. Health-related quality of life in a multicenter randomized controlled comparison of telephonic disease management and automated home monitoring in patients recently hospitalized with heart failure: SPAN-CHF II trial. *J Card Fail.* 2011;17(2):151-157.
29. Rosenzweig JL, Taitel MS, Norman GK, Moore TJ, Turenne W, Tang P. Diabetes disease management in Medicare Advantage reduces hospitalizations and costs. *Am J Manag Care.* 2010;16(7):e157-e162.
30. Dall TM, Askarinam Wagner RC, Zhang Y, Yang W, Arday DR, Gantt CJ. Outcomes and lessons learned from evaluating TRICARE's disease management programs. *Am J Manag Care.* 2010;16(6):438-446.
31. Schwartz SM, Day B, Wildenhaus K, Silberman A, Wang C, Silberman J. The impact of an online disease management program on medical costs among health plan members. *Am J Health Promot.* 2010;25(2):126-133.
32. Bott DM, Kapp MC, Johnson LB, Magno LM. Disease management for chronically ill beneficiaries in traditional Medicare. *Health Aff* (Millwood). 2009;28(1):86-98.
33. Brown R, Peikes D, Chen A, Schore J. 15-site randomized trial of coordinated care in Medicare FFS. *Health Care Financ Rev.* 2008;30(1):5-25.
34. Maciejewski ML, Chen SY, Au DH. Adult asthma disease management: an analysis of studies, approaches, outcomes, and methods. *Respir Care.* 2009;54(7):878-886.
35. Buntin M, Jain A, Mattke S, Lurie N. Who gets disease management? *J Gen Intern Med.* 2009;24(5): 649-655.
36. Pazin-Filho A, Peitz P, Pianta T, et al. Heart failure disease management program experience in 4,545 heart failure admissions to a community hospital. *Am Heart J.* 2009;158(3):459-466.
37. Buntin MB, Jain SH, Blumnethal D. Health information technology: laying the infrastructure for national health reform. *Health Aff.* 2010;29(6):1214-1219.
38. Patrick DL, Burke LB, Powers JH, Scott JA, Rock EP, Dawisha S, O'Neill R, Kennedy DL. Patient reported outcomes to support medical product labeling claims: FDA perspective. *Value Health.* 2007;10(Suppl 2):125-137.

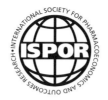

# PART 1

## Claims Databases

CHAPTER 1   Administrative Claims Databases to Evaluate Health
            and Disease Management Programs ........................................ 13

CHAPTER 2   Characteristics of Claims Databases ........................................ 15

CHAPTER 3   Scope of Claims Databases ........................................ 28

CHAPTER 4   Using Claims to Guide Decision Making ........................................ 45

CHAPTER 5   Retrospective Drug Utilization Review for Generating,
            Evaluating, and Benchmarking Health and Disease
            Management Data ........................................ 53

CHAPTER 1

# Administrative Claims Databases to Evaluate Health and Disease Management Programs

Renée J.G. Arnold, PharmD, RPh; and Iftekhar Kalsekar, PhD

This section discusses the use of administrative health insurance claims databases (medical and pharmacy) to evaluate health and disease management (HDM) programs. These data are well suited for the evaluation of HDM initiatives largely due to their longitudinal nature, enabling researchers, employers, insurers, and other stakeholders to assess how HDM interventions can, or have, affected health care utilization and other outcomes over time.

Health insurance claims databases are maintained primarily for billing and administrative purposes. They typically include information on the utilization of outpatient, inpatient, emergency room, and pharmacy services. Chapter 2 presents details on the characteristics of claims datasets and their components, including the use of terminology and diagnosis in addition to procedure codes for capturing specific services and events. The chapter also describes the common sources of claims data and issues to consider when evaluating HDM programs using these data.

Administrative claims data are an important source of information on processes of care. These data are useful for describing outcomes used to evaluate HDM programs such as health care utilization, patterns of care, medication adherence, and cost of care. Chapter 3 outlines the scope of claims databases and provides a practical approach to using these data for HDM program evaluation. The chapter focuses on ways to assess the potential impacts of HDM programs on health care outcomes. Issues of reliability and validity associated with the measurement of these outcomes are also addressed.

Researchers can use health care claims data to help guide decision making for HDM programs, such as identifying prevalent chronic conditions among members of a study population, gaps in quality of care, and variations in medical practice.[1] These issues are discussed in Chapter 4, including how to select a target population, identify outcomes of interest, determine if a comparator group is sufficiently similar to an intervention group, and measure costs. This chapter will also address the use of pay-for-performance incentives to improve patient outcomes.

Claims data are also used to compare health care outcomes to internal and external performance measures, a process known as *benchmarking*.[2] The systematic organization of claims data lends itself to comparisons of various measures, such as treatment patterns, typically examined in HDM programs. As described in Chapter 5, medication-use evaluation (also known as retrospective drug utilization review) is a mechanism for generating, evaluating and benchmarking HDM data. This process can identify gaps in HDM programs and provide insight into how a disease is treated in a real-world setting, allowing assumptions to be made regarding use or misuse of a medication within a defined patient population.[3] For example, if an employer has implemented a diabetes education program, then employee claims, such as the number of prescription drug fills indicated for diabetes or hospitalizations for diabetes-related complications, can be reviewed to determine the incidence and/or prevalence of diabetes and health care utilization among that employer's workforce.

Researchers may also use benchmarking to help determine where limited resources for HDM programs might be directed, investing in areas where clinical benefits and costs are relatively more certain. Moreover, benchmarking can identify patient populations for which HDM programs are more likely to be successful.[4] For example, Buntin and colleagues found that patients enrolled in a diabetes program differed significantly from those who did not in terms of their number of prescriptions per year and their A1C HEDIS scores.[4]

Although administrative claims databases are useful in the evaluation of HDM programs, there are also inherent biases related to using these data when employing nonexperimental methods to identify program impacts. Limitations, such as selection bias, must be addressed with statistical methods, such as propensity scores and multivariable regression.[5,6] These methods are detailed in Part 5: Statistical Approaches and Methods.

## References

1. Solz H, Gilbert K. Health claims data as a strategy and tool in disease management. *J Ambul Care Manage*. 2001;24(2):69-85.
2. DeLise DC, Leasure AR. Benchmarking: measuring the outcomes of evidence-based practice. *Outcomes Manag Nurs Pract*. 2001;5(2):70-74.
3. Eisenberg SS. Usefulness of database studies as applied to managed care. *J Manag Care Pharm*. 2005;11(1 suppl A):S9-S11.
4. Buntin MB, Jain AK, Mattke S, Lurie N. Who gets disease management? *J Gen Intern Med*. 2009;24(5):649-655.
5. D'Agostino RB Jr. Propensity score methods for bias reduction in the comparison of a treatment to a non-randomized control group. *Stat Med*. 1998;17(19):2265-2281.
6. Takemoto S, Arns W, Bunnapradist S, et al. Expanding the evidence base in transplantation: the complementary roles of randomized controlled trials and outcomes research. *Transplantation*. 2008;86(1):1-8.

CHAPTER 2

# Characteristics of Claims Databases

Iftekhar Kalsekar, PhD; Lisa Mucha, PhD;
and Sanjeev Balu, PhD, MBA, BPharm

---

This chapter describes the different components of claims datasets and the uses of various codes, such as International Classification of Diseases, Current Procedural Terminology (CPT), National Drug Classification (NDC), and Diagnosis-Related Group (DRG) codes, for identifying specific health care service use and events. The chapter provides a brief explanation of the claims submission process and the data commonly found in outpatient, inpatient, pharmacy, and demographic and eligibility files. The chapter also describes inpatient DRGs and those based on severity, the MS-DRG. Lastly, common commercial and noncommercial sources of claims data and issues (encountered with many types of datasets for example, missing data or coding issues) to consider when evaluating programs using claims data are also discussed.

## 1. The Claims Process

Health insurance administrative claims data are derived from claims forms that health care providers submit, usually electronically, to a payer when a patient utilizes services, including inpatient care, emergency room visits, or outpatient care such as physician visits, prescription drug fills, and laboratory or radiology tests. The payer then reviews the claim and, if accepted, processes the payment to the provider for services rendered. Researchers frequently use these data to conduct outcomes research (such as, an analysis of health care practice patterns or an epidemiologic study of disease progression), to predict the rate of adverse events in a patient population, to conduct formulary evaluation, or to supplement prospective datasets, among other uses. Such data are also potentially useful for the evaluation of health and disease management (HDM) programs.

Health insurance claims databases are maintained largely for billing and administrative purposes and not for research studies. Nevertheless, claims databases are useful for describing health care utilization, patterns of care, disease prevalence and incidence, drug and disease outcomes, medication adherence, and cost of care, among other outcomes. These datasets capture comprehensive health care utilization information for individuals and are often used for conducting research in the fields of epidemiology, health economics, and health services research. Claims data enable researchers to examine data from actual practice settings, and provide access to information on the health care used by large numbers of patients.

## 2. Components of Claims Databases

Administrative health care claims databases include many common components, also called files, although the specific details of any one database can vary from one source of claims data to another. The most common files in administrative claims data include patient demographic and health care claims files. To link information contained in one file to others, these databases include patient identification numbers in each file.

Patient demographic files help to characterize the patient population and include information, such as patient health insurance eligibility, date of birth, date of death, sex, race, and location of residence. Some demographic files may also include data on marital status, ethnicity, and type of health plan or insurance arrangement. Claims data for public health insurance programs, such as Medicaid and Medicare, might also indicate an individual's aid category or whether the person was enrolled in a waiver program or other health care demonstration program.

Health care claims files store information specific to processed claims for medical and pharmacy services. For each medical claim, the file typically contains fields such as a patient identification number, provider number, International Classification of Disease, Ninth Revision (ICD-9) codes of diagnosis for which the service was provided, CPT codes for procedures and services provided, DRG codes, dates of service, location of service (for example, outpatient, emergency room, or inpatient), total amount billed, and total amount paid. For pharmacy claims, files typically contain fields such as number of days' supply, metric quantity, NDC code, provider identification number, date of the prescription fill, total billed amount, and total amount paid.

When conducting research and evaluating the potential impact of HDM programs, it is important to understand how health care information from an outpatient setting, inpatient setting, or pharmacy is identified with the use of specific codes. The following provides a summary of each of these data components to offer insight into the appropriate use of these databases for evaluating HDM programs.

## Outpatient Claims

Outpatient files contain claims data submitted by institutional outpatient providers that primarily reflect services conducted during physician office visits or diagnostic and laboratory tests conducted in an outpatient setting. Outpatient claims provide information on these health care visits including the date of service, site of service, provider specialty, type of service (based on CPT codes), medical diagnosis (based on ICD-9 codes), total amount billed, and total amount paid.

### Medical Diagnosis

Each outpatient claim submitted by a provider includes medical diagnoses that identify the reason for the visit or encounter. These medical diagnoses are identified with ICD-9 codes that classify diseases and a variety of signs, symptoms, and external injuries, and are the international standard diagnostic classification for epidemiological health management and insurance purposes.[1,2] Most health conditions diagnosed by a health care provider are assigned to a unique category and provided an ICD-9 code. Each outpatient claim includes a primary diagnosis code (the primary reason for the claim or visit) and as many as 8 other diagnosis codes, depending on the source of the dataset. In late 2010, the diagnosis coding convention in use globally was the ICD-9 (ninth revision), which was originally published by the World Health Organization (WHO) in 1977.

The United States National Center for Health Statistics, jointly with the Council on Clinical Classifications, created an ICD-9 extension in 1979 to capture additional morbidity data referred to as ICD-9-CM where the *CM* stands for *Clinical Modification*. These codes make up the official system of assigning codes to various diagnoses and procedures associated with hospital utilization in the United States.[1,2] ICD-9-CM diagnosis codes are composed of 3 to 5 digits. Three-digit codes are headings of a category of codes that may be further subdivided by the use of fourth and/or fifth digits, which provide greater detail. Documentation about ICD-9-CM codes and a listing of codes are available from the Centers for Disease Control and Prevention (CDC).[3]

## Type of Service

CPT codes on outpatient claims identify the type of service or procedure performed during an outpatient visit. These codes describe medical, surgical, and diagnostic services, thereby providing a uniform data source and communication tool to health care providers, patients, and third parties. The American Medical Association (AMA) developed CPT codes in 1966. The fourth edition of CPT is used throughout the United States as the preferred system of coding and describing health care services.

There are 3 categories of CPT codes. Category I codes describe a procedure or service with 5 primary digits. For example, a code of 10060 indicates that a procedure involving "Incision and drainage of abscess" was performed. Category II codes are supplemental, alphanumeric tracking codes used for performance measurement consisting of 4 digits followed by the letter *F*. For example, the code 1220F indicates that a provider conducted a depression screen. Category III codes are temporary tracking codes for new and emerging technologies. For example, the code 0198T is assigned to "Measurement of ocular blood flow by repetitive intraocular pressure sampling, with interpretation and report." These codes are useful for data collection and the assessment of new technologies, services, and procedures.

## Date of Service

Each outpatient claim also includes the date on which a patient visits a hospital outpatient department or other outpatient clinic setting. This data element enables a researcher to identify when a particular service was used in relation to other services. However, a potential limitation of this data element is that the dates of visit could be coded incorrectly. Another related issue regarding capturing an accurate visit date is that claims data are usually organized around a billing event rather than an actual visit. This might lead to several visits being submitted on one claim, particularly from health care providers who provide repetitive services (for example, chiropractors or physical therapists). There might also be duplicate data if a second visit to the same health care provider occurred on the same day.

## Provider Information

Each outpatient claim includes identifying information for providers, usually in the form of a number that a researcher can link to a reference file to identify the provider rendering the service, his or her specialty, and licensing information. Providers can be physicians or other health care professionals, such as chiropractors, dentists, nurses, nurse practitioners, physical therapists, psychologists, or technicians. The reference file may also provide details about physician specialty.

Similar to issues with service date coding, provider information can lead to incorrect information about patient care if these data are documented incorrectly. This is especially significant when there are many provider categories to be coded. For example, on some claims, rather than being an individual, the provider might be a pathology or radiology laboratory or an outpatient clinic. However, as there are multiple claims generated for each outpatient visit, other claims for the visit may provide the needed information about provider specialty and type.

Analyses based on physician specialty, for example, are usually possible only for a subset of the entire research population. The type of codes used to identify physicians varies between datasets. In addition, use of the universal provider identification numbers (UPINs) to identify physician specialty must be viewed with caution in longitudinal analyses, as these numbers may be reused and assigned to different specialties. Identification of physicians becomes complex for studies that include data from year 2007 or earlier. At that time, UPIN codes were replaced by national provider identifiers (NPIs), so datasets may potentially have 2 different types of codes to identify physicians. Other potential physician identification numbers are license or DEA numbers, although these are usually in specialty datasets such as pharmacy-specific databases.

## Cost of or Charge for a Service

Outpatient claims typically include fields that identify an amount billed or an amount paid, which can be used to compute health care costs. The amount billed, or charged, does not necessarily reflect the amount the insurance company is contracted to cover, but may provide a more accurate measure of total resources used because charges, such as uncollected liability, bad debt, charitable care, discounting, and outpatient expenditures, are usually calculated based on amount paid. The amount paid, or reimbursed, by the insurance company for an outpatient service may depend on other factors that may not be available in the database, including patient cost-sharing requirements, such as deductibles, copayments, or coinsurance amounts.

Because the amount billed or the amount paid may not be standard across a variety of providers and payers, researchers may choose to ignore the amounts provided in claims data and use CPT codes to calculate expenditures. These codes are frequently used in conjunction with the Resource-Based Relative Value Scale (RBRVS) to determine the amount medical providers are paid. RBRVS assigns procedures provided by a physician a relative value that is adjusted by geographic region. This value is then multiplied by a fixed conversion factor (that is updated annually) to estimate the final payment amount. The RBRVS for each CPT code is usually estimated using 3 factors: physician work (physician time, mental effort, and technical skill, among others), practice expense (comprises the direct expenses related to supplies, nonphysician labor, and *pro rata* cost of the medical equipment used), and malpractice expense.

## Inpatient Claims

Administrative claims data for hospitalization episodes are valuable for assessing the incidence and frequency of hospitalization episodes and severity of episodes as measured by length of stay and costs. Inpatient claims data are also useful to assess the costs associated with a condition or disease in a population, aiding in the identification of patient populations for HDM programs. Each inpatient claim typically includes patient identifiers, provider identifiers, ICD-9-CM diagnosis codes, CPT codes, DRG codes, date of hospital admission, date of discharge, total amount billed, and total amount paid. Most variables in an inpatient dataset are similar to those in outpatient files, but rather than a date of service, inpatient claims have admission and discharge dates for each episode. In some databases, the type of services and procedures performed during hospitalizations are identified with ICD-9-CM procedure codes rather than CPT codes.

## Diagnosis-Related Groups

Diagnosis-Related Group (DRG) codes are groupings of hospital cases that are relatively similar in terms of clinical conditions and their impact on hospital resources.[4] Every hospitalization episode is assigned a DRG code based on the primary diagnosis, presence of comorbid conditions or complications, patient age, use of a surgical procedures, and patient discharge status (living or deceased).

Each DRG code has an associated relative weight that is used for the purpose of reimbursement under the prospective payment system.[5,6] A relative weight of 1 indicates that the hospitalization episode resulted in average resource consumption across all other episodes. The weights are multiplied by a hospital-specific, per case payment rate to arrive at the reimbursement rate. The hospital-specific, per case payment rate is designated for each hospital based on its teaching status, case-mix, size, the percentage of its patient population classified as indigent, and location. Based on these parameters, a blended rate is determined for each hospital for reimbursement purposes. Additional adjustments are made for hospitalization episodes that accrue substantially higher costs than the average costs for a specific DRG code.

In October 2007, the Centers for Medicare & Medicaid Services (CMS) adopted a severity-based DRG system called Medicare Severity DRG (MS-DRG) codes to provide a more accurate reflection of the patient's severity and medical condition. This system provides 745 severity-adjusted codes instead of the 538 codes in the original system.[7] A significant change in this version was to refine older DRG codes based on the presence of complications or comorbidities or major complications or comorbidities. For example, the DRG code for heart failure and shock was expanded into 3 different codes to accommodate the presence, or lack thereof, of complications or comorbidities.

DRG codes can be useful for studies that assess the cost of illness or a condition, or evaluate the impact of an HDM program on economic outcomes. With the aid of DRG codes and their relative weights, standardized methods can be used for computation of hospitalization costs in research studies. DRG codes can also be used to identify the exact clinical scenario of the hospitalization episode as the codes may provide more detailed information than ICD-9-CM or CPT codes alone.

## Pharmacy Claims

Prescription drug files contain information that is captured when a patient fills a prescription and results in a claim filed by a pharmacy. Similar to how the primary purpose of a medical claim is reimbursement, the primary focus of the pharmacy claim is the fill transaction. Thus, pharmacy claims identify that prescriptions were filled, but not that patients actually took the medications received. Although claims can serve as a proxy for compliance and adherence, primary data collection (for example, through a survey) could be used as an adjunct to determine if patients actually used the medications. The following describes specific data elements in a pharmacy claims dataset.

### Medication Information

Information on the drug dispensed is provided in the form of an NDC code which is a 10-digit number that uniquely identifies the specific agent that was dispensed. Some claims databases include an American Hospital Formulary Service number rather than an NDC code, but the latter is a universally accepted coding system used to identify medications found at the end of all drug labels.[†] Because each NDC code

---

[†] The United States Food and Drug Administration (FDA) maintains a website where researchers can search NDC codes: http://www.fda.gov/cder/ndc/database/default.htm.

is unique to each formulation of a medication, the code identifies whether the medication is a brand name or generic version, the primary drug ingredient, the drug dose, and the dosage form.

## Other Prescription Information

Other information on a pharmacy claim includes descriptors of the fill itself, such as the date of the fill and quantity supplied. Although days' supply is not included on the claim form, it is generally provided as an additional field in pharmacy claims data. Days' supply can also be calculated by dividing the quantity supplied by the dosing regimen for the drug. For example, if a prescription quantity was 90 pills for a drug to be used 3 times a day, the days' supply could be computed as 30 days' worth of medication. However, there are many agents with multiple dosing regimens, which make assignment of a specific regimen challenging. In these cases, the researcher should enlist the help of a clinical expert to assess which dosing schedule is the most commonly used.

## Provider Information

Other descriptors in pharmacy claims data are for the pharmacy provider and prescriber. Data on the pharmacy provider can be used to identify the type of pharmacy (such as mail order, chain, or independent) and its location. Information on the provider who wrote the prescription is similar to the physician information in outpatient claims; however, prescriber information might not be available in all pharmacy claims datasets.

## Cost Information

Pharmacy claims also include the amounts billed and paid. Often, both are present, but this will vary depending on the dataset being used. The amount paid is usually a percentage of the amount billed or is an absolute number after a copayment is made. In order to calculate the total cost of a fill, coinsurance and copayments should be added to the amount paid when this information is available.

## **Demographic and Eligibility Files**

Demographic and eligibility files contain much information that can be useful for research purposes. The patient demographic file contains information such as patient identifiers, sex, race, date of birth, date of death, and patient residential information. These files may also contain data on marital status, race/ethnicity, type of health plan, and aid category. Eligibility files enable researchers to determine when patients were enrolled in the plan or employed, and covered by payers. These files can be used to assure that the analysis identifies patients who were eligible during the study period of interest. As claims are reimbursed only during periods when a patient has health insurance eligibility, assessing eligibility information is critical to ensure comprehensive evaluation of health care utilization data.

For many research studies, selecting a population of patients who are continuously enrolled in their health plans allows for the comparison of a consistent cohort of patients across time. Thus, one can identify, in an HDM framework, changes in health care utilization in the same cohort of patients before and after an intervention. However, there are times when continuous enrollment criterion may be relaxed. For example, Medicaid beneficiaries tend to regularly enroll and disenroll from health insurance. In this case, an algorithm can be established, with clinician input, on the minimum amount of time—either in absolutes such as 6 months, or a percentage such as 50%—of the study time period that eligibility is required. Of course, the exact rule one might use will depend on the research question being addressed and the disease area being examined.

In disease areas in which the mortality rate may be high, a decision should be reached on when the absence of enrollment indicates a gap, death, or other reason. If the enrolled patient has no claims appearing from a specific time to the end of available data, the decision of how to designate the patient must be made. One of the limitations of enrollment data is that in a number of datasets, if patients switch plans or employers, they cannot be followed across the plans.

## 3. Sources of Claims Data

The source or sources of claims data included in any given database vary and depend primarily on the type of insurance that covers the patient population included in the database. In this section, we describe commercial and noncommercial sources of claims. Additionally, we highlight some issues with a particular noncommercial data source (Medicaid claims data) of which researchers should be aware when conducting research.

### Commercial Sources of Claims Data

Claims data from private insurers or employers are usually referred to as commercial claims and are typically deidentified for research purposes so that the identity of individual patients cannot be determined. These are large datasets that comprise claims from a single insurer, usually a managed care organization, or multiple insurers, which may include managed care or fee-for-service plans. Claims databases comprised of data from employers may also have data from single or multiple sources.

Single-sourced claims are typically derived from insured populations of employees of a large corporation. Multiple-sourced claims are derived from vendors that have pooled several employers' claims for research purposes. In employer-based files, there is customarily a field that allows identification of the type of plan, such as a fee-for-service plan or preferred provider organization (PPO) under which the employee was covered. This enables analyses that control for plan type.

## Noncommercial Sources of Claims Data

The most common noncommercial databases in the United States include health care utilization information of Medicare and Medicaid beneficiaries. The infrastructure of the Medicaid program, acquisition of these data, and some program-specific issues for data analysis will be discussed later. Additional information on the Medicare program can be found in Part 4 Alternative, Population-Based Data Sources.

## Medicaid

Medicaid is a federally sponsored health insurance program for low-income individuals, individuals with disabilities, and families with dependent children. While the federal government provides fiscal assistance and the basic framework of regulations, guidelines, and operation policies, state governments are responsible for administration of Medicaid programs. Benefits provided by Medicaid include coverage for physician visits, inpatient and outpatient hospitalizations, laboratory testing, nursing home care, family-planning services and supplies, and home health care. The federal government mandates these health care benefits. Optional services are left to the discretion of each state. Although optional, all states provide prescription drug coverage.[8]

## Utilization of Medicaid Claims Data for Research

Medicaid claims data have been used extensively for research purposes.[9, 10] These data can be obtained directly from the individual states or the Centers for Medicare & Medicaid Services (CMS) via the Medicaid Analytic eXtract (MAX) files. These data can be requested for a fee by specific states and/or by year. Assistance with these data is provided by the Research Data Assistance Center (ResDAC).[11] The CMS subjects the data that it receives from individual states to multiple reliability and validity checks.

MAX data contain elements that are similar to typical administrative claims data. The data are available in the following 5 files: (1) a personal summary file that contains demographic and eligibility information; (2) an inpatient file; (3) a prescription file; (4) a long-term care file that provides claims for services provided by long-term care facilities, such as nursing homes and intermediate care facilities; and (5) other therapy including outpatient physician office visits and associated diagnostic tests.

## Medicaid-Specific Issues

Because Medicaid data are overrepresentative of pregnant women, young children, and racial and ethnic minorities, it is useful as a data source to examine research questions or diseases of specific importance to these populations and also to examine research related to health disparities. However, studies that use these data might also have limited generalizability as they may not be representative of a national population.

Medicaid data are also useful to study diseases or conditions that have relatively higher prevalence in patients with conditions associated with low socioeconomic status, such as schizophrenia and HIV. The option of using data from multiple states also aids in conducting research on rare medical conditions. A challenge for researchers and practitioners in using Medicaid data is managing the potential incompleteness of data for specific populations. Health care utilization for enrollees not reimbursed by Medicaid in a traditional fee-for-service system may not be available in the dataset. For example, some state psychiatric hospitals do not bill Medicaid for expenses, but not having these data may lead to underestimates of health care utilization.

Researchers should also be cautious when working with the population of Medicaid-eligible who are enrolled in managed care. Depending on the source of the Medicaid data, claims are restricted only to enrollees in the traditional fee-for-service program. The same applies to beneficiaries dually enrolled in Medicaid and Medicare (dual eligibles) as their health care utilization reimbursed by Medicare is not available in Medicaid claims data. Researchers have the option of restricting the study to enrollees in a traditional fee-for-service system and those who are not eligible for Medicare. Another option is to obtain the additional claims information from Medicare (see Part 4) or specific managed care organizations to have access to comprehensive health care utilization data.

## 4. Limitations of Claims Data

Although there are many advantages to using medical claims data, researchers and practitioners should be aware of their limitations as well.

- *Lack of clinical information.* Clinical information, such as creatinine clearance rate, ejection fraction, blood pressure levels, blood glucose levels, or other diagnostic test results given during an outpatient visit or a hospitalization, is not available in claims data. However, studies have indicated that proxies generated from administrative claims data may be comparable to clinical data for predicting health outcomes.[12, 13]

- *Preexisting conditions or complications.* Most diagnosis codes listed on inpatient claims data are processed and entered at discharge and are classified as discharge diagnosis codes. As a result, it is difficult to discriminate between preexisting conditions and complications that develop during the hospitalization. Also, disparities have been found in the frequency and type of complications recorded in an administrative database compared to a detailed review of medical charts.[14, 15] Inpatient data also fail to document the rate and type of infections occurring during hospitalization.[16] To overcome this limitation, a clinical judgment can be made on the likelihood of a condition being comorbidity or a complication or by examining claims data prior to the hospital admission.

- *Potential coding issues.* Patient identification through ICD-9-CM diagnosis codes from claims data may suffer from errors in coding and documentation. Also, if databases use ICD-9 codes instead of the fully specified ICD-9-CM codes, there might be issues related to underestimation of the particular medical conditions. ICD-9 codes are less finely grained than 4- or 5-digit codes in accurately identifying a condition, thus the codes are sometimes not specific enough to characterize a patient's condition adequately.

- *Incomplete documentation.* In order for claims data to be useful for research purposes, such as estimating disease prevalence in a study population, providers must properly document patients' conditions. However, if such documentation is incomplete, the use of claims data might be limited. For example, individuals with elevated blood pressure or HbA1c levels might not have medical claims that indicate that they have hypertension or diabetes, respectively, underestimating their prevalence in a population. Because inpatient reimbursement is determined on DRGs, there are few incentives for hospitals to document all of the procedures and diagnostic testing performed during a hospital episode. Therefore, although these data are available in inpatient claims in CPT codes, there is a potential for undercoding for laboratory services and diagnostic tests. On the other hand, because all the codes in an administrative claims database are collected for reimbursement purposes, there is potential for up-coding to increase reimbursement.[17]

- *Lack of information on medications provided during hospitalizations.* Lack of information on medications provided during a hospitalization can lead to problems with misclassification of exposure and also prevent researchers from controlling adequately for confounders. If the hospitalization is long, this can also lead to an underestimate of drug utilization and adherence if they are provided in a hospital setting.

- *Comprehensiveness of drug utilization information.* Some types of medications, such as those delivered by infusion, may not be documented in all types of datasets. Specialty datasets, such as those found in system- or hospital-specific settings, may be sought out to obtain this information. Relatively inexpensive drugs (those less expensive than typical copayments) and over-the-counter (OTC) medications may not be documented in pharmacy data, highlighting a drawback of claims data in terms of their inability to capture services or benefits not covered by the insurer that generates the claims.

- *Correction/Duplication claims.* Use of claims to assess medication adherence can be complicated because of claims that are filed for purposes other than reimbursement of care. This problem applies to all types of health care claims, but is critical to address in pharmacy data, especially when it is used to calculate drug adherence. For example, correction claims may be filed after a prescription is filled. A pharmacy claim with a value in the quantity field that is less than zero might be an error or a correction claim used to adjust the quantity on an existing claim. By checking for duplicative dates, NDC codes and other information such as patient identifier, it may be possible to assess if it is an error (for example, if there is no match to existing claims) or a correction (if many fields match an existing claim). Duplicate claims can also be filed to correct text fields, such as a name change or correction of a misspelling on the original field.

- *Changes in NDC codes.* NDC code recycling may cause problems when analyzing prescription claims data. If the claims data include a number of consecutive years, it is possible that NDC codes for some medications change over time. Therefore, it is imperative that the drug dictionary be kept up to date and that each listed NDC code be kept date-sensitive as well.

# References

1. Centers for Disease Control and Prevention. Classifications of diseases, functioning and disability. Available at: http://www.cdc.gov/nchs/icd.htm. Accessed September 17, 2012.
2. Centers for Disease Control and Prevention. ICD-9 CM official guidelines for coding and reporting. Available at: http://www.cdc.gov/nchs/data/icd9/icd9cm_guidelines_2011.pdf. Accessed September 17, 2012.
3. Centers for Disease Control and Prevention. ICD-9 CM 2008 dataset. Available at: http://www.cdc.gov/nchs/icd/icd9cm.htm#ftp. Accessed September 17, 2012.
4. United States Congress, Office of Technology Assessment. Diagnosis Related Groups (DRGs) and the Medicare Program: Implications for Medical Technology. University of North Texas (UNT) Digital Library. http://digital.library.unt.edu/ark:/67531/metadc39505/. Accessed August 12, 2008.
5. Beaty L. A primer for understanding diagnosis-related groups and inpatient hospital reimbursement with nursing implications. *Crit Care Nurs Q*. 2005;28(4):360-369.
6. US Department of Health and Human Services, Centers for Medicare & Medicaid Services. Acute inpatient prospective payment system (PPS). Available at: http://www.cms.hhs.gov/AcuteInpatientPPS/. Accessed July 10, 2008.
7. US Department of Health and Human Services, Centers for Medicare & Medicaid Services. Medicare programs: changes to the hospital inpatient prospective payment systems and fiscal year 2008 rates. Available at: http://www.cms.hhs.gov/AcuteInpatientPPS/downloads/CMS-1533-FC.pdf. Accessed July 11, 2008.
8. US Department of Health and Human Services, Centers for Medicare & Medicaid Services. Medicaid. Available at: http://www.cms.hhs.gov/home/medicaid.asp. Accessed July 13, 2008.
9. Strom BL, ed. *Pharmacoepidemiology*. 4th ed. Hoboken, NJ: John Wiley & Sons, Inc.; 2005: 219-222.
10. Crystal S, Akincigil A, Bilder S, Walkup JT. Studying prescription drug use and outcomes with Medicaid claims data: strengths, limitations, and strategies. *Med Care*. 2007;45:S58-S65.
11. Research Data Assistance Center (ResDAC). Available at: http://www.resdac.umn.edu/. Accessed July 15, 2008.
12. Krumholz HM, Wang Y, Mattera JA, et al. An administrative claims model suitable for profiling hospital performance based on 30-day mortality rates among patients with an AMI. *Circulation*. 2006;113:1683-1692.

13. Landon B, Iezzoni LI, Ash AS, et al. Judging hospitals by severity adjusted-mortality rates: the case of CABG surgery. *Inquiry*. 1996;33(2):155-166.
14. Wray NP, Ashton CM, Kuykendall DH, Hollingsworth JC. Using administrative databases to evaluate the quality of medical care: a conceptual framework. *Soc Sci Med*. 1995;40(12): 1707-1715.
15. Iezzoni LI, Foley SM, Daley J, Hughes J, Fisher ES, Herin T. Comorbidities, complications, and coding bias: does the number of diagnosis codes matter in predicting in-hospital mortality? *JAMA*. 1992;267:2197-2203.
16. Massanari RM, Wilkerson K, Streed SA, Hierholzer WJ. Reliability of reporting nosocomial infections in the discharge abstract and implications for receipt of revenues under prospective reimbursement. *Am J Pub Health*. 1987;77:561-564.
17. Iezzoni LI. Using administrative diagnostic data to assess the quality of hospital care: pitfalls and potential of ICD-9-CM. *Int J Technol Assess Health Care*. 1990;6:272-281.

CHAPTER 3

# Scope of Claims Databases

Tao Fan, PhD, MS; Iftekhar Kalsekar, PhD; Sanjeev Balu, PhD, MBA, BPharm; Hans Petersen, MS; Bijal M. Shah, BPharm, PhD; and Mireya Diaz, PhD

This chapter describes the scope of claims databases and a practical approach to using claims databases for Health and Disease Management (HDM) program evaluation. It focuses on understanding how the methodologies used to assess the impact of HDM programs on outcomes, such as clinical events, medication adherence, and expenditures, constructed from claims databases affect the reliability and validity of these outcomes and how to address common challenges with claims data.

## 1. Assessment of the Validity and Reliability of Claims Data and Research Studies that Use These Data

Claims-based outcome measures are valuable tools for understanding patient behavior, the course of disease, and the costs and effectiveness of interventions. However, claims databases depend upon data generated by systems designed for other, often competing purposes (such as billing systems that ensure that providers are paid for services rendered), thus creating potential challenges when constructing outcomes from these data. The unique advantages and disadvantages of a particular database must be identified before constructing claims-based outcomes and interpreting findings.

In reviewing a study that uses administrative claims databases as a primary data source, it is important to assess whether or not the database is suitable for addressing the stated research question(s), and whether or not the investigators have used an appropriate methodology in reaching their conclusions. A Checklist for Retrospective Database Studies—Report of the ISPOR Task Force on Retrospective Databases is one guideline that researchers can use to evaluate the quality of published studies that use retrospective claims databases.[1] The checklist was developed for commonly used medical claims or encounter-based databases. However, it could also be used to assess studies that use other types of databases, such as disease registries and survey data.

An initial step in research involving claims data must be an assessment of the validity and reliability of the data source for the particular research question. However, even before this step, applying basic data integrity checks constitutes an accepted practice in the design, execution, and dissemination phases of a project.

Database validity consists of 2 components: internal and external validity. Internal validity is a measure of database integrity; it is a minimum, but not sufficient, requirement for either a retrospective study or its supporting database. A study's internal validity can be gauged by the extent to which bias and confounding factors have been reduced or eliminated, resulting in an expectation that the observed association between a treatment and outcome of interest is a valid measure of the true association. External validity refers to the extent to which a study's findings are extrapolated to other populations. External validity of a claims database is gauged by the extent to which the reports gathered from the data mirror the actual health care experiences of the patients they describe. Data reliability depends heavily on the particular application.

Data that are not valid in some aspects may still provide reliable answers to certain research questions. Nevertheless, some perfectly valid datasets may be inappropriate and, thus, unreliable. Again, prior to any assessment of validity and reliability specific to the study question, applying basic data integrity checks constitutes good practice.

## Reviewing Claims for Missing Data

When using a claims database to evaluate an HDM program, the data will typically arrive in the form of text files generated as a series of reports from a health plan billing system. Upon examining the file sizes, an investigator must determine whether or not these files are comparable between years. In other words, it is necessary to check the file sizes to ensure that there are not large differences in the volume of data represented from one year to the next. Assuming that there are not large disparities in file sizes between and across the available years of data, the next step is to ensure that there are no gaps in the dates and time periods represented. Finally, if the data represent multiple delivery sites (for example, hospitals or pharmacy locations), one must check that none of these is omitted.

## Reviewing Claims for Consistency

Once the researcher has decided that the data appear to be complete, it is useful to check for the presence of data anomalies such as evidence of male pregnancies; prostate exams performed on females; births for women aged 60 and older; and encounters with patients thought to be deceased. The presence of any of these may indicate a patient identifier mismatch or other problems such as shifting birth dates or genders changing over time, although each of these can have other plausible, patient-specific explanations. Identifier mismatch can occur for a number of reasons, but it is often the result of coding a dependent's health care charges under the guarantor's patient identifier. It is up to the researcher to determine the acceptable level of anomalies before proceeding with the analysis.

## Identifying Mortality

Basic demographics, including birth date, sex, and patient location of residence, are standard data included in claims databases. However, whether or not a member is living or deceased is not always available. The identification of a death record can be accomplished by linking a member's name to the National Death Index, but such a procedure is costly and might take several months to accomplish.

Even then, such links can provide only a snapshot of the deaths for the enrolled population at the time of submission. Although it may be tempting to rely solely on observed inpatient deaths, by definition these will be missing records of accidental or sudden deaths, as well as deaths that occur out-of-area or in hospice (unless captured). Hence, even for a simple mortality study based on claims data, the validity of such data is not readily ascertained.

## 2. Identification of Target Population for Health and Disease Management

When evaluating the impact of HDM interventions with administrative claims data, it is critical to identify the appropriate cohort of patients targeted by the interventions. A well-designed and successful evaluation of an HDM program should have had a clearly defined target population. With comprehensive inclusion and exclusion criteria, a target population can be selected using information contained in administrative databases.

### Identifying Target Population Based on Medical Conditions

Criteria used to identify patients vary extensively from one study to another, depending on the objectives of the HDM programs or investigations and characteristics of the therapeutic area. Identifying target populations can be achieved from administrative claims data, often among patients: (1) who are diagnosed with certain conditions, (2) who have a specific demographic profile, (3) who utilized certain health care resources, and/or (4) who received care under certain practice patterns. The identification from medical claims is accomplished by the use of codes indicating diagnoses (ICD-9 or -10), procedures (CPT), drugs (NDC), hospital revenue, or others. It is straightforward when a definitive diagnosis is possible, and the records for such events are complete and accurate, such as for major medical life events. However, identifying cases from claims databases is not always straightforward. In this regard, it is important to remember the underlying philosophy of claims coding. Codes are used to support medical necessity and, thus, the corresponding reimbursement for procedures performed and/or services rendered.

For claims records with multiple fields for diagnoses, the first or primary diagnosis is typically the underlying reason for the specific medical encounter. The secondary diagnoses complement the primary diagnosis to provide a more complete picture of the severity of illness and required intensity level of treatment in decreasing order of importance. Whether the target population is sought using the primary diagnosis only or both primary and secondary diagnoses only, or both will determine the degree of sensitivity and specificity of the cohort used for the condition in question. As a general rule, using more diagnoses (primary and secondary) for the condition of interest will increase the sensitivity of capturing these cases, but also will increase the number of false positives, thus reducing the specificity.

## Undiagnosed Conditions

Sometimes the objective of an HDM program is to improve the awareness of underdiagnosed diseases, such as atherosclerosis, hypertension, or osteoporosis among high-risk populations. Osteoporosis, for example, should be diagnosed with bone mineral density screening, an examination method that may not be readily available. Many patients may not even be aware that they have this condition and, as a result, no osteoporosis-related medical services or any medical claims would be available in their records. Therefore, it is not possible to identify these patients from claims data alone.

For other patients, diagnoses were made in the past, perhaps before these patients enrolled in the health plan or prior to the availability of data to researchers; therefore, individuals may be misclassified as free of disease. Sometimes patients are identified based on risk factors, which might also be a challenging task for claims-based patient identification. Many common risk factors, such as family history, behavioral risk factors, or dietary intake, will not be available in the databases. In these cases, claims data may not be a reliable source for these objectives and other methods, such as proxy measures, surveys and examinations, must be used to identify these patients who are eligible for an HDM program.[1]

## Uncertain Diagnosis

Identifying patients with diseases that lack clear-cut diagnostic criteria is challenging. For example, there are no standardized diagnostic criteria for asthma disease severity; thus, claims databases alone will not be a reliable source of identifying patients with severe asthma. Such a circumstance requires the HDM program to have a well-defined target population. Sometimes, patients must be examined and screened in person or a chart review may need to be undertaken. Before these steps are taken, an analysis of diagnosis codes and medications used in claims data may help narrow the population to be evaluated.

## Misleading Diagnoses

Diagnosis codes associated with an encounter record may represent either a condition with which the patient was diagnosed or a condition the provider wishes to rule out. Therefore, it is common to insist on evidence of multiple encounters on different days or of an inpatient admission with the associated diagnosis code of interest to establish the reliability of the identification algorithm. Such stringent requirements are sometimes further restricted to those patients who filled prescriptions for condition-associated drugs or who received condition-specific procedures.

## Up-coding of Diagnoses

Another problem with diagnosis information in claims data is the practice of *up-coding*,[2] or inflating the severity of a patient's condition. This practice is sometimes deliberate, but often may be a subconscious result of a health care system that has long reinforced the notion that it will reimburse most generously those providers who care for its sickest patients, and less so those who keep the healthier ones well. Obviously, such a practice, if widespread, will cause enrolled populations to appear in poorer health than they are, bias any resulting claims data analysis, and cause the HDM programs based on those analyses to become less reliable. Solutions to this problem, where they exist, involve complicated, clinician-guided algorithms to adjust for the potential bias.

## Coding Issues with Medications

National Drug Classification (NDC) code recycling is an additional coding issue that one might encounter with claims data. If the claims data represent a number of consecutive years, the NDC codes of some drugs might have changed over time. It is therefore imperative that a drug reference file be kept current and that each listed NDC code be kept date-sensitive as well. Other coding problems include an inability to capture new drugs, which are often classified under existing codes while they await assignment of their own, and difficulty in capturing cancer drugs and cancer *line of therapy*, typically administered via infusion in outpatient clinics often lacking unique associated Healthcare Common Procedure Coding System (HCPCS) codes.

## Prevalence and Incidence of Cases

*Prevalence* refers to the proportion of a population with evidence of a disease at a given time, while *incidence* refers to the proportion of the population that has newly developed the disease at a given time. Both the rates of prevalence and incidence are common targets of HDM programs, and they may be identified from claims data based on a variety of methods. For example, in a study validating an algorithm to identify patients with vertebral clinical fractures based on claims data, researchers were trying to identify incident and prevalent vertebral compression fractures (VCFs), which are often diagnosed with radiographs or other types of spine imaging in conjunction with a physician's clinical assessment.[3] Prevalent cases were defined as patients with an ICD-9 code indicating VCFs, given that the exact time of diagnosis was unknown, while incident cases were cases newly diagnosed with determinative spine imaging during the study period.[4]

Most administrative claims databases are unable to identify health care utilization or the health of a person before his or her period of enrollment in a health plan, making the identification of the first instance of a disease difficult. For example, in a study that assesses the impact of macrovascular cardiovascular diseases (CVD) on the medical expenditures of patients with type 2 diabetes mellitus, patients with CVD were identified by medical claims labeled with ICD-9 diagnosis codes during the study period.[4] However, based on claims data, researchers could not identify the duration of the CVD diagnosis, which affects evaluation of the disease progression and its impact on outcomes and medical costs.[5]

The prevalence of the target disease also affects the reliability and validity of HDM program evaluations. For highly prevalent conditions or procedures, it is more likely that a sufficient number of patients can be identified, providing a sample size large enough to evaluate the impact of programs or interventions reliably. However, for rare conditions or procedures, researchers may end up with a small number of patients from claims data, which makes it difficult or impossible to make a statistically reliable evaluation. Merging multiple claims databases or applying relaxed inclusion and exclusion criteria could increase the sample size, but may sacrifice the internal validity.

## Validity of Identification Algorithms

Crystal and colleagues[6] describe an intuitive method of examining the validity of algorithms to identify cohorts via diagnoses and procedures. Their method corresponds to the contingency table framework used for the performance assessment of screening and diagnostic tests. As such, it generates the corresponding true and false positives and negatives and, with them, measures of sensitivity, specificity, and positive and negative predictive values. Since this validation process is crucial to establishing the validity of claims-based analyses, there is a wealth of literature on the subject for many disease conditions, particularly prevalent ones. Although a thorough review of this literature is out of the scope of this chapter, we provide a brief synopsis and some examples to illustrate the process as well as interesting aspects the practitioner may want to consider.

The first step for these validation assessments is to define which source will serve as the gold standard against which the other source of information will be compared. For this purpose, it is customary to use medical records or disease registries. Using a disease registry has led to one of the most successful endeavors of claims-based outcomes research, that is, the linkage of the National Cancer Institute's Surveillance Epidemiology and End-Results (SEER) program registry with Medicare claims. One example study for which SEER data were used was conducted by Cooper and colleagues.[7] This work assessed the sensitivity of Medicare inpatient diagnoses and procedures and the incremental gain of outpatient claims in identifying 6 of the most common cancer sites among elderly patients (invasive breast, colorectal, endometrial, lung, pancreatic, and prostate) against the cases identified by the SEER registry during the years 1984 and 1993. In a subsequent study, the same researchers examined the concordance on treatment administered between the SEER files and Medicare claims for the same cohort of beneficiaries.[8] They found that the level of concordance between the 2 sources was high (85-90%) for procedures involving resection and radical surgery, but was low (≤50%) for biopsy or local excision.

Validation studies regarding identification of incident and prevalent cancer cases from claims have marked the potential complementary role of claims to registries in terms of identifying additional cases (especially those who have gone untreated or without a hospital admission), as well as other treatments not captured by the registry. With regard to identifying additional cases, Penberthy et al[9] examined the role of various case definitions to complement the detection of incident cancer cases by the Virginia Cancer Registry. They also examined the validity of the claims data against medical records in physician offices for a sample of patients. They evaluated the individual and combined roles of inpatient and outpatient claims in addition to the position where the cancer diagnosis appeared. The study suggests that one of the advantages of using an inpatient-only based approach, although not the most sensitive, is that it would be more practical to implement for tumor registries given the similarities between the reporting mechanism of the Medicare inpatient claims and the state's hospital discharge file.

Similar efforts of linking to a disease registry have also been attempted by other authors in the context of the Medicaid system for HIV-AIDS. Identifying HIV-AIDS cases through claims data highlights one of the major advantages of research based on Medicaid claims, that is, the ability to capture treatment based on prescription medications. Initial AIDS case-finding algorithms included ICD-9-CM codes for AIDS specifically, and for opportunistic conditions mimicking the 1993 CDC definition. The existence of highly specific medication, such as the antiretrovirals used for the management of AIDS, increases substantially the mechanisms by which these cases can be identified. To assess the effectiveness of the case-finding algorithms in claims databases that do not capture prescription claims, Walkup and colleagues[10] examined algorithms with and without medications.

## 3. Eligibility and Enrollment Data

Researchers use patient insurance eligibility and/or enrollment data to determine the appropriate research sample with which to evaluate an HDM intervention over a fixed observational period. These data are vital to the development of a valid and reliable evaluation because they identify the time intervals during which it can be assumed that the data representing all or most of the health care a given member received was faithfully captured by the health plan's billing system. Unfortunately, these data also are subject to errors, typically of omission, and should be cross-checked with other encounter and pharmacy data to ensure validity.

The primary challenge that enrollment data bring to patient identification is incomplete information. Events that can cause discontinuous medical claims include switching health insurance plans, loss of health insurance, changes of residence and changes of marital and employment status (for example, unemployment or retirement). The prior medical history of patients who switch in a relatively short time to a health plan is unknown. In addition, researchers are not able to identify patients diagnosed with certain target conditions before the person switches to another plan. Finally, these events may occur in another insurance plan after patients have switched to the new plan.

Missing data can have significant consequences for the reliability of a research sample chosen with claims data. For example, a missing or omitted termination date can cause a departed member to be counted among the denominator of all enrolled patients. One method for overcoming this problem and establishing enrollment status is to insist that at least one prescription is filled or one encounter with the health plan's delivery system is recorded per year. Even this practice though can have the undesirable effect of biasing the data of the newly designated enrolled population against that of its healthiest members by excluding them.

Another problem with enrollment data is that of dual coverage. Working couples sometimes have the option to receive care or fill prescriptions using their spouse's group health insurance rather than their own. In this case, the health plan's claims data appear to describe the complete health care experience for such members, but do not. Dual coverage is also observed among individuals in Medicare who have disabilities and whose incomes are below the poverty level, possibly qualifying them for benefits under Medicaid. Problems with dual coverage lie in the incomplete information in any single system's claims. Depending on the type of services, these may appear in one or the other. Dual coverage is an inherent bias in claims data that cannot be fully compensated for without access to additional plan data.

## 4. Episodes of Care

Administrative claims data are useful for identifying episodes of care for a number of chronic and acute medical conditions. An *episode of care* refers to the duration of time between the diagnosis and resolution of a medical condition.[11] Analyses based on episodes of care are appealing because this approach assists: (1) in measuring the appropriateness of services for the medical condition from a clinical perspective; (2) with managing the uncertainty accompanying differing patterns of coding; (3) with adjusting for case-mix; and (4) in evaluating costs and effectiveness within the same framework.[12]

The time horizon is a critical concept for economic analysis. However, the length of a clinically defined episode of care might be different from the economic definition of an episode of care.[13] An episode of care can be defined in a subjective way, in which expert opinion determines its duration. It can also be defined using empirical approaches, in which utilization can be measured and quantified. The latter is a definition most useful to the analysis of episodes of care using claims.

Previous studies have used average weekly charges and proportions of patients with charges to quantify the episode of care based on claims databases.[14] A variety of software programs have been developed based on the *grouper* approach to help identify the specific unit of care for individual patients with particular conditions. Grouper software is designed to use complex hierarchical logic to separate a large amount of group administrative data into episodes based on billing.[15]

## 5. Use of Claims Data for Medication Adherence Studies

Claims data are useful for studying patients' adherence to prescribed drug regimens. Effectiveness of medications at treating an illness depends on many factors, including patients' medication compliance and persistence. When the prescribed dosing regimen is deviated from and the patient becomes less adherent to his or her medication regimen, there are several risks of varying degrees to which a patient is exposed. These include altering the medication's efficacy, increasing the likelihood of greater morbidity or mortality, and increasing the overall costs to the health care system.[15-21] Assessment of medication compliance and persistence is critical to an appropriate understanding and accurate measurement of therapeutic effectiveness and cost-effectiveness.

### Compliance or Adherence and Persistence

Researchers typically refer to the terms *adherence*, *compliance* and *persistence* in a similar fashion. Medication compliance or adherence refers to "the act of conforming to the recommendations made by the provider with respect to timing, dosage, and frequency of medication taking."[18] Therefore, medication compliance may be defined as "the extent to which a patient acts in accordance with the prescribed interval and dose of a dosing regimen."[18]

The word *adherence* is preferred by many health care providers as the word *compliance* is perceived to be more passive in terms of a patient's behavior in following the provider's instructions. In contrast, *medication persistence* refers to whether or not a patient stays on the prescribed therapy and, thus, is time-sensitive.[15,17] Adherence rates are typically higher among acute medical conditions. Medication adherence can be calculated in several ways; however, the first methodology developed by Sclar and his colleagues that has become standard is the medication possession ratio (MPR).[7,8]

### Calculation of the Medication Possession Ratio

The medication possession ratio is defined or calculated as the sum of the days' supply of medication divided by the number of days between the initial fill and the last refill plus the days' supply of the last refill. Thus, this calculation includes 2 important variables that need to be identified from administrative claims databases: days' supply and the number of days between the initial prescription fill and the last refill that can be obtained from the specific database. For example, if the sum of days' supply for a particular medication for a patient identified from a database is 180 days and the number of days between the initial fill and the last refill plus the days' supply of the last refill is 360 days, then the medication possession ratio for this patient for this specific medication is 50%.

When the patient deviates from the prescribed regimen, the possession ratio calculation through the above procedure results in a ratio or percentage of less than 1.0 or 100%, respectively. However, there are instances when the patient refills early that might lead to MPR being greater than 1.0 or 100%. In such instances, the value is truncated to 1.0 or 100%, denoting full adherence. Additionally, the ratio can be calculated by dispensing the days' supply for the last prescription refill. Thus, the medication possession ratio in this instance would be defined as sum of days' supply divided by the number of days from the first dispense date to the date of the last prescription refill.

In the literature a medication possession ratio greater than or equal to 80% is often considered the cutoff for the determination of persistence. However, there is no consensus about this cutoff across therapeutic areas due to variations in characteristics of disease progression, medication use, symptoms, and patient populations.[18] For example, for symptom-associated treatments, such as arthritis or migraine, it is very challenging to differentiate from claims data alone the patients who stopped medication due to nonadherence or from relief of symptoms.

## Medication Possession Ratio Calculation Issues

The use of administrative claims databases to calculate the medication possession ratio has its own limitations and issues. The value obtained from administrative data for this ratio does not provide information on medication consumption; rather, it provides information on medication possession. Whether or not a patient actually ingests the medication is not identified. Moreover, when databases do not provide information on days' supply, the measurement of medication adherence using the medication possession ratio becomes somewhat cumbersome.[19] Identifying days' supply in an administrative claims database accurately and defining the number of days to classify or categorize a gap in therapy are 2 important issues to deal with in the calculation of this ratio.

### Accurately Identifying Days' Supply in Claims Data

The days' supply variable is available in most administrative claims databases on each prescription claim.[20] In instances when the days' supply field is missing, one can estimate days' supply by applying the defined daily dose to the quantity dispensed. In many cases, one cannot reliably depend on the values recorded under the days' supply field seen in most claims databases due to several issues such as errors in entering the right data or missing information. Thus, as a validation step, researchers should recalculate the days' supply by multiplying the daily dose of each medication by the quantity dispensed. However, accuracy of days' supply might be hampered by dosage form (for example, in medications such as ointments and creams) where a perceivable quantity is not available.[7] In addition, if the prescribed dosage varies during the length of the study period then multiple calculations might be required.[21] Other means of calculating days' supply are also available, including standard practice estimates for prescribed dosage assumptions; however, these methods are less accurate and reliable.[22]

## Determining Number of Days to Define Gap in Therapy

When calculating the medication possession ratio, once the target population has been identified and an analytic start date of the prescribed medication has been noted, an appropriate selection of gaps in therapy must be defined. This is critical in accurately estimating the medication possession ratio as not every patient refills prescriptions in a timely manner. The gaps in refilling prescriptions, also known as the *grace period*, depend on several unrelated factors, including medication half-life, clinical efficacy, dosage titration, or the source of refilling.[23]

The usual practice of selecting a grace period in calculating gaps in therapy is to base the decision on the number of days in the previous prescription's supply or 1.5 multiplied by the number of days' supply, as proposed by McCombs and colleagues.[24] For example, a retail medication with a days' supply of 30 days will have a grace period of 15 days. However, this strategy might be complicated to use, especially if the prescription is obtained through a mail-order pharmacy, where the usual days' supply is 90 days. In such cases, a permissible grace period of 45 days (half of 90 days) would be a long enough period to be assigned as an appropriate gap in therapy. Also, a fixed estimation of gap in therapy would lead to an already low-adherence rate (30 days/45 days = 66%).

There is no consensus in the published literature as to what should be considered an appropriate gap in therapy when calculating the medication possession ratio. This gap has varied from 15 days to 120 days if a fixed length of time independent of the days' supply of the previous refill is considered. When the gap in therapy is based on the previous refill's days' supply, then the gap has varied from one-half to 3 times the days' supply of the previous prescription refill.[25] One way to ensure robust analyses around an appropriate gap in therapy, depending on the therapeutic disease and the medication(s) used, would be to perform sensitivity analyses around different therapy gaps. This would enable a judgment on the effect of varying the therapy gap on adherence rates.

## 6. Economic Analysis and Cost-of-Illness Studies

Administrative claims data are an essential resource for conducting cost-of-illness studies, which are useful for assessing relative resource utilization associated with medical conditions or diseases and establishing cost-effectiveness of interventions. Estimating the cost of illness with specific disease states and conditions can also aid in identifying medical conditions that should, perhaps, be targeted for an HDM program.

Comprehensive cost-of-illness studies calculate the total direct and indirect costs associated with a medical condition.[26,27] Direct costs include medical expenses attributable to medications, hospitalizations, outpatient visits, other services, and nonmedical costs, such as the costs of transportation to health care providers. Indirect costs are those related to lost productivity due to morbidity and mortality. The type of costs to be included in a cost-of-illness study depends on the perspective of the analysis. Using the societal perspective requires us to include indirect, as well as direct, costs in the analysis, whereas using the payer perspective typically encompasses only direct costs.[28]

## Cost Attribution

A primary challenge in calculating cost of illness from administrative claims data is identifying the specific costs related to a medical condition. Although debatable, utilization of prescription medications can be attributed to a condition based on the clinical indication of the drugs. However, attribution of hospitalization episodes, nursing home costs, and outpatient visits can be complex as there are generally multiple diagnosis codes associated with these claims. The following strategies are used to identify specific costs attributable to a medical condition:

- The most straightforward option is to identify a sample of individuals with the specific medical condition and then calculate the total health care costs, irrespective of the type of diagnosis for specific claims or the type of medication used. This approach works well for conditions such as HIV/AIDS or cancer, where the costs related to the comorbid conditions are generally inconsequential compared to the primary condition itself. However, for other conditions that may not be as resource intensive, such as pneumonia or arthritis, or conditions with the presence of multiple comorbid conditions, such as depression, this method may result in overestimation of the cost of illness.

- Another option is to identify a sample of patients with the medical condition in question and sum up the costs related to all the claims with a primary diagnosis code for that condition. This method leads to conservative estimates as claims with the medical condition listed as a secondary diagnosis are not taken into consideration. This is especially important for conditions, such as diabetes, that not only directly promote resource utilization, but also add financial burden by being a major risk factor for cardiovascular complications. To account for this potential underestimation, cost of illness can be calculated by summing up the costs related to all the claims with primary or secondary diagnosis codes for the medical condition.

- Another approach used to identify the incremental costs that are attributable exclusively to a medical condition is through matching or regression.[22] This approach generally involves identifying a population with the condition in question and a comparison group of people without the condition. These 2 groups could be matched simply by demographic parameters, such as age and gender, or by multiple factors through the process of propensity matching. The additional cost in the group with the disease/condition could be attributable to the medical condition. Regression methods employ a similar procedure of identifying a group with the condition and a group without the condition.

In addition to the issue of appropriate allocation of resources to a medical condition, it is important to decide whether one computes prevalence- or incidence-based cost of illness. Prevalence-based cost of illness calculates the cost of illness in a patient population during a specific year, regardless of the duration of the disease or time since diagnosis. On the other hand, incidence-based cost of illness accounts for the duration of the disease. It provides estimates of the costs of a medical condition that estimate lifetime costs, measuring the costs of an illness from onset to conclusion for cases beginning within the study period. Incidence-based cost of illness is useful in tracking the cost of disease over time and is especially informative when studying diseases for which patients' costs vary over time.

From the perspective of identifying a patient population or a disease for implementation of an HDM program, it might be enough to know the prevalence-based cost of illness. However, if the HDM program incorporates prevention components, then the incidence-based cost-of-illness approach may be particularly useful to target conditions that have a high initial incidence cost.

## Challenges Associated with Duplicate, Zero Dollar and Charge-Based Claims

### Duplicate Claims

Determining the validity of claims data is critical to the accuracy of a cost-of-illness study. If multiple claims exist for the same service on the same day for a single patient, they need to be examined to identify duplicate claims. Claims may be valid if a patient is seen for a specific condition, and presents later in the day for the treatment of a new condition, or for worsening of the prior condition. In such cases, multiple claims may be generated for the same patient for the same service. These claims are usually valid and should be included in the analysis.

Multiple claims may also be generated when an edit is made to an existing claim as part of the coding/billing process. For example, updating the patient's address or age may result in the generation of a new claim for the same patient. Further examination of the duplicate claims must be conducted to identify claims that are meaningful and warrant inclusion in the analysis.

### Zero Dollar Claims

Zero dollar claims must be investigated before inclusion in any cost-of-illness analysis. Typically, such claims are those deemed ineligible for reimbursement by the payer.[25] However, these claims may also be noted in the patient out-of-pocket payment cost if the plan includes a preset threshold for patient copays. Until this threshold is reached, the payment field may represent a zero dollar value on a valid claim. Once the threshold is reached, the field will contain positive dollar values.

In addition, some health plans have zero dollar copays on some medications to encourage their use.

## Charge Data

Limitations inherent with cost information included in administrative claims data are well documented. Claims data typically include the amounts the health plan bills for reimbursement for services provided. However, claims data rarely include (a) the adjudicated reimbursement amounts or agreed-upon fraction of the billed amount, and (b) the actual cost to the health plan for the service. Complicated algorithms may be applied by researchers in an attempt to impute true costs for health care services and drugs. Such miscodings and charges lead to some of the most difficult problems one can encounter when working with claims data.

Since claims data exist as a byproduct of the billing system, an unavoidable artifact of this is the audit trail, that is, mistakes in the billing record being discovered, but not erased and corrected. Instead, they are compensated for and adjusted through the insertion of correcting records. This method satisfies the bottom line, but for the HDM program evaluator it creates a complexity of duplicate records and negative charges. To generate an accurate picture of the true services provided and the true costs, the researcher must resolve each of these duplicate records and attendant negative charges.

## Assessment of Costs over Time

Researchers typically conduct cost-of-illness studies using claims databases that extend across several years. However, because the cost of an item or service changes over time due to either inflation or a change in the availability of such resources, researchers must adjust their analyses to account for such changes. Two adjustment strategies include accounting for the differential timing of costs and annualization.

## Adjusting for the Differential Timing of Costs

When data on costs are estimated from different time periods, it becomes essential to account for the effects of inflation to allow for meaningful comparisons from year to year. In such cases, data are converted to a common time period, usually their current monetary value, before any comparisons are made. Data from past years can be adjusted to represent the current dollar value using the Consumer Price Index (CPI). However, since health care costs typically rise faster than the rate of inflation of other goods and services, the medical component of the CPI may be a more appropriate choice for making adjustments. The medical CPI inflation rate measures changes in the prices of medical care commodities and services and is available from the Bureau of Labor Statistics.

Similar to how cost estimates from previous years must be inflated to their present dollar values, cost projections for future years must be discounted to reflect their current dollar values. This practice refers to the time preference or time value associated with money. Most people would prefer to receive money now rather than later since future costs and benefits are worth less. Costs as well as benefits accrued in future years need to be discounted to their present value using a discount rate. Discounting is usually carried out using rates between 3% and 5%.[29,30]

## Annualization of Costs

The annual costs for each year of the program can be summed up to determine the overall costs for an HDM program or service. The overall cost is usually composed of program costs, which recur on an annual basis, and capital costs, which differ from year to year. In these situations, an equivalent annual cost can be obtained by an amortization or annualization procedure. For example, capital goods such as an X-ray machine may be purchased at the beginning of an HDM program, but will be useful for several years. However, the costs for capital items are reflected only in the early years when they were incurred. On the other hand, recurrent or variable program costs such as salaries or prescription drugs are reflected in each year's costs. To determine the equivalent annual costs, the capital and recurrent costs are combined in the annualization procedure.

There are 2 approaches to annualizing the cost of a capital item—the financial and the economic. In the financial approach, the annual cost can be determined by the straight line depreciation method. This method assumes that the services from the capital goods are uniformly divided over the useful life of the capital item. The current or replacement cost of the capital item is divided by its expected useful life to determine the annual (financial) costs.[31]

In the economic approach, to annualize the cost of a capital item, we need to know its replacement cost (or the original cost indexed to current dollars), the useful life of the item (to determine depreciation), the discount rate and the annuity factor. The useful life of capital goods, especially clinical equipment, is highly dependent on technological change. Choosing the appropriate discount rate is critical since it can influence the relative cost estimates. The annualization rate can be determined based on the discount rate and the useful life of the item in a standard table. The annual cost can then be determined by dividing the current value of the capital item by the annualization factor.

# References

1. Strom BL, ed. *Pharmacoepidemiology*. 4th ed. Hoboken, NJ: John Wiley and Sons; 2005.
2. Retchin SM, Ballard DJ. Commentary: establishing standards for the utility of administrative claims data. *Health Serv Res*. 1998;32(6):861-866.
3. Curtis JR, Mudano AS, Solomon DH, Xi J, Melton ME, Saag KG. Identification and validation of vertebral compression fractures using administrative claims data. *Med Care*. 2009;47:69-72.
4. Gandra SR, Lawrence LW, Parasuraman BM, Darin RM, Sherman JJ, Wall JL. Total and component health care costs in a non-Medicare HMO population of patients with and without type 2 diabetes and with and without macrovascular disease. *J Manag Care Pharm*. 2006;12:546-554.
5. Monane M, Matthias DM, Nagle BA, Kelly MA. Improving prescribing patterns for the elderly through an online drug utilization review intervention: a system linking the physician, pharmacist, and computer. *JAMA*. 1998;280:1249-1252.
6. Crystal S, Akincigil A, Bilder S, Walkup JT. Studying prescription drug use and outcomes with Medicaid claims data. *Med Care*. 2007;45(suppl 2):S58-S65.
7. Cooper SG, Yuan Z, Stange KC, Dennis LK, Amini SB, Rimm AA. The sensitivity of Medicare claims data for case ascertainment of six common cancers. *Med Care*. 1999;37:436-444.
8. Cooper SG, Yuan Z, Stange KC, Dennis LK, Amini SB, Rimm AA. Agreement of Medicare claims and tumor registry data for assessment of cancer-related treatment. *Med Care*. 2000;38:411-421.
9. Penberthy L, McClish D, Manning C, Retchin S, Smith T. The added value of claims for cancer surveillance: results of varying case definitions. *Med Care*. 2005;43:705-712.
10. Walkup JT, Wei W, Sambamoorthi U, Crystal S. Sensitivity of an AIDS case-finding algorithm: who are we missing? *Med Care*. 2004;42:756-763.
11. Rattray MC. Measuring healthcare resources using episodes of care. http://carevariance.com/images/Measuring_Healthcare_Resources.pdf. Accessed April, 2009.
12. Physician Advocacy Institute, Inc. Understanding Episodes of Care: An Educational Video for Physicians and Self-Study Continuing Education Course. Presented June 22, 2007. Chicago, IL http://www.ncmedsoc.org/non_members/pai/PAI-FinalWorkbookforVideo.pdf. Accessed October 20, 2012.
13. Shah BR, Laupacis A, Hux JE, Austin PC. Propensity score methods gave similar results to traditional regression modeling in observational studies: a systematic review. *J Clin Epidemiol*. 2005;58:550-559.
14. Schulman KA, Yabroff KR, Kong J, et al. A claims data approach to defining an episode of care. *Pharmacoepidemiol Drug Saf*. 2001;10:417-427.
15. Cramer JA, Roy A, Burrell A, et al. Medication compliance and persistence: terminology and definitions. *Value Health*. 2008;11:44-47.
16. Gerth WC. Compliance and persistence with newer antihypertensive agents. *Curr Hypertens Rep*. 2002;4:424-433.
17. ISPOR Medication Compliance Special Interest Group. Available at: http://www.ispor.org/sigs/medication.asp. Accessed July 12, 2008.
18. Andrade SE, Kahler KH, Frech F, Chan KA. Methods for evaluation of medication adherence and persistence using automated databases. *Pharmacoepidemiol Drug Saf*. 2006;15:565-574.
19. Cooper WO, Arbogast PG, Hickson GB, Daugherty JR, Ray WA. Gaps in enrollment from a Medicaid managed care program: effects on emergency department visits and hospitalizations for children with asthma. *Med Care*. 2005;43:718-725.
20. Peterson AM, Nau DP, Cramer JA, et al. A checklist for medication compliance and persistence studies using retrospective databases. *Value Health*. 2007;10:3-12.
21. Hess LM, Raebel MA, Conner DA, Malone DC. Measurement of adherence in pharmacy administrative databases: a proposal for standard definitions and preferred measures. *The Annals of Pharmacotherapy*. 2006;40:1280-1288.

**Part 1: Claims Databases**

22. Sikka R, Xia F, Aubert RE. Estimating medication persistency using administrative claims data. *Am J Manag Care*. 2005;11:449-457.
23. McCombs JS, Nichol MB, Newman CM, Sclar DA. The costs of interrupting antihypertensive drug therapy in a Medicaid population. *Med Care*. 1994;32:214-226.
24. Hodgson TA, Meiners MR. Cost-of-illness methodology: a guide to current practices and procedures. *Milbank Mem Fund Q Health Soc*. 1982;60:429-462.
25. Scitovsky AA. Estimating the direct cost of illness. *Milbank Mem Fund Q Health Soc*. 1982;60: 463-491.
26. Clabaugh G, Ward MM. Cost-of-illness studies in the United States: a systematic review of methodologies used for direct cost. *Value Health*. 2008;11:13-21.
27. Akobundu E, Ju J, Blatt L, Mullins CD. Cost-of-illness studies: a review of current methods. *Pharmacoeconomics*. 2006;24:869-890.
28. Kumar RN, Gupchup GV, Dodd MA, et al. Direct health care costs of 4 common skin ulcers in New Mexico Medicaid fee-for-service patients. *Adv Skin Wound Care*. 2004;17:143-149.
29. Gold M, Siegel J, Russell L, Weinstein M. *Cost-Effectiveness in Health and Medicine*. Oxford, UK: Oxford University Press; 1996.
30. Drummond M, Sculpher M, Torrance G, O'Brien B, Stoddart G. *Methods for the Economic Evaluation of Health Care Programmes*. Oxford, UK: Oxford University Press; 2005.
31. Walker D, Kumaranayake L. Allowing for differential timing in cost analyses: discounting and annualization. *Health Policy Plan*. 2002;17:112-118.

CHAPTER 4

# Using Claims to Guide Decision Making

Heidi C. Waters, MS, MBA

The era of health care reform in the early 21st century brought many changes to health care systems. One specific change is that health and disease management (HDM) programs are commonly offered by health plans and employers. Typically, these programs identify members with a particular disease and develop interventions to improve health. Interventions range from developing treatment guidelines to guiding care, to providing educational information to physicians or enrollees, and to monitoring enrolled members' health status.[1] These programs are not always intended to reduce costs. In fact, higher costs may be warranted if quality of care or clinical outcomes improve.[1]

For a successful HDM portfolio, health plans must decide how to target appropriate populations, track the interventions provided, monitor adherence to the programs, measure outcomes, and provide feedback to patients and providers.[2] This chapter provides guidance for this decision-making process. It discusses populations to target, how to identify outcomes of interest, how to incorporate a comparator group when evaluating the program, how to measure costs, how to evaluate program performance, and how to use pay-for-performance incentives to improve patient outcomes.

## 1. Decision Making in Health and Disease Management Programs

### Identifying Target Populations

An important decision that health plans considering an HDM program must make is how to identify a target population. Claims data are an important source of information when determining possible target populations as these data provide information on the incidence and prevalence of various diseases within a plan's enrolled population. These data also enable the researcher to stratify patients by demographic characteristics, such as age, gender or race, and to understand the risk factors and outcomes associated with specific disease states.[1,3]

In many HDM programs, eligible participants are chosen from all enrolled members based on evidence available in claims data as identified with ICD-9-CM codes. For example, in an HDM program that targets patients with congestive heart failure (CHF), an ICD-9 code of 428.xx can be used to identify eligible participants. However, using these diagnosis codes to choose eligible members may lead one to overestimate the size of the eligible population, as physicians often document patients' medical conditions based on a speculative diagnosis, or one to be ruled out, rather than one that has been confirmed.[4]

HDM programs are usually targeted at patients with chronic medical conditions who account for a disproportionate share of health care costs among a plan's population. When HDM programs are implemented without randomly assigning eligible patients to treatment and control groups, it may be difficult to determine whether the changes in clinical course, utilization, and cost are due to the HDM intervention, the natural disease course, or other factors.[4] HDM programs also may not have enough statistical power to assess program-related changes. Developers of HDM programs should identify the number of patients needed to ensure adequate statistical power during the program development stage so that meaningful statistical conclusions can be drawn at the end of the study.[4] The outcomes assessed and conclusions drawn should be clinically meaningful, as well, in order to determine which programs are most beneficial to patients.

Unfortunately, program administrators sometimes withdraw members from the analysis of program effects for a number of reasons such as death or a concurrent severe or costly illness that may confound the results. This results in a select subset of eligible members being evaluated, which further affects the validity of results unless identical criteria are applied in both the pre- and post-periods and to all comparator groups.

## Identifying Outcomes of Interest

It is not only imperative to identify the appropriate target population, but also to identify the appropriate outcomes on which researchers will evaluate the HDM program. Typically, outcomes fall into the following categories: process, clinical, utilization, financial return on investment, patient-reported outcomes, quality of care, and others that bring value to stakeholders involved, such as measures of productivity.[5]

Even when choosing appropriate outcomes for measurement, results can still be confusing. For example, in an analysis of clinical, cost, and quality outcomes of HDM programs in coronary artery disease, diabetes, asthma and heart failure, Fireman and colleagues[6] found that the percentage of patients receiving recommended tests and medications increased following implementation of the HDM program and patient costs rose for each of the 4 conditions during the study period after adjusting for age, sex, and inflation. In comparison, costs also increased (on a percentage basis) among adults without any of the 4 conditions.

While quality improved in terms of the percentage of patients receiving recommended tests and medications, costs increased. The levels and trends of quality and costs varied greatly across program sites with no systematic correlations. For example, there was no tendency for costs to increase less at medical centers where quality improved more. Nor did costs at the end of the study period tend to be lower at centers where quality indicators were higher. Thus, when making choices based on program evaluation results, it is necessary to distinguish which costs are attributable to the disease and which to the HDM program.

## Evaluating Effectiveness of Health and Disease Management Programs Using Claims Data

HDM programs should be evaluated to determine whether or not changes in the population are attributable to the designed intervention. If the program is shown to improve outcomes, it is useful to discern which components of the intervention are valuable and should be sustained.[6]

### Cost Measurement

Directly measuring the impact of HDM programs on health care costs is potentially difficult because factors such as reimbursement fees or member benefit design might change between the initial and follow-up measurement periods. Changes in cost may not be easy to identify and control for in an evaluation. If an evaluation of an HDM program utilizes the total population approach methodology, in which all eligible members are included in the analysis, then a concurrent control group must be used, in which costs are measured at the same points in time. The historical control design would be inadequate due to the time difference and potential cost differences between the measurement periods for each cohort.[7,8]

Researchers could use time series analysis to estimate the impact of an intervention on costs. Following each measurement period, a comparison of normalized aggregate costs to forecasted costs can be conducted to determine if the intervention resulted in monetary savings.[9] However, this method might also be subject to bias if the cost variables were measured differently from period to period, if inflation occurred and was not accounted for in the analysis, or if there is not a comparable control group.[7]

### Utilization Measurement

An alternate measure of cost outcomes would be resource use as a proxy for cost. Measurement of the utilization of resources such as hospitalization, ER visits, and physician visits would not be subject to the same level of variation over time as would costs.[4] When using control group designs such as the total population approach or historical controls, the utilization measures will reflect more accurately differences between the intervention cohort and the comparator group, since utilization is less susceptible to bias than cost over time.

If necessary, present day cost data may be applied to changes in the utilization of services to model estimated financial benefit of the program. Furthermore, increased knowledge about a disease, improvements in technology, changes in the health care delivery system, changes in payment structures, contracting cycles, physician fee schedule changes, coding practice modifications and other nonprogram factors might change utilization measures for patients with chronic illness.

When applying health care utilization measures to determine program success, one must take care to choose those measures that are directly associated with the intended impact of the intervention. When designing the intervention, it is important to make certain that the program has the potential to result in utilization improvements consistent with the claimed cost impact. Moreover, some increases, rather than decreases, in utilization may be logically expected as a result of the intervention.[7] For example, a program aimed at decreasing cardiac-related hospitalizations may result in an increased use of beta-blockers. The increased utilization of prescriptions would be offset by reduced inpatient utilization. These trade-offs must be taken into account during analysis as well.

## Pay for Performance

The number of pay-for-performance measures in HDM programs has grown exponentially. As of 2007, there were 148 different pay-for-performance programs in the United States that covered more than 55 million patients.[8] The purpose of these programs is to create incentives for providers to use a common set of quality measures that will ultimately improve patient care. Payment systems are then based on how physicians perform against the quality measures.[10] Pay-for-performance initiatives often focus on the underuse of therapies that are widely viewed as medically essential.

As with the other methods of assessing impact of HDM programs, the outcome measures chosen in pay-for-performance programs should be realistically achievable, clinically relevant, and readily measurable. The outcomes chosen should be meaningful to the different stakeholders, including health plans, physicians and patients.[10]

Clinical practice guidelines have been designed to define the best practices for more than 1,000 specific clinical situations. However, studies report that fewer than half of physicians actually use these guidelines in their practice.[11] One method of improving performance against guidelines is to implement pay-for-performance measures aimed at guideline adherence. Recent evidence from the National Committee for Quality Assurance (NCQA) revealed findings from a Medicare demonstration project that rewards Medicare Advantage health plans for improvements in member health under the Affordable Care Act of 2010 (ACA). Under this demonstration project, improvements in smoking cessation, adult body mass index assessment, colorectal cancer screening, and controlling high blood pressure were realized. Furthermore, health plans that participated in NCQA accreditation programs over time consistently performed at a higher level in a variety of performance measures than plans that did not participate.[12]

Provider profiling may improve the quality of care. Casalino and colleagues[13] determined that the presence of external incentives to improve quality of care was most strongly associated with use of care management programs. When all other variables, including other incentives, are held constant, physicians who were publicly recognized for scoring well on quality-of-care measures used 1.3 times more care management programs and physicians who received better contracts for scoring well used 0.74 times more care management programs than those who did not receive external incentives. Requiring physicians to report quality-of-care data and activities to outside organizations also was significantly associated with increased care management program use.[13]

A study by Costanti demonstrated that a program in which physicians who adopted an active care management approach was superior to clinical practice guidelines alone for improving quality and efficiency of care in hospitalized patients with congestive heart failure. Implementation of this program was associated with improvement in the use of recommended therapies and diagnostic studies, as well as with decreased resource utilization.[11]

A meta-analysis of HDM and provider programs indicated that of 24 programs that included provider education, improvement in provider adherence to guidelines was observed in 50% and disease control was improved in 38%. Of programs incorporating direct feedback to providers, provider adherence to guidelines improved by 56%, with 39% of all providers showing improvement in disease control. Those programs that incorporated provider reminders led to the largest improvement in provider adherence to guidelines (60%) and disease control (43%).[14]

## 2. Limitations of Claims Data for Evaluation of Health and Disease Management Programs

While claims data are extremely useful for informing decision making in HDM, there are important limitations that researchers and policy makers must consider. For HDM programs that use both electronic medical records and claims data for evaluation, there may be a lack of synchronization between the 2 systems. Changes in financial outcomes tracked through claims data would therefore appear lower, but would not be due necessarily to an improvement in clinical outcomes.[4] In addition, a plan may define enrollment by monthly increments rather than measuring incremental enrollment. If member turnover rates are high, incomplete matching of claim timeframes and month participation designations may change cost outcomes. A variety of data reviews should be built into the HDM program evaluation, where feasible, to avoid methodological errors with claims data analysis.[4]

While claims data can be used to measure changes in utilization and to estimate changes in cost, clinical outcomes of an HDM program cannot be ascertained from claims data. These databases often do not include clinical outcomes, laboratory test results, or patient quality-of-life data. In addition, most health system databases consist of data from discrete systems that are not easily compatible with one another. Modifying these datasets to obtain improved data is also time-consuming and costly.

In addition to the limitations due to the scope of the datasets, within chronic disease populations severity of illness is distributed among members. For example, those patients with greatest disease severity will typically remain at higher risk for increased morbidity in the future compared to those who are less severe at the same time. In general, those patients at the extreme ends of the severity spectrum will move further to the mean disease severity over time.[4] Thus, it may be difficult to assess if HDM programs have improved outcomes or the natural course of the disease has played a role. One study found that regression to the mean may account for 20% to 30% of the reduction in care costs in some HDM programs, and may be shown within 6 to 12 months of initiation of a program.[4]

The design of the HDM program itself may result in regression to the mean. Commonly, eligible patients are selected into the program based on claims during a certain period of time containing specific ICD-9 codes (for example, members hospitalized for cardiovascular disease during the past year). By definition, these members have more clinically active disease than those who have not been hospitalized during the same time period. Because hospitalization is chosen as the trigger event, the members selected to participate are less likely to be hospitalized during the measurement period than prior to it. Regression to the mean is particularly likely when the identification event is included in the baseline measurement.[4] Regression to the mean is a particular concern in pre-post studies when a comparison group is not randomly allocated. Such design issues should be considered to avoid the issues of statistical regression.

## 3. Ongoing Challenges and Future Directions

As health care becomes more expensive and a greater cost burden is shifted to employers and patients, the demand for proof of quality will increase. HDM programs must provide evidence that informs the choices confronting employers, patients, and clinicians. For clinical decisions, the programs' evidence should closely align with the sequence of decisions faced in the treatment of illness.[15]

There are still many challenges to building successful HDM programs. HDM programs may cause patient care to become more fragmented if the program directs patients to certain specialists who, in turn, do not communicate with the patients' primary care doctors.[16] Furthermore, there is a lack of standardization among managed care plans on standards of practice, and this can lead to confusion during implementation. Physicians participating in multiple programs must attempt to remember the rules, protocols, benefit coverage, procedures, paperwork, and compensation levels for the different programs, which may affect outcomes and patient care.[16]

HDM programs have traditionally focused on a small number of high-cost diseases. However, there are many other diseases that could benefit from standardized HDM. Expanding the numbers and types of conditions for which programs exist may result in either greater-than-expected savings or just more administrative burden on providers.[16] Systems that will enable physicians and managed care plans to track outcomes over longer periods of time should continue to be implemented, but these must be correctly evaluated to determine if they are effective. This will enable outcomes and health status data to be reliable enough to support conclusions showing desired results from HDM programs. Unfortunately the cost to integrate data may be large, and the startup costs of programs can be a barrier to implementation.[16]

One of the greatest opportunities for HDM is a shift in focus from managing care to managing health.[17] To shift focus from disease management to disease prevention, at-risk members would need to be easily identified and programs would be designed to intervene before the disease process took hold. Achieving this can be difficult because of the lack of data that can be correlated to early disease detection for many conditions. Current disease management and disease prediction techniques are built from what we know about disease processes, and this information is only available for a small percentage of the population.[17] Better early disease modeling techniques and access to more complete medical history data to build these models will be essential to future disease prevention efforts. In addition, focusing on subsets of groups who are most at risk and/or most ready to make changes to their lifestyle will impact the success, and therefore the return on investment, for HDM programs.[18]

Patient cohort stratification must go beyond the current risk adjustment for disease level, while taking into account other factors, such as socioeconomic status and level of social support.[19] HDM interventions should also shift to become more inclusive. Reference groups such as family, friends, coworkers, church, support or advocacy groups, and other interpersonal communities have a large influence over patient behavior.[20] How patients, families and communities cope with illness and experience disease is essential to proper treatment.[21] Unfortunately, traditional disease management programs do not include these other extended groups. Especially in chronic care management, health professionals must understand how patients and families perceive the meaning of illness, suffering, recovery, and death.

Not only will understanding patients help improve care, but the patterns that illness takes differ from person to person based on the interaction of the disease, its consequences, and the social context.[21] Understanding these complex relationships may help target HDM interventions based on community and psychosocial characteristics. Interventions that include a patient's reference groups could have a great impact on the outcomes of a HDM program.[20] Examples may include interventions aimed at improving patient compliance through family or caregiver education.

When looking to the future, HDM programs must be prospectively managed, cost-effective and well coordinated.[18] Measurement and evaluation of HDM programs must also be tightened. The use of external reviewers would be one way to improve both study design and measurement. In addition to the program sponsors and clinical personnel involved, the study design and all subsequent results should be reviewed and signed off by actuarial, finance, and informatics experts.[4] Involvement of those whose performance will be measured in program design will help create incentives for providers and patients alike.[12]

## References

1. Armstrong EP. Disease management: state of the art and future directions. *Clin Ther.* 1999;21(3): 593-609.
2. Summers KH. Measuring and monitoring outcomes of disease management programs. *Clin Ther.* 1996;18(6):1341-1348.
3. Zhan C, Miller MR. Administrative data based patient safety research: a critical review. *Qual Saf Health Care.* 2003;12:58-63.
4. Fetterolf D, Wennberg D, Devries A. Estimating the return on investment in disease management programs using a pre-post analysis. *Dis Manag.* 2004;7(1):5-23.
5. Fitzner K, Sidorov J, Fetterolf D, et al. Principles for assessing disease management outcomes. *Dis Manag.* 2004;7:191-201.
6. Fireman B, Bartlett J, Selby J. Can disease management reduce health care costs by improving quality? *Health Affairs.* 2004;23:63-75.
7. Linden A, Adams JL, Roberts N. Evaluation methods in disease management: determining program effectiveness. *Dis Manag.* 2003;6(3):93-102.
8. Linden A, Adams JL, Roberts N. An assessment of the total population approach for evaluating disease management program effectiveness. *Dis Manag.* 2003;6(2):93-102.
9. Linden A, Adams JL, Roberts N. Evaluating disease management program effectiveness: an introduction to time-series analysis. *Dis Manag.* 2003;6(4):243-255.
10. Roache K. Healthcare transitions: trends in quality outcomes and performance measures pay for performance. *Journal of Managed Care Medicine.* 2008;11(1):24-28.
11. Costantini O, Huck K, Carlson MD, et al. Impact of a guideline-based disease management team on outcomes of hospitalized patients with congestive heart failure. *Arch Inter Med.* 2001;161: 177-182.
12. NCQA (National Committee for Quality Assurance). The State of Health Care Quality: Focus on Obesity and on Medicare Plan Improvement 2012. Available at: http://www.ncqa.org/Portals/0/State%20of%20Health%20Care/2012/SOHC%20Report%20Web.pdf. Accessed November 16, 2012.
13. Casalino L, Gillies RR, Shortell SM, et al. External incentives, information technology, and organized processes to improve health care quality for patients with chronic diseases. *JAMA.* 2003;289(4):434-441.
14. Weingarten SR, Henning JM, Badamgarav E, et al. Interventions used in disease management programmes for patients with chronic illnesses. Which ones work? *BMJ.* 2002;325:925-932.
15. Clancy CM. Getting to smart health care. *Health Aff.* 2006;25:589-592.
16. DMAA. The top six challenges in disease management. Available at: http://www.dmaa.org/pdf/TopSixChallengesinDM.pdf. Accessed March 3, 2008.
17. Stehno CE. An innovative health risk measurement technique for disease management. *Dis Manag.* 2007;10:1-5.
18. Edlin M. Total population management reduces future treatment costs. *Managed Healthcare Executive.* 2002:46-48.
19. Wennberg JE, Fisher ES, Skinner JS, et al. Extending the P4P agenda, part 2: how Medicare can reduce waste and improve the care of the chronically ill. *Health Aff.* 2007;26(6):1575-1585.
20. Turpin RS, Blumberg PB, Sharda CE, et al. Patient adherence: present state and future directions. *Dis Manag.* 2007;10(6):305-310.
21. Soubbi H. Toward an ecosystemic approach to chronic care design and practice in primary care. *Ann Fam Med.* 2007;5:263-269.

CHAPTER 5

# Retrospective Drug Utilization Review for Generating, Evaluating, and Benchmarking Health and Disease Management Data

Mireya Diaz, PhD; and Bijal M. Shah, BPharm, PhD

Health and disease management (HDM) evolved in the 1990s as a mechanism to avoid preventable complications, reduce morbidity, and improve mortality rates, while simultaneously reducing health care costs of individuals with chronic illnesses. At the core of HDM is a patient-centered and integrated mode of care to improve patients' quality of life. In an effort to improve quality of care, HDM programs implement benchmarking practices, employing a continuous evaluation process by which an organization compares internal components of its performance in relation to best practices put forth by national or international organizations. Complementary to this perspective, the federal government instituted drug utilization reviews (DURs) in the same spirit of performance improvement, but also focused on patient safety and cost containment. Within this context, retrospective DURs (rDURs) function by identifying trends and outliers in medication utilization patterns, upon which HDM programs can be developed and benchmarked.

DUR programs have been defined as "the ongoing study of the frequency of use and cost of drugs, from which patterns of prescribing, dispensing, and patient use can be determined."[1] DUR programs can be conducted using data from patient medical records or administrative claims. Given their convenience, we will focus on the role of administrative claims data as the source for these reviews; thus, it is the aim of this chapter to illustrate how DURs based on claims data can help support the analysis of the effectiveness of HDM programs.

This chapter presents basic definitions and methodological issues that should be considered when performing an rDUR. The chapter also presents conceptual frameworks and algorithms for some components of these reviews available in the literature in addition to examples of claims-based rDUR studies. Finally, we provide examples of strategies based on rDURs that have worked in improving providers' prescribing patterns, as well as unresolved issues as part of future directions in the topic.

## 1. Definition and Scope of a Retrospective Drug Utilization Review Study

A DUR assesses patterns of drug prescribing and use against predefined criteria[1,2] and engages providers in interventions that aim to reduce medication errors and improve patient outcomes and quality of care.[3] Qualified health professionals, including physicians and pharmacists, develop the predefined criteria used in the first stage of a DUR based on the labeling approved by the US Food and Drug Administration (FDA), peer-reviewed literature, standards, and guidelines.[3] The assessment of concordance between actual utilization and recommended guidelines is generally conducted using claims data, given the availability of such data and the relative ease of conducting population-based research using these data.

Retrospective DUR is synonymous with drug-use evaluation (DUE) and medication-use evaluation (MUE).[4] Although these terms may be used interchangeably, some researchers confer a more all-encompassing character to MUE because it requires a multidisciplinary approach to patient care.[5] The focus on administrative claims as the source for the review and its direct bearing on US public insurance led us to use the term *DUR* or *rDUR*, as it is preferentially called at the federal level, throughout the chapter.

Retrospective DUR studies based on claims data exclusively assess the adherence of prescribing or dispensing patterns of providers, *not* the adherence of patients to treatment. In order to examine adherence to prescription treatment in the setting of rDUR, measures of biological effect of the medication would be necessary, such as reduction or control of blood pressure in a hypertensive patient. Typically, this kind of information is not available in claims data; however it could be ascertained in studies that combine claims data analysis with medical records review.[6]

DURs are mandated by the 1990 Omnibus Budget Reconciliation Act, which contributed to their widespread adoption by public insurer programs. In addition to the participation of Medicaid programs in these DURs, a substantial portion of the retrospective reviews are performed by private firms.[2]

Despite the greater evidence level provided by prospective DURs, retrospective studies are nonintrusive and provide more data at a lower cost.[7] They can provide information to health care providers and payers about one, some, or all of the following: therapeutic appropriateness, underutilization and overutilization, appropriate use of generic drugs, drug-disease contraindications, drug-drug interactions (DDI), therapeutic duplication, incorrect drug dosage, duration of drug treatment, and clinical abuse/misuse. For further details regarding the conceptualization, history and implementation of these programs, the reader is referred to the review by Peterson and colleagues.[4]

## 2. Methodological Issues when Dealing with Prescription Databases for rDUR

General challenges that arise during the analysis of administrative claims databases have been reviewed in earlier chapters. Here we describe some challenges inherent to these databases within the context of an rDUR. Retrospective DUR studies may be conducted on pharmacologic treatments to identify adverse event rates or to assess favorable health outcomes. Studies also may be conducted to assess prescribing patterns for a disease state, trends in utilization over time, or as a surveillance tool to assess the incidence or prevalence of a health state to provide guidance for future interventions.

## Specificity of Drugs

In an rDUR, specificity refers to the ability to identify and evaluate medications restricted to the disease in question. Poor specificity may render prescribing measures invalid. Examples of such a problem are some measures of quality treatment for asthma, such as the percentage of corticosteroids prescribed or the ratio of inhaled corticosteroids to bronchodilator drugs.[8] Himmel and colleagues found that corticosteroids were frequently prescribed for COPD, rendering the marker invalid if the purpose was to assess prescribing behavior for asthma exclusively. In the more general sense, the study found that the marker function of drugs for chronic airflow disease is rather limited.

## Study Designs for Retrospective Drug Utilization Reviews

There are a wide range of rDUR study designs. The selection of a design should be guided by the aims of the study research questions; however, resource constraints frequently determine what can actually be implemented. Some rDUR studies are cross-sectional in nature, providing a *snapshot* of current treatment patterns. For example, Laumann and colleagues used claims data from Iowa Medicaid to compare asthma medication utilization patterns with prescribing guidelines.[9] These studies are useful for determining the prevalence of disease or specific outcomes. Associations between exposure and outcome status can be determined relatively quickly and inexpensively using existing data; however, these studies cannot be used to determine causality.

Retrospective cohort study designs are often used with administrative claims data and are conducted by identifying a group of patients with a specific disease or those using a specific drug class. This study design is useful for assessing multiple outcomes that may be associated with a single exposure or for determining if patients are receiving appropriate treatment. For example, Ye and colleagues used a retrospective cohort study design to determine the proportion of patients who received outpatient statin therapy after hospitalization for coronary heart disease.[10] This type of study design is able to control for confounding by using multivariable analysis. However, these studies are more time and resource intensive compared to cross-sectional studies.

Case-control studies are useful when determining the risk for an adverse event, particularly when multiple factors or exposures are suspected, and when examining rare diseases or drugs of low use. For example, Graham and colleagues used a nested case-control study design with claims data from Kaiser Permanente to determine the risk of myocardial infarction and sudden cardiac death in patients using cyclo-oxygenase enzyme (COX-2) inhibitors.[11] The strength of the association between exposure and outcome can be determined using multivariable regression analyses. Matching and propensity score analysis can also be used as techniques to control for confounding effects. In addition, data can be stratified to assess the effects of the exposure at different dosages of the drug or varying lengths of exposure. These techniques are further addressed in Part 5 of this book.

The case-crossover study is another design that may be used when confounding is a cause for concern. In this study design, case patients serve as their own control (before initiation of study medication), thus minimizing the effect of confounding within each individual.

## Controlling for Comorbidities

In rDUR studies, comorbid conditions function as methodological diagnostic tools. That is, they can be used to determine whether or not prescribing patterns follow guidelines, as well as to explain whether exceptions in such patterns are due to exclusion criteria supported by the presence of concomitant conditions or are, in fact, prescribing errors. For example, unidentified comorbid conditions in studies that examine prescribing patterns of nonsteroidal anti-inflammatory drugs (NSAIDs) for management of pain may lead to incorrect interpretations. It may appear that for a given sample of patients with arthritis, NSAIDs are underutilized.

Identifying the underlying comorbid conditions in this sample may show that it contains a large number of individuals with a risk for, or with a history of, gastrointestinal bleeding, precluding the use of nonselective NSAIDs.[12] Alternatively, nonselective NSAIDs may appear to be prescribed more frequently than selective NSAIDS, despite their purported higher risk for gastrointestinal bleeding. Closer analysis could reveal that within this sample there is a high prevalence of individuals with cardiovascular disease or its risk factors in which selective NSAIDs are contraindicated. In both scenarios, knowledge of the comorbid status of the individuals would allow one to adjust accordingly, leading to a correct interpretation that patterns of use are due to concomitant disease and not due to limited knowledge of the provider.

Comorbidities can be assessed using instruments such as the Charlson Comorbidity Index, the Elixhauser index, the Cumulative Illness Rating Scale, the Index of Coexisting Disease, and the pharmacy claims-based RxRisk V score, among others.[13] The Charlson index measures 19 disease conditions and was originally developed for use with patient charts but has been adapted for use with claims databases. It is the most extensively studied comorbidity measure and has been shown to be a reliable and valid predictor of patient outcomes, such as mortality, disability, readmissions and length of hospital stay. The Elixhauser index is a relatively newer instrument that measures 30 comorbidities associated with mortality. Instruments such as the Charlson and Elixhauser indices have become widely used with either ICD-9 or ICD-10 diagnosis codes, as available in prescription claims databases.[14]

## Over-the-Counter Medications

Drugs that can be acquired over the counter (OTC) may alter rDUR evaluations because OTC drug users will be misclassified as unexposed, leading to underestimation of drug use. Moreover, OTC use could induce or explain some of the observed side effects of medication errors; mainly interactions between drugs. Nonetheless, the evaluator would be unable to measure such an effect. To this end, Ulcickas and colleagues estimated the potential bias of the use of OTC medications in claims-based evaluations using the case study of NSAIDs and their association with colorectal cancer incidence.[15] To determine such bias, they assessed the sensitivity of estimates to the overall prevalence of NSAID exposure, the proportion of NSAID exposure due to OTC use exclusively, and the true risk ratio. They found that under the setting of nondifferential exposure of the OTC formulation (that is, exposure is the same for diseased and nondiseased individuals), OTC drug exposure would not be a large source of bias. For higher overall use of the drug, OTC exposure should be small in order for the bias to remain contained, and thus make claims-based rDUR valid.

## Prescription Benefits by Insurers

Other issues to consider when executing an rDUR are the benefits established by the patients' insurance provider. The effect of pharmacy benefit designs on drug utilization and outcomes is largely unexplored except for the impact of patient cost sharing.[16] Pharmacy benefits can vary considerably across and even within insurance programs. For example, Medicaid programs differ in a number of ways: whether or not prior authorization is required to dispense a given prescription, the number of prescriptions allowed on a monthly basis, copayment and reduced fees, drug rebate programs, OTC coverage, and preferred drug lists.[17] All of these have potentially high impact in terms of the information that can be found within the claims, as well as the internal and external validity of the analysis performed. For example, limited or no utilization of a given drug may be an artifact of its exclusion from the corresponding formulary.

Another example of the complexities surrounding insurance plans is the more recent outpatient prescription drug benefit instituted within the Medicare program, Part D. Three issues related to this program impact rDURs: (1) effects of Part D implementation are more tangible for evaluations pertaining to those insured by Medicaid in the dually eligible category (that is, those receiving benefits from both Medicaid and Medicare), prior to the establishment of Part D these beneficiaries had their prescriptions covered through Medicaid, but shifted to Medicare for most medications;[18] (2) reaching the drug benefit threshold imposes financial constraints to certain beneficiaries, which translates into features that may mimic medication errors (for example, lack of adherence and medication discontinuation may be interpreted instead as underutilization);[19] and (3) high variability in pharmacy benefits covered by the programs implementing Part D leads to confusion among providers who may prescribe drugs that are not covered.[20]

## 3. Survey of the Retrospective Drug Utilization Reviews Literature

State Medicaid agencies in the United States have conducted the vast majority of rDURs. However, very few of these are published, perhaps because they were done primarily for the purpose of internal review. In this section, we present an overview of published research on rDURs based on claims data that are mainly representative of the prescription patterns in the United States health care system. For further detail on these issues, the reader is referred to the monograph by De Smet and colleagues.[21]

Based on the focus of the review, the published literature on rDUR can be organized into 7 different categories: therapeutic appropriateness, underutilization/ overutilization, appropriate use of generic drugs, drug-drug and drug-disease contraindications, therapeutic duplication and incorrect drug dosage. Table 1 summarizes the conceptual frameworks used to perform specific rDURs, the added value of the review, and examples encountered in the literature for each of the 7 categories.

The selected examples were chosen to illustrate the different medication events trying to cover a wide range of medical conditions, settings, and insurance providers. Also, the reader is advised to consult these examples directly since they contain a considerable amount of detail regarding the execution of the particular rDUR, which is beyond the scope of this review. It is important to highlight that the prevalence or incidence of these different medication events will vary considerably across studies depending on the population's distribution of underlying conditions and the setting under assessment.

### Therapeutic Appropriateness

Retrospective DUR studies are often conducted to determine the appropriateness of drug therapy being used for the treatment of a chronic or acute condition. Pre-defined criteria or practice guidelines are used to determine the appropriateness of care against which patterns of care are compared. These patterns aid researchers in examining the rate of adoption of medical guidelines related to medication management, factors favoring such adoption, as well as their effectiveness.

Elderly patients are a population of particular interest due to the many chronic conditions that afflict them. Inappropriate prescribing in the elderly may occur due to the absence of an indication or due to the lack of evidence for effectiveness under the presence of an indication.[22] Two different indices are frequently used to assess inappropriate prescribing in this population: the Beers criteria[23] and the Medication Appropriateness Index (MAI).[24,25,26]

The Beers criteria have been used extensively to document potentially inappropriate medication use in the elderly. For example, Curtis and colleagues assessed inappropriate prescribing among elderly patients using claims data from a large national pharmaceutical benefit manager.[27] The study found that more than 21% of patients filled a prescription for a medication that would be considered inappropriate based on the Beers criteria. A large proportion of the inappropriate medications (41%) were found to be psychotropic medications. In another study using data from 10 HMOs, 29% of elderly patients were found to be using inappropriate medications, with women being more likely to receive these medications compared to men.[28]

A systematic review assessed the relationship of medication errors as measured by the Beers criteria and specific health outcomes in the elderly.[29] This review highlights the utility of the criteria when the outcomes of interest are adverse drug reactions and costs. However, it also cautions the reader about the high dependence of the association on other outcomes within the particular health care setting. Despite their widespread use, the Beers criteria have been criticized for their lack of comprehensiveness given that the criteria do not consider measures such as underutilization of drugs, drug-drug interactions or drug duplications.[30]

The MAI is a patient interview technique used in tandem with retrospective review. It solves the lack of comprehensiveness of the Beers criteria. Nevertheless, it has been found to be time and resource intensive, requiring more than 10 minutes per drug evaluated. It is important to highlight that inappropriate use—defined in the narrow sense of prescribing without an indication or based on the wrong indication, particularly when measured through the MAI—encompasses most of the other medication prescribing errors as well. Thus, the literature overview of the following sections corresponds to articles that have addressed very specific components of an rDUR. Also, separate sections have been created to illustrate individual frameworks that allow a systematic rDUR for a particular component.

## Underutilization and Overutilization

Underutilization of medications, and in some cases overutilization, is another focus of rDUR programs that center on HDM. The level of appropriate utilization is generally based on available management guidelines, including expert consensus. Similar to an rDUR focused on therapeutic appropriateness, an rDUR focused on utilization rates can inform the adoption of guidelines and factors associated with them.

Underutilization of effective medications to treat chronic medical conditions, despite rDUR evidence to support their use, is an important issue for HDM programs. For example, numerous trials have demonstrated the effectiveness of statins in reducing rates of coronary heart disease (CHD) recurrence, stroke, myocardial infarction, peripheral vascular disease, and overall mortality. However, therapies for the treatment and prevention of CHD continue to be underutilized. For example, the study by Ye and colleagues found that less than half of patients with CHD had received outpatient statin therapy within 6 months of a hospital discharge. In another study using claims data from Medicaid beneficiaries, elderly patients, ethnic minorities and patients with a poor health status were found to be underutilizing therapies for congestive heart failure.[31]

Underuse of efficacious therapies has also been observed for antithrombolytic therapy after hospital discharge,[32] antiviral treatment in chronic hepatitis C infection,[33] and use of renoprotective therapy among patients with diabetes.[34] In the case of antithrombolytic therapy, in a study among the dually eligible (that is, individuals receiving benefits from both Medicare and Medicaid), it was found that 23% of patients discharged after a venous thromboembolic event received fewer than 90 days of anticoagulants. Shorter duration of therapy was more common among African Americans and those with deep venous thrombosis.

Sometimes, a medication utilization analysis can be limited by the availability of certain information in claims data, making the validation of rDUR evidence challenging. For example, a study using claims from a commercial health plan, it was found that only 30% of those in whom antiviral treatment for hepatitis C was advisable received the indicated therapy. Nonetheless, antiviral therapy is not recommended in individuals with certain comorbidities or health states (mental health problems, pregnancy, autoimmune disease, diabetes, heart disease), risky behavior (alcohol consumption or intravenous drug use), or advanced disease. Similarly, if blood tests and liver biopsy show chronic infection, but no liver damage, treatment may not be indicated. Of course, much of this information might not be available in administrative claims data, making the assertion that only 30% of the population received indicated therapy a challenging one.

In the case of renal protection for diabetic patients,[34] there is evidence indicating the efficacy of ACE inhibitors and angiotensin II receptor blockers (ARBs). A study conducted using Medicare patients found that half of patients who had a clear indication for renoprotection did not receive treatment as per the national guidelines. However, the authors cautioned that even in the ideal setting of clinical trials it has been found that up to 46% of patients discontinue treatment during 3 years of follow-up. Nonetheless, the authors also indicated that those who do not tolerate ACE inhibitor therapy could use an ARB, noting that protective renal therapy should reach 90% utilization. The examples cited illustrate the limitations of rDUR findings based on claims data when potential confounders (see Table 2) cannot be controlled. Most of these confounders have been examined in the context of rDUR within the Medicaid program.[35]

## Appropriate Use of Generic Drugs

A generic drug is a drug product that contains the same active ingredient as the brand drug, in identical strength, dosage, and route of administration, and prescribed for the same indications.[36] As such, generic drugs offer an opportunity for cost containment. Four main issues need to be considered when reviewing the appropriate use of generic drugs: (1) whether or not the particular prescription allows for generic drug use, (2) the potential modifying roles of prescriber and pharmacist characteristics, drug insurance coverage, patient characteristics, and drug characteristics, (3) if the aim is the financial rather than the patient outcomes perspective, and (4) generic substitution. The last issue deserves further consideration.

Generic substitution refers to the power conferred to pharmacists to override a doctor's choice for the brand product and dispense any approved generic version instead. In the US every state has the authority to implement its own rulings[37] regarding generic substitution and, thus, we encounter states that identify generics that can be substituted, while others indicate which drugs cannot be substituted. Likewise, there are states that allow the pharmacist to substitute a brand-name drug, while others mandate such substitution.

Other aspects of state legislation include whether or not notification of the substitution to the patient is required and if substitutions should be done for a cheaper product. Thus, when conducting rDURs involving generic utilization, it is critical to know the legal requirements of the particular state to interpret results adequately. Within this same context, it is clear that rDURs offer additional gains as they allow one to examine the effectiveness of generics versus brand-name drugs under scenarios of high levels of substitution and variability across practices. This has great public health implications given that very few blinded and controlled studies compare generic to brand versions.[38]

Mott and Cline[39] proposed a conceptual framework that can be used to explore the appropriate use of generic drugs within an rDUR. In situations in which the prescribing behavior of the physician and the dispensing behavior of the pharmacist can be observed, this model allows one to assess both separately. However, the separation of these 2 factors cannot be achieved if the review is based on administrative claims alone.

An example of evaluating generic prescribing within an rDUR is the work by Labiner et al,[40] that examined the association between generic substitution for antiepileptic drugs and medical resource utilization in the US. A key issue in this case study was that antiepileptic drugs illustrate the potential consequences of generic substitution of a drug with a narrow therapeutic index, that is, one in which there is very little difference between lethal and therapeutic doses. This study utilized a database containing commercial health insurance claims for over 90 health plans. The authors implemented an open-cohort design in which patients were classified into mutually exclusive periods of brand versus generic use of antiepileptic drugs. The resource utilization in terms of hospitalization and outpatient visits between these periods was compared. The authors found that during periods when generics were used there was an increase in the medical utilization rate as well as in risk of injury even among patients defined as stable.

## Drug-Disease Contraindications and Drug-Drug Interactions

The potential interactions of the medication under assessment with another drug or with a coexisting disease are 2 additional drug utilization issues of interest within rDURs. These 2 types of interactions may be of special interest for particular conditions (for example, HIV, diabetes, renal or hepatic insufficiency) and drug classes. Retrospective DURs in this scenario mainly aid in determining the factors that contribute to contraindicated prescribing. Knowledge of those factors may assist in the implementation of corrective measures and programs that help to minimize such negative practices.

## Drug-Disease Contraindications

This interaction illustrates the potential of the medication to exacerbate other conditions present.[41] Medications that may be beneficial for most patients may be contraindicated in others based on their disease state. This is especially true for the elderly who might suffer from renal or hepatic dysfunction, thus altering the metabolism and excretion of drugs. The section of the Beers criteria that links contraindicated medications to specific conditions can assist in the pertinent rDURs.

Findings of errors related to drug-disease contraindications highlight the limitations of existing management guidelines developed for a single condition without considering the role of comorbid disease. Examples of claims rDURs focused on contraindicated drugs include the assessment of contraindicated long-term use of benzodiazepine among elderly patients with depression,[23] and beta-blockers use in contraindicated disease states (eg, hypotension, bradycardia, AV block) found to be prescribed to approximately 6% of post-MI Medicaid patients who had these contraindications.[42]

## Drug-Drug Interactions

This interaction indicates a drug pair that has the potential to exert a generally harmful clinically significant event in an individual.[41] In some circumstances the interaction results in reducing or nullifying the effect of one or both drugs (for example, antibiotics and contraceptive pills). Peng and colleagues, present 51 drug pairs of potential DDIs, which can serve as a good stepping point from which an algorithm can be devised to identify these interactions.[43] When conducting an rDUR focused on DDIs, additional care should be given to OTC products. A study performed within the Iowa Priority Prescription Savings Program identified that OTC products contributed to 35% of the DDIs.[44]

Three American studies have assessed the prevalence of DDIs based on claims data.[26,45,46] Such prevalence has ranged between 0.2% (based on 65,000 prescription claims) and 6% (within 756,000 patient-years). These studies uniformly indicate polypharmacy (that is, the use of multiple drugs in the same patient) as a risk factor in the occurrence of DDIs, and as a risk factor for most of the medication errors. A review article[47] identified other factors contributing to an increased risk for DDIs.

These factors are: (1) a high number of primary care physicians and multiple dispensing pharmacies; (2) extreme signaling of medication surveillance software (that is, too many or too few), as well as poor knowledge, training and supervision of technicians who are the first ones in judging these signals; and (3) a high workload of the pharmacy services when accompanied by low intervention rates.

## Therapeutic Duplication

Therapeutic duplication refers to the use of more than 1 drug from the same class or different brands of the same drug. Similar to DDIs, therapeutic duplication rates are increased with polypharmacy and with multiple indication drugs. Other factors that contribute to the duplication of medication are miscommunication between patient and providers, providers' deficit in knowledge of drug classes, poor tracking of drugs within a given practice and/or during transitions within the health system, and formulary issues.[48] Similarly to DDIs, additional care should be paid when conducting rDURs focused on duplication with regard to OTC products. OTC products have been found to be involved in approximately 50% of duplication errors.[44]

The following studies conducted in the United States exemplify the assessment of the efficacy of interventions targeted at reducing medication errors, including therapeutic duplication, via a retrospective review of prescription claims data. The first study examined the efficacy of generating alerts from prescription claim profiles, in addition to the usual regimen reviews, in order to control polypharmacy in the elderly.[49] Using North Carolina Medicaid claims data, the authors found a reduction in errors with a corresponding reduction in costs. The second study[50] assessed the efficacy of providing 6 months of claims data to primary care physicians on the day of a scheduled appointment with a patient. These data assisted physicians in identifying medication nonadherence and therapeutic duplication, and reduced the time required to obtain the patient's medication history. The third study[51] assessed the efficacy of an early implementation of prospective DUR targeted at therapeutic duplication and DDIs for beta-agonist inhaler use among elders with chronic lung disease. The authors found no significant changes in the occurrence of such errors after the implementation of the prospective DUR.

## Incorrect Drug Dosage

A prescription is given in excess (that is, overdose) if its daily dose exceeds the defined maximum value. Likewise, it is an underdose if its daily dose is below the defined minimum value. Both exert negative effects: one by increasing the risk of adverse events (that is, safety), the other by providing a medication that basically may not work (that is, effectiveness). Correct drug dosage is more complex for certain conditions, such as in the presence of renal disease[52] or impaired hepatic function.

The method employed by Seidling and colleagues[53] could be used as an algorithm to assess appropriate drug dosage. Factors to consider are those related to the variability in the dose required to achieve a maximum therapeutic response across individuals. These factors correspond to patient characteristics (age, genetic markers, comorbidities, use of other medications), and drug characteristics (approved indication, active ingredient, route of administration). The dose variability pointed out is the one providing opportunities for benchmarking. To assist in this task, lists containing information on thousands of active ingredients, without linking them to specific indications or brands, are compiled by the FDA and the World Health Organization in the Anatomical Therapeutic Chemical Classification System and the Defined Daily Doses for different routes of administration.

Briesacher and colleagues [54] offer an example of claims data used in assessing incorrect dosage of antipsychotic drugs for elders in nursing homes. Using a representative sample of Medicare beneficiaries, the author found that 35% received overdoses of antipsychotics, contrary to nursing home guidelines. With this study the authors highlight the gaps between clinical evidence and care delivery.

## 4. Interventions Based on DURs: What Works and What Does Not

Once an rDUR study has been conducted to document inappropriate medication use, health plans use this information to design programs aimed at educating health care providers and/or patients with the ultimate goal of improving patient quality of care. Among successful strategies based on communication with and education of providers is the implementation or use of:

- Standardized physician orders to increase adherence with treatment guidelines. Reingold and Kulstad[55] demonstrate the effective use of this strategy with congestive heart failure, in which data from the postintervention period show a substantial increase in the utilization of ACE inhibitors and nitroglycerin.

- Education programs and/or letters to promote appropriate prescribing to eligible patients. This approach was successfully used to improve: (1) calcium and vitamin D supplementation among residents of long-term care institutions;[56] (2) prescribing of beta-blockers among post-AMI Medicaid beneficiaries,[57] and (3) prescribing of prophylactic enoxaparin. This latter case used preprinted stickers placed in patient charts for easy identification of eligible individuals, in addition to the education program.[58] Letter interventions have shown some improvement in prescribing patterns despite the large variability in the response rates with pharmacists and prescribers.[59] This is a strategy used by more than half of the state Medicaid rDUR programs.[60]

- Report cards and training in order to change providers' prescribing patterns of generic medications. The combined strategy of training and feedback resulted in an increase in the prescription of generic drugs by 12 to 15% points from a baseline of 38% among providers.[61] Other strategies that marginally increased the use of generic prescribing by about 1 to 5% are step therapy, 3-tier plan design and increased differentials between the generic and brand copayments.[62]

- Follow-up calls to community pharmacists, in addition to educational letters to physicians and pharmacists, to reduce overutilization of unnecessary long-term therapy. This was the approach formally tested with control groups by the Idaho Medicaid program regarding prescribing of antiulcer medications.[63] This resulted in significant cost-savings for the program.

- Prior authorization requirements for coverage to decrease inappropriate utilization of medications, known as the *sentinel effect*.[64] This was the case of cefuroxime tablet prescriptions within a managed care organization in Israel. Prescription for the antibiotic decreased in the 3-month period of the authorization intervention from 8% to 1% to rise again during the 3-month period postintervention to 4%.

However, it is important to bear in mind that rDURs may not always be effective. This may be the case when the effectiveness of rDURs is compared to that of concurrent prospective DURs. Gregoire and colleagues designed a controlled study aimed at assessing the effectiveness of both modalities on the quality of in-hospital prescribing in Canada.[65] The study showed that the concurrent DUR program significantly improved prescribing practices while the retrospective DUR program had no significant effect. This may also be the case when the intervention does not provide sufficient exposure to the training material. It also may explain the ineffectiveness of an automatic alert system for DDIs implemented in the California Veterans system.[66] That is, due to the low incidence rate of the DDI events, prescribers were not exposed long enough for the educational intervention to work.

## 5. Future Work

As described in the sections above, there are examples in the literature of the uses and progress of rDUR. Most of the time these reviews are comprehensive (ie, they evaluate most of the components of medication errors). However, some studies have evaluated only particular components and, for that reason, only the particular theoretical framework and/or algorithm used to examine it has been illustrated. Potential venues for improvement in the field follow.

For example, it would increase the efficiency of these reviews if the Beers criteria could be updated on a regular basis, as well as if the Beers criteria and the MAI were combined to generate a more comprehensive and robust instrument. The inclusion of providers' characteristics in these evaluations, as well as controlling for factors known to increase confounding errors, would account for a potential source of heterogeneity, neglected by the rDUR literature so far. In addition, there is room for the development of formal conceptual frameworks or algorithms for examining underutilization and overutilization, and therapeutic duplication.

The major advantages of prescription claims, in particular those generated by public US insurance, make them ripe for establishing benchmarks for HDM and, therefore, should play a major role in such endeavors. They are relatively easy to acquire and low cost with respect to other data sources. They include a large number of individuals, in particular those with chronic conditions and the elderly. Finally, they are easy to link to sources indicating the patient's health risk profile and undergo

## Part 1: Claims Databases

a strict scrutiny process. Furthermore, developing systems and processes for rDUR based on claims data and learning from their complexities and deficiencies may facilitate implementation of rDURs encompassing perhaps a more inclusive dataset of electronic medical records.

**TABLE 1:** Drug Utilization Review Focus, Conceptual Frameworks, Added Value, and Their Representation in the Published Literature

| Drug Utilization Focus | Framework | Added Value | Examples |
|---|---|---|---|
| Therapeutic appropriateness | Beers criteria[23,26] Medication Appropriateness Index (MAI)[24,25,26] | Assess medical guidelines adoption, associated provider/health system factors | Asthma prescribing practices in Iowa Medicaid, prescribing for elderly patients |
| Underutilization/Overutilization | Not developed yet | Assess medical guidelines adoption, associated provider/health system factors | Therapy for coronary heart disease, congestive heart failure, venous thromboembolism, chronic hepatitis C, renoprotection in diabetes |
| Use of generic drugs | Mott and Cline[39] | Assess effectiveness of generic substitution and derived cost-savings | Generic substitution of antiepileptic drugs |
| Drug-drug interactions | Peng, et al.[43] drug pairs of potential interactions | Identify points of care requiring integration | Long-term benzodiazepine use in depressed elders, beta-blockers among post-MI patients |
| Drug-disease contraindications | Beers criteria[23,26] | Inform guidelines about effectiveness of medications in multiple comorbidities scenario | Polypharmacy and other risk factors |
| Therapeutic duplication | Not developed yet | Identify conditions more susceptible to polypharmacy, and points of care requiring integration | Alerts generation in N.C. Medicaid, provision of prior claims to primary care physicians, evaluation of success of prospective DUR |
| Incorrect drug dosage | Seidling, et al.[53] | Assess effectiveness of different therapeutic regimens (timing, dosage, duration) | Antipsychotic overdosage in nursing homes |

**TABLE 2:** Potential Confounders to Consider for Retrospective DURs

*Supply variables*

- List of approved/reimbursable drugs (formularies among Medicaid programs)
- Pharmacy program's reimbursement policy (could include drug cost and dispensing fee)
- Relative representation of main interest groups measured by per capita physicians and per capita pharmacists, percentage of physician members of American Medical Association
- Hospital beds per capita (for evaluations including hospital pharmacy services)

*Direct demand variables*

- Number of medication recipients
- Percentage of recipients in specific age categories (practical surrogate for health status and need for medications)
- Socioeconomic status (poverty level, employment), program benefits, drug copayments

*Indirect demand variables* (nondrug cost-containment policy variables, appropriate to assess spillover effects)

- Limitations in coverage for hospital inpatient services, hospital outpatient services, and skilled nursing facilities
- Use of Medicare principles for reimbursement of inpatient hospital services, outpatient hospital services, physicians
- Requirement of prior authorization to enter intermediate care facility for mentally disabled, or for physicians before performing certain procedures
- Limitations on physicians' inpatient hospital visits
- State's nominal physician copay adjusted by annual Consumer Price Index for multiyear evaluations

*Federal policy variables*

Specifics of federal policies mandating services or coverage for specific patient groups

*State variables*

Dummy state or health system variables used as surrogates for unobservable state or health system characteristics that could influence supply or demand for drug services, as well as the effectiveness of the program

# References

1. Brodie DC. Drug utilization review/planning. *Hospitals.* 1972;46:103-112.
2. Soumerai SG, Lipton HL. Computer-based drug-utilization review—risk, benefit, or boondoggle? *N Engl J Med.* 1995;332:1641-1645.
3. Fulda TR, Lyles A, Pugh MC, Christensen DB. Current status of prospective drug utilization review. *J Manag Care Pharm.* 2004;10:433-441.
4. Peterson AM, Chan V, Wilson MD. Drug utilization review strategies. In: Navarro RP, ed. *Managed Care Pharmacy Practice.* 2nd ed. Sudbury, MA: Jones & Bartlett Publishers Inc.; 2009.
5. Phillips MS, Gayman JE, Todd MW. ASHP guidelines on medication-use evaluation. *Am J Health Syst Pharm.* 1996;53(16):1953-1955.
6. Vincze G, Barner JC, Bohman T, et al. Use of antihypertensive medications among United States veterans newly diagnosed with hypertension. *Curr Med Res Opin.* 2008;24:795-805.

**Part 1: Claims Databases**

7. Sax MJ. Essential steps and practical applications for database studies. *J Manag Care Pharm.* 2005;11(1 Suppl A):S5-S8.
8. Himmel W, Hummers-Pradier E, Schumann H, et al. The predictive value of asthma medications to identify individuals with asthma: a study in German general practices. *Br J Gen Pract.* 2001;51:879-883.
9. Laumann JM, Bjornson DC. Treatment of Medicaid patients with asthma: comparison with treatment guidelines using disease-based drug utilization review methodology. *Ann Pharmacother.* 1998;32:1290-1294.
10. Ye X, Gross CR, Schommer J, et al. Initiation of statins after hospitalization for coronary heart disease. *J Manag Care Pharm.* 2007;13:385-396.
11. Graham DJ, Campen D, Hui R, et al. Risk of acute myocardial infarction and sudden cardiac death in patients treated with cyclo-oxygenase 2 selective and non-selective non-steroidal anti-inflammatory drugs: nested case-control study. *Lancet.* 2005;365:475-481.
12. Dominik KL, Bosworth HB, Jeffreys AS, Grambow SC, Oddone EZ, Horner RD. Nonsteroidal anti-inflammatory drug use among patients with GI bleeding. *Ann Pharmacother.* 2004;38:1159-1164.
13. deGroot V, Beckerman H, Lankhorst GJ, et al. How to measure comorbidity: a critical review of available methods. *J Clin Epidemiol.* 2003;56:221-229.
14. Li B, Evans D, Faris P, et al. Risk adjustment performance of Charlson and Elixhauser comorbidities in ICD-9 and ICD-10 administrative databases. *BMC Health Serv Res.* 2008;8:12.
15. Ulcickas M, Campbell UB, Rothman KJ, et al. Using prescription claims data for drugs available over-the-counter (OTC). *Pharmacoepidemiol Drug Saf.* 2007;16(9):961-968.
16. Roebuck MS, Liberman JN. Impact of pharmacy benefit design on prescription drug utilization: a fixed effects analysis on plan sponsor data. *Health Serv Res.* 2009;44:988-1009.
17. Crowley JS, Ashner D, Elam L. Medicaid outpatient prescription drug benefits: findings from a national survey, 2003. Kaiser Commission on Medicaid and the Uninsured. December 2003. Technical Report. http://www.kff.org/medicaid/upload/Medicaid-Outpatient-Prescription-Drug-Benefits-Findings-from-a-National-Survey-2003.pdf. Accessed August 3, 2010.
18. Bruen BK, Miller LM. Changes in Medicaid prescription volume and use in the wake of Medicare Part D implementation. *Health Aff (Millwood).* 2008;27:196-202.
19. Bayliss EA, Ellis JL, Delate T, Steiner JF, Raebel MA. Characteristics of Medicare Part D beneficiaries who reach the drug benefit threshold in both of the first two years of the Part D benefit. *Med Care.* 2010;48:267-272.
20. Tseng C-W, Brook RH, Keeler E, Dudley RA. Identifying widely covered drugs and drug coverage variation among Medicare Part D formularies. *JAMA.* 2007;297:2596-2602.
21. De Smet PAGM, Denboom W, Kramers C, Grol R. A composite screening tool for medication reviews of outpatients: general issues with specific examples. *Drugs Aging.* 2007;24:733-760.
22. Hajjar ER, Hanlon JT, Sloane RJ, et al. Unnecessary drug use in frail older people at hospital discharge. *J Am Geriatr Soc.* 2005;53:1518-1523.
23. Beers MH, Ouslander JG, Rolingher J, et al. Explicit criteria for determining inappropriate medication use in nursing home residents. *Arch Intern Med.* 1991;151:1825-1832.
24. Hanlon JT, Schmader KE, Samsa GP, et al. A method for assessing drug therapy appropriateness. *J Clin Epidemiol.* 1992;45:1045-1051.
25. Beers MH. Explicit criteria for determining potentially inappropriate medication use by the elderly. *Arch Intern Med.* 1997;157:1531-1536.
26. Fick DM, Cooper JW, Wade WE, et al. Updating the Beers criteria for potentially inappropriate medications use in older adults: results of a US consensus panel of experts. *Arch Intern Med.* 2003;163:2716-2724.
27. Curtis LH, Ostbye T, Sendersky V, et al. Inappropriate prescribing for elderly Americans in a large outpatient population. *Arch Intern Med.* 2004;164:1621-1625.

28. Simon SR, Chan KA, Soumerai SB, et al. Potentially inappropriate medication use by elderly persons in U.S. Health Maintenance Organizations, 2000-2001. *J Am Geriatr Soc*. 2005;53:227-232.
29. Jano E, Aparasu RR. Healthcare outcomes associated with Beers' criteria: a systematic review. *Ann Pharmacother*. 2007;41:438-448.
30. O'Mahony D, Gallagher PF. Inappropriate prescribing in the older population: need for new criteria. *Age Ageing*. 2008;37(2):138-141.
31. Bagchi AD, Esposito D, Kim M, et al. Utilization of, and adherence to, drug therapy among Medicaid beneficiaries with congestive heart failure. *Clin Ther*. 2007;29:1771-1783.
32. Ganz DA, Glynn RJ, Mogun H, Knight EL, Bohn RL, Avorn J. Adherence to guidelines for oral anticoagulation after venous thrombosis and pulmonary embolism. *J Gen Intern Med*. 2000;15:776-781.
33. Shatin D, Schech SD, Patel K, McHutchison JG. Population-based hepatitis C surveillance and treatment in a national managed care organization. *Am J Manag Care*. 2004;10:250-256.
34. Winkelmayer WC, Fischer MA, Schneeweiss S, Wang P, Levin R, Avorn J. Underuse of ACE inhibitors and angiotensin II receptor blockers in elderly patients with diabetes. *Am J Kidney Dis*. 2005;46:1080-1087.
35. Moore WJ, Gutermuth K, Pracht EE. Systemwide effects of Medicaid retrospective drug utilization review programs. *J Health Polit Policy Law*. 2000;25(4):653-687.
36. US Food and Drug Administration. Understanding Generic Drugs. http://www.fda.gov/Drugs/ResourcesForYou/Consumers/BuyingUsingMedicineSafely/UnderstandingGenericDrugs/default.htm. Accessed August 3, 2010.
37. Vivian JC. Generic-substitution laws. US Pharm. 2010;35(8):60-63. Available at: http://www.uspharmacist.com/content/d/pharmacy%20law/i/1166/c/22033/. Accessed August 3, 2010.
38. Schachter SC. Generic and Brand Name AEDS: Considerations for Clinicians. PowerPoint presentation. http://professional.epilepsy.com/pdfs/generic_aeds.ppt#585. Accessed August 3, 2010.
39. Mott DA, Cline RR. Exploring generic drug use behavior: the role of prescribers and pharmacist in the opportunity for generic drug use and generic substitution. *Med Care*. 2002;40:662-674.
40. Labiner DM, Paradis PE, Manjunath R, et al. Generic antiepileptic drugs and associated medical resource utilization in the United States. *Neurology*. 2010;74:1566-1574.
41. Hastings SN, Sloane RJ, Goldberg KC, Oddone EZ, Schmader KE. The quality of pharmacotherapy in older veterans discharged from the emergency department or urgent care clinic. *J Am Geriatr Soc*. 2007;55:1339-1348.
42. Fernandes AW, Madhavan SS, Amonkar MM. Evaluating the effect on patient outcomes of appropriate and inappropriate use of beta-blockers as secondary prevention after myocardial infarction in a Medicaid population. *Clin Ther*. 2005;27:630-645.
43. Peng CC, Glassman PA, Marks IR, et al. Retrospective drug utilization review: incidence of clinically relevant potential drug-drug interactions in a large ambulatory population. *J Manag Care Pharm*. 2003;9:513-522.
44. Farris KB, Ganther-Urmie JM, Fang G, et al. Population-based medication reviews: a descriptive analysis of the medication issues identified in a Medicare not-for-profit prescription discount program. *Ann Pharmacother*. 2004;38:1823-1829.
45. Hellinger FJ, Encinosa WE. Inappropriate drug combinations among privately insured patients with HIV disease. *Med Care*. 2005;43(9 suppl):III53-III62.
46. Solberg LI, Hurley J, Roberts MH, et al. Measuring patient safety in ambulatory care: potential for identifying medical group drug-drug interaction rates using claims data. *Am J Manag Care*. 2004;10:753-759.
47. Becker ML, Kallewaard M, Caspers PWJ, et al. Potential determinants of drug-drug interaction associated dispensing in community pharmacies. *Drug Saf*. 2005;28(5):371-378.
48. Singh R. How a series of errors led to recurrent hypoglycemia. *J Fam Prac*. 2006;55 (6):489-497.

**Part 1: Claims Databases**

49. Trygstad TK, Christensen D, Garmise J, et al. Pharmacist response to alerts generated from Medicaid pharmacy claims in a long-term care setting: results from the North Carolina polypharmacy initiative. *J Manag Care Pharm*. 2005;11:575-583.
50. Bieszk N, Patel R, Heaberlin A, et al. Detection of medication nonadherence through review of pharmacy claims data. *Am J Health Syst Pharm*. 2003;60:360-366.
51. Stuart B, Fahlman C. Outcomes of prospective drug-use review of beta-agonist inhaler use in an elderly Medicaid population. *Clin Ther*. 1999;21:2094-2112.
52. Long CL, Raebel MA, Price DW, Magid DJ. Adherence with dosing guidelines in patients with chronic kidney disease. *Ann Pharmacother*. 2004;38:853-858.
53. Seidling HM, Al Barmawi A, Kaltschmidt J, et al. Detection and prevention of prescriptions with excessive doses in electronic prescribing systems. *Eur J Clin Pharmacol*. 2007;63:1185-1192.
54. Biesacher BA, Limcangco MR, Simoni-Wastilla L, et al. The quality of antipsychotic drug prescribing in nursing homes. *Arch Intern Med*. 2005;1280-1285.
55. Reingold S, Kulstad E. Impact of human factor design on the use of order sets in the treatment of congestive heart failure. *Acad Emerg Med*. 2007;14:1097-1105.
56. Munir J, Wright RJ, Carr DB. A quality improvement study on calcium and vitamin D supplementation in long-term care. *J Am Med Dir Assoc*. 2007; 8(3 suppl 2):e19-e23.
57. Zucherman IH, Weiss SR, McNally D, et al. Impact of an educational intervention for secondary prevention on myocardial infarction on Medicaid drug use and cost. *Am J Manag Care*. 2004;10:493-500.
58. Davis RG, Hepfinger CA, Sauer KA, et al. Retrospective evaluation of medication appropriateness and clinical pharmacist drug therapy recommendations for home-based primary care veterans. *Am J Geriatr Pharmacother*. 2007;5:40-47.
59. Coleman CI, Reddy P, Laster-Bradley NM, et al. Prescriber and pharmacist responses to intervention letters for Connecticut Medicaid beneficiaries with asthma. *Am J Health Syst Pharm*. 2003;60:1142-1144.
60. Sleath B, Collins T, Kelly HK, et al. Effect of including both physicians and pharmacists in an asthma drug-use review intervention. *Am J Health Syst Pharm*. 1997;54:2197-2200.
61. Wadland WC, Farquhar L, Priester F, et al. Increasing generic prescribing: a resident educational intervention. *Fam Med*. 2005;37:259-264.
62. Mager DE, Cox ER. Relationship between generic and preferred-brand prescription copayment differentials and generic fill rate. *Am J Manag Care*. 2007;13:347-352.
63. Culbertson VL, Force RW, Cady PS, et al. Positive impact of a follow-up phone call to community pharmacies in a Medicaid drug utilization program. *Ann Pharmacother*. 1999;33:541-547.
64. Kahan NR, Chinitz DP, Waitman DA, et al. When gatekeepers meet the sentinel: the impact of a prior authorization requirement for cefuroxime on the prescribing behaviour of community-based physicians. *Br J Clin Pharmacol*. 2006;61:341-344.
65. Gregoire JP, Moisan J, Potvin L, et al. Effect of drug utilization reviews on the quality of in-hospital prescribing: a quasi-experimental study. *BMC Health Serv Res*. 2006;6:33.
66. Glassman PA, Belperio P, Simon B, et al. Exposure to automated drug alerts over time: effects on clinicians' knowledge and perceptions. *Med Care*. 2006;44:250-256.

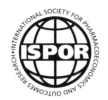

# PART 2

## Electronic Health Records

| | | |
|---|---|---|
| CHAPTER 6 | Introduction to Electronic Health Records | 73 |
| CHAPTER 7 | Uses of Electronic Health Records for Health and Disease Management | 84 |
| CHAPTER 8 | Strengths and Weaknesses of Using Electronic Health Records for Health and Disease Management | 98 |
| CHAPTER 9 | Electronic Health Record Implementation Challenges at the Practice Level | 107 |
| CHAPTER 10 | Real-Time Applications of Electronic Health Record Data | 115 |
| CHAPTER 11 | Policy Maker Perspectives on Electronic Health Records | 122 |

CHAPTER 6

# Introduction to Electronic Health Records

Ryung Suh, MD, MPP, MBA, MPH; Andrew B. Einhorn, MS;
Richard Hartman, PhD; Edward Kim, MD, MBA;
Jaspal Ahluwalia, MD, MPH; Carla Zema, PhD;
Sam Ho, MD; and Steven R. Simon, MD, MPH

This chapter has 3 primary goals: to examine the functions of the medical record and its evolution from paper to electronic form; to define the terminology used to describe the electronic exchange of health information, including electronic medical records (EMRs), electronic health records (EHRs), electronic health record systems (EHR-S), and personal health records (PHRs); and to provide a summary of the remaining chapters in this section.

Because of difficulties storing, communicating, and abstracting data from paper medical records, paper-based data exchange and records systems have been and continue to be replaced by electronic health records at every level of the health care system, ranging from drug prescriptions to clinical decision support tools. Research indicates that EHRs exhibit considerable potential for improving health and disease management (HDM). Supporters of EHRs argue that the health care system will benefit from improved care coordination among providers, billing accuracy, records management, medical test ordering, diagnostic accuracy, and patient access to services through secure online portals.[1]

Providers and administrators at all levels of the health care system rely on detailed health reporting and records management to initiate, administer, track, and analyze patient care. Each piece of data provides insight into the nature of a patient's problem, disease presentation, and prognosis. Collectively, these data provide researchers, health care providers, and other health care decision makers the opportunity for continual improvement of health and disease management at the patient and population levels. Ultimately, electronic medical record data might also enable enhanced analysis and the potential to improve health outcomes.

Health care systems rely heavily on the exchange of information between different health system components or stakeholders. Each piece of health data exchanged—as often occurs between patients and providers, providers and institutions, patients and institutions, and among providers—affords a chance to improve patient health. Prescriptions, lab test results, recommendations from health care specialists, and reimbursements or coverage for medical expenses are all made possible through the exchange of medical data. EHRs promise to make these exchanges more efficient and accurate.

## 1. Functions of Medical Records

The documentation of patient care has evolved from a simple journal of patients' problems and their treatments to a complex, multipurpose document designed to detail clinical care; manage population health; ensure compliance with clinical, accreditation, and certification standards; justify reimbursement and care decisions; protect providers from liability; and conduct research. These functions of the medical record are critical to the understanding of paper-based and electronic records used for conducting health services research and disease management evaluations.

## Clinical Communications

In ambulatory settings, the medical chart or record comprises the paradigm for clinical documentation and is a longitudinal account of a patient's medical care. The medical chart is considered the gold standard for documenting the process of patient care and results of clinical decisions. In this capacity, it is used by the provider to observe the results (or lack thereof) of clinical interventions across time. It also represents a scientific *sample size of one* analysis in which the practitioner makes a diagnosis (scientific hypothesis), initiates an intervention (hypothesis testing), and observes an outcome.

In hospital settings, the medical record documents patients' care across an acute episode of care rather than multiple visits over time. Unlike the ambulatory setting in which records typically include care from a certain type of provider, such as primary care or specialist, hospital medical charts enable health care providers of different disciplines to assess patients' medical history and treatments to make decisions. Because care is delivered continuously over a hospital stay, multiple types of providers might coordinate care to improve patients' health and minimize the risk of adverse events, signaling that the role of the hospital medical record is to communicate across silos. Medical records enable nurses, allied health professionals, and subspecialty consultants to assist the primary medical or surgical team to make informed decisions for patient care. In teaching hospitals, medical charts can also serve as a means of communication between trainees and faculty who may append or amend entries to reflect subtleties of diagnostic and therapeutic relevance not observed by the trainee.

## Management of Population Health

Although providers use medical records to document patients' care, other common uses of medical records extend beyond patient care, and providers are only one of many groups of users. Many other stakeholders, such as payers, employers, researchers, and regulators, also use medical records to manage the health of populations. These stakeholders use medical records to review care across populations and subgroups to determine how care is delivered and to examine population health outcomes. Subgroups of patients can include patients at a certain practice, facility, or location; patients with a certain condition or treatment; or patients in a certain geographic location.

## Compliance with Clinical, Accreditation, and Certification Standards

In addition to care management, stakeholders use medical records to evaluate clinical quality and effectiveness. Medical records provide the documentation of care provided to patients to determine compliance with clinical standards, such as evidence-based medicine and guidelines. The reviews can be focused on individual providers for the purposes of pay for performance, professional certification, or provider credentialing as typically sponsored by payers and professional organizations. Reviews can also be focused on provider groups, facilities, and health plans. Measures of clinical quality and effectiveness used for these purposes often require data that can only be found in medical records.

## Reimbursement and Care Decision Justification

Payers use medical record information to ensure providers' practices meet guidelines for appropriate care. For example, utilization review, also referred to as utilization management, is a tool used by many payers to encourage evidence-based care and to limit unnecessary care. Payers typically request portions of patients' medical records (from ambulatory care and inpatient settings) to review the care that is being provided. This documentation is used to examine the acuity of the case, complexity of decision making, and the extent of counseling and education provided to patients. Based upon the information provided, payers make decisions on whether or not certain aspects of care will be reimbursed, such as additional days in the hospital, the need for tests, and the appropriateness of treatments. These reimbursement decisions can have a significant impact on patient care because reimbursement is a primary driver of care delivery. The Centers for Medicare & Medicaid Services (CMS), health insurance plans, employer groups, and other public and private payers have developed documentation guidelines to ensure that reimbursement is consistent with the level of service delivered.

## Risk Management

The influence of medical liability on the practice of medicine is an unfortunate necessity, ranging from an increase in diagnostic tests to err on the side of caution to professionals restricting their caseload to reduce exposure to high-risk cases. A 2010 study estimated medical liability costs, including defensive medicine, to be $55.6 billion in 2008 dollars or 2.4% of total health care spending.[2] This practice may result in considerable variability in documentation as physicians selectively document high-risk cases at the expense of low-risk cases.

Most importantly, while trying to mitigate legal risk, a health care provider might introduce reporting biases. For example, if a clinician feels that a case involves unnecessary risk, he or she may spend a considerable amount of time documenting the clinical rationale for the decision. This may include outlining alternatives that were considered, or documenting the discussion held with the patient and/or caregivers and their decision. It may also include whether the patient or caregiver made an informed decision. In a case of lower perceived risk, the clinical decision-making process might be more straightforward. As a result, the provider may document less information and detail about the encounter. In a time-constrained environment, the physician may adopt the *documentation by exception* rule, in which he or she only documents those elements that present a perceived legal risk.

## Research

Although not a primary function of medical records, researchers use medical record data in a variety of ways because these records are often the only source of some types of medical data. Most studies that use such data involve a retrospective review of medical records such as observational studies for which randomization of research subjects is oftentimes not feasible. Moreover, studies that are not practical to conduct prospectively are conducted with medical record data.

## 2. Paper Medical Records

The ability to use medical record information for the functions described above can be dependent on the format in which the data are available. Providers have traditionally relied upon paper medical records to record illnesses, track patient progress, report test results, and communicate information between different health care providers and facilities. Today, clinicians, health care facilities, and health insurers are steadily supporting, and in some cases, replacing paper-based systems with EMRs due to inherent problems and risks associated with paper medical records. Still, as of 2008, only 38.4% of office-based physicians in the US reported using full or partial EHR systems (not including billing records), and use of specific EMR features varied substantially.[3] Thus, the majority of physicians remain exposed to the disadvantages of paper health records, of which there are several that might prohibit researchers from using these data to study health and disease management programs.

### Financial Cost of Medical Record Review Abstraction

The cost of paper medical record review abstraction—the process of converting data from paper to electronic form—can add considerable costs to research. Consider a national health system abstracting paper health record data for health and disease management research from 50 or more patients from each of 200,000 physicians. Even with a conservative estimate of $100 per medical chart abstraction, the total cost of this effort would be approximately $10 billion. Moreover, this excludes costs associated with auditing or developing an abstraction tool, and likely underestimates the actual expense to the health care system due to opportunity costs. This significant financial barrier makes such comprehensive medical record review initiatives unrealistic. As a result of this lack of feasible data collection, major gaps persist in the scientific literature concerning health and disease management of populations.

## Time Cost of Medical Record Review Abstraction

Other factors also contribute to the prohibitive cost of using paper medical record data for health and disease management. For example, records for one patient may reside in as least as many locations as that patient has providers. Paper records might also be lost, damaged, or misfiled, thereby limiting access to them. Consequently, finding the appropriate medical record can be resource intensive.

Significant time is also necessary for the data entry into an electronic format, and data preparation, including identifying appropriate medical and therapeutic codes using appropriate coding dictionaries, and data cleaning. While specialized computer software can facilitate data abstraction and reduce the time necessary to collect the data, the resource needs are still significant limiting factors when paper records are used.

## Documentation Quality and Completeness

Although the paper medical record contains unique clinical data, their validity is contingent upon documentation in the record itself. Moreover, the level of documentation in the medical record by a health care provider is dependent upon the information the provider chooses to document. While providers generally agree and are trained to document key pieces of information in the medical record, such as medical and family history, chief complaints, physical exam, medications and allergies, the level of documentation can be highly variable.[4]

Information that is critical to health and disease management, such as health risk assessment, education, and counseling may be missing from the records. Such omissions may indicate that the provider did not discuss the issue or perform the task with the patient; or these omissions may simply represent incomplete documentation. Although the former can be a serious quality-of-care issue and the latter less serious, differentiating between the 2 is not possible if information in the medical record is missing. Providers will record data that are pertinent to their role in the clinical process; therefore, if more or different data are necessary to fulfill other uses for the data, providers may require an incentive to record such information.

Data quality is also an issue. The Institute of Medicine (IOM) report, *To Err Is Human: Building a Safer Health System*, cites illegible handwriting as a source of patient safety error that has the potential to cause significant patient harm or even death.[5] Although many health plans and professional organizations have developed medical record documentation standards, variability in documentation levels persists often due to time pressures on providers.

## Medical Record Abstractor Validity and Reliability

Medical record abstractors transferring data from paper to electronic form for the purposes of a study or to store the data electronically can also influence the quality of the medical record data. Despite efforts to standardize abstracted data elements, and training to ensure reliability in what is abstracted, medical record reviews still rely on abstractor judgment. Given the variability of documentation by the health care providers, it is impossible to specify every type of documentation that could be encountered during the abstraction process.

For example, consider determining whether or not a physician provides anticipatory guidance—a proactive, developmentally based counseling technique that focuses on the needs of a child at each stage of life—during a well-child visit. Specifically, during the visit, the provider administers preventive care by assessing a child's physical, behavioral, developmental, and emotional well-being. Following the visit, data abstractors must determine whether or not the physician provided appropriate anticipatory guidance, even if the provider did not capture the anticipatory guidance relayed on any medical record forms.

Although abstractors are typically provided guidance and some examples, their judgment plays a role in how data are recorded. Moreover, abstractors must often describe how best to interpret paper medical records. In this example, they might have to decide if a copy of an information sheet provided to the patient counts as anticipatory guidance. Or abstractors might have to make judgments on partially complete data. For instance, a provider might note that anticipatory guidance was given without any other information about the content of that guidance. Similarly, there may be evidence of developmental guidance but not prevention. Variation across abstractors could result in different interpretations of the same data. The degree of difference between such interpretations is known as inter-rater reliability, the lower the inter-rater reliability, the poorer the quality of the medical record data.

## Care across Multiple Providers

The reliability of medical record data is limited by the consistency with which care coordinated by, or received from, multiple health care providers is documented. Consider a patient with diabetes who receives care from both a general practitioner and an endocrinologist. Additionally, the patient sees an ophthalmologist for annual eye exams to screen for diabetic retinopathy and was recently hospitalized for ketoacidosis. Even in this simple example, health care relevant for the patient's diabetes would be spread across 4 different providers, all of whom maintain their own medical records for the same patient that they may or may not share with one another. Information on laboratory results, prescriptions, and other ancillary services may or may not be included in the medical records at these providers. Consequently, it would be difficult to examine episodes of care given the nature and availability of data from paper medical records.

## Availability of Information from Ancillary Providers

A related and final disadvantage of paper records stems from the frequency of incomplete data derived from lab, X-ray, emergency department, consultant, or ambulance services. These records may be lost, damaged, accidentally destroyed, never received, or never sent. In contrast, electronic administrative claims data can identify such diverse sites of services, and more importantly, may be used for disease management identification in some cases.

## 3. Definitions and Differentiation among Electronic Health Records/Electronic Medical Records, Electronic Health Record Systems, and Personal Health Records

Given the drawbacks of paper medical records, it should come as no surprise that the United States government and the health care industry have actively sought ways to increase the use of electronic medical records. The passage of the Health Information Technology for Economic and Clinical Health Act (HITECH) as part of the American Recovery and Reinvestment Act of 2009 (ARRA) represented a significant federal investment in health information technology, including incentives for adopting electronic medical records.[6] Before delving into the many applications of electronic data management for health and disease management programs, it is useful to establish some baseline definitions.

### Electronic Health Record and Electronic Medical Record

The term *electronic health record (EHR)* is often used interchangeably with *electronic medical record (EMR)* to mean an electronic analog of the paper medical record. Yet, standardization of their definitions and potential differences between EHRs and EMRs has yet to be completely resolved. For example, the International Standard Organization (ISO) defines an EHR as:

> "A repository of information regarding the health status of a subject of care in computer processable form, stored and transmitted securely, and accessible by multiple authorized users. It has a standardized or commonly agreed logical information model, which is independent of EHR systems. Its primary purpose is the support of continuing, efficient and quality integrated health care, and it contains information which is retrospective, concurrent, and prospective."[7] (ISO/TC 215, 2005).

In contrast, ISO defines an EMR as a special case of the EHR that is "restricted in scope to the medical domain or at least very much medically focused." Thus, EHRs take on the broader definition of all electronic patient data, while EMRs refer only to the electronic medical data.

The term *EMR* is widely used in the United States, Canada, and a number of other countries. But despite the efforts of ISO and other organizations to standardize the definition and use of the terms *EMR* and *EHR*, variability persists. For instance, the National Alliance for Health Information Technology (NAHIT) established definitions for electronic medical records (EMR) and electronic health records (EHR) that differ from the ISO descriptions. The group defines an EMR as:

> The electronic record of health-related information on an individual that is created, gathered, managed, and consulted by licensed clinicians and staff from a single organization who are involved in the individual's health and care.

But like the ISO, they also classify the EHR as a broader category of electronic information, referring to an EHR as:

> The aggregate electronic record of health-related information on an individual that is created and gathered cumulatively across more than one health care organization and is managed and consulted by licensed clinicians and staff involved in the individual's health and care.[8]

This definition deviates from the ISO definition in its suggestion that EHRs, by nature, contain information from disparate sources, while an EMR is derived at a single point of contact or facility.

In this section, the term *EHR* refers broadly to any and all forms of electronic data that contain useful information about an individual patient's health care. Given the direction of technology development and the push to incorporate many different health data points inside an electronic health record, we use the term EHR throughout this chapter and section as a broader term that also incorporates the EMR. Moreover, usage of the term *medical* implies physician-centered usage while *health* encompasses other clinicians.

## Electronic Health Record System

Whether *EHR* or *EMR* eventually becomes the preferred term for electronic medical data is perhaps less important than the distinction between an EHR/EMR and an EHR system. An EHR system (EHR-S) is a larger network that links together important functional units of health-related data. Fischetti defines an *EHR-S* as "the tools and applications that facilitate the use of the data from the EHR by the end user. The EHR-S thus becomes a more comprehensive application consistent with what many mean by the term EHR."[9]

From another perspective, based on her previous work developing an EHR System Functional Model as a Draft Standard for Trial Use with Health Level Seven (HL7 is an ANSI-accredited Standard Developing Organization (SDO) working in the health care arena), Fischetti describes the functional specifications for an EHR-S. These are grouped into 3 areas: (1) *direct care* (subdivided into care management, clinical decision support, and operations management and communication); (2) *supportive* (subdivided into clinical support; measurement, analysis, research, and reporting); and (3) *administrative, financial, and information infrastructure* (subdivided into EHR security; EHR information and records management; unique identity, registry and directory services; support for health information and terminology standards; interoperability; management of business rules; and workflow).[9]

The Institute of Medicine (IOM) provides additional clarity as it defines 8 functionalities of an EHR-S, as noted in the box to the right.

The IOM further defines the primary uses of an EHR-S: patient care delivery, patient care management, patient care support processes, financial and other administrative processes, and patient self-management. Secondary uses include education, regulation, research, public health and homeland security, and policy support.[10]

> Functionalities of EHR-S as defined by the IOM
> 1. Health information and data
> 2. Results management
> 3. Order entry/management
> 4. Decision support management
> 5. Electronic communication and connectivity
> 6. Patient support
> 7. Administrative processes
> 8. Reporting and population health

## Personal Health Record

The *personal health record (PHR)* is a collection of health information specifically useful to and managed by the patient. This information might be stored on a home computer, smart card, mobile device, or on the internet. PHRs can contain a diverse range of data, but they typically include information about allergies and adverse drug reactions; medications (for example, dose and how often taken), including over-the-counter medications and herbal remedies; illnesses and hospitalizations; surgeries and other procedures; vaccinations; laboratory test results; and family history.

## 4. Conclusion

Data constitute the core of any health care or disease management system. Without accurate, accessible data, it is more difficult to coordinate patient care between providers and health care facilities, manage health care risks, conduct research studies, or run medical financial management systems. For decades, the US health care system revolved around paper medical records. As a result, many records were lost or damaged, records were stored at disparate facilities and inaccessible as a single medical history, and large medical research efforts were stalled or abandoned due to the exorbitant costs of compiling data from paper sources.

Following the advent of the personal computer and the Internet, it became possible, and in some cases necessary, to collect, store, manage, and communicate medical data in electronic formats. EHR-S, EMRs, and EHRs may be employed to enhance the coordination of care, safeguard medical data from destruction, more accurately track billing information, and facilitate groundbreaking research in health and disease management.

## 5. Chapter Summaries

Each subsequent chapter in this section will address various issues related to electronic data sources in greater detail, in an effort to provide a holistic picture of the uses, benefits, opportunities and drawbacks of electronic health records and systems.

Chapter 7 reviews the role of EHRs in health and disease management, including specific uses of EHR data, such as in research studies and health surveillance. This chapter also describes the advantages and disadvantages of using EHR data in health and disease management programs.

Chapter 8 provides a foundation for understanding the strengths and weaknesses of using electronic data sources for health and disease management. Benefits addressed in the chapter include the standardization of data categories, accurate diagnostic and procedural coding, technology-driven health applications (for example, decision support software), enhanced opportunities for research analysis, and the detection of rare sentinel events. Limitations of EHRs addressed include difficulties accessing data stored on disparate systems, interoperability gaps of disparate EHR systems, the biasing of electronic records, and general ways in which even electronic data may be rendered less reliable.

Chapter 9 examines the challenges to EHR implementation specific to providers. It explores barriers to EHR adoption including the cost and selection of a system as well as the cost of implementation. The chapter also addresses postadoption challenges encountered by practices, including the availability, use, and limitations of EHR features. Policy implications specific to providers are also summarized.

Chapter 10 explores innovative approaches to EHR data management, such as real-time monitoring of trends in disease and illness within a population, automated epidemiological systems, and enhancing reimbursement tracking. An in-depth analysis of the continuous monitoring process follows by examining the sampling and reporting criteria.

Chapter 11 addresses the role of policy making in establishing electronic data systems, electronic data exchanges, and standardizing EHRs. Various statewide, provincial, national, and international EHR initiatives to overcome electronic interoperability issues are discussed. As the nation moves toward increasing EHR use, policy makers work to address problems indirectly imposed by EHRs through research and analytic programs; however, many barriers to legislating experimental and pilot programs exist. These barriers, including fears about data privacy, loss, theft, or corruption, are also discussed.

# References

1. Miller R, Sim I. Physicians' use of electronic medical records: barriers and solutions. *Health Aff.* 2004;23(2):116-126.
2. Mellow MM, Chandra A, Gawande AA, Studdert DM. National costs of the medical liability system. *Health Aff.* 2010;29(9):1569-1577.
3. Hsiao CJ, Burt CW, et al. Preliminary estimates of electronic medical record use by office-based physicians: United States, 2008. US Department of Health and Human Services, CDC, National Center for Health Statistics; 2008. Available at http://www.cdc.gov/nchs/products/pubs/pubd/hestats/physicians08/physicians08.pdf. Accessed September 23, 2012.
4. Soto CM, Kleinman KP, Simon SR. Quality and correlates of medical record documentation in the ambulatory setting. *BMC Health Serv Res.* 2002;2(1):22.
5. Institute of Medicine. *To Err Is Human: Building a Safer Health System.* Washington, DC: National Academy Press; 1999.
6. Buntin MB, Jain SH, Blumenthal D. Health information technology: laying the infrastructure for national health reform. *Health Aff.* 2010;29(6):1214-1219.
7. ISO/TC 215. Health informatics: electronic health record: definition, scope, and context. Geneva: ISO; 2005.
8. The National Alliance for Health Information Technology. Report to the Office of the National Coordinator for health information technology on defining key health information technology terms. Washington, DC: Department of Health and Humand Services; April 28, 2008. Available at: www.hhs.gov/healthit/documents/m20080603/10_2_hit_terms.pdf. Accessed September 23, 2012.
9. Fischetti LF, Schloeffel P, Blair JS, Henderson ML. Standards. In: Lehmann H, ed. *Aspects of Electronic Health Record Systems.* New York, NY: Springer; 2006:chap 12.
10. Institute of Medicine. *Key Capabilities of an Electronic Health Record System: Letter Report.* Washington, DC: National Academies Press; 2003.

CHAPTER 7

# Uses of Electronic Health Records for Health and Disease Management

Andrew B. Einhorn, MS; Carla Zema, PhD; Steven R. Simon, MD, MPH; Ryung Suh, MD, MPP, MBA, MPH; and Sam Ho, MD

This chapter describes how electronic health records (EHRs) and electronic medical records (EMRs) are used in health and disease management (HDM), as well as considerations for the use of these data. Although the potential value of medical records data to HDM has been known for some time, using these data was often infeasible, especially for population studies, due to the limitations of and challenges involved with using paper medical records. EMRs, EHRs, and electronic health record systems (EHR-S) make these data accessible for the purposes of studying and evaluating HDM programs.

In reviewing the fundamental components of HDM, the usefulness of electronic data records becomes evident quickly. Nearly every component of HDM, from identifying a target population to providing feedback to patients and providers, relies on data. Because data are nearly always more easily stored, located, and read using electronic means, using EMRs and EHRs for disease management serves as a best practice. For instance, electronic data are particularly helpful in integrating practice or treatment guidelines into clinical encounters. Compliance tracking, medical surveillance, and the monitoring of provider and patient activities are also greatly enhanced, if not dependent upon, electronic data management in population-based HDM initiatives.

## 1. The Role of Electronic Sources in Disease Management

Exploring the many ways in which electronic data may be used to improve disease management remains an interesting, fast-growing, and well-funded sector of health care. The rapid influx of public and private sector funding for research and development projects within this area signifies an evolving perception of the usefulness of electronic medical data. However, barriers to the implementation of these new technologies still remain. In particular, issues of data protection, privacy, and interoperability continue to challenge researchers, academics, public officials, and technicians in the health care field.

Although solutions for many of these issues have yet to be discovered, the diverse ways in which electronic data are being used to improve patient care continue to grow. For instance, electronic data affect health care delivery and disease management through the documentation of vital signs, medications, and lab results; the organization of data queries for outcomes studies; and the electronic coordination of care delivery. Broadly, the uses of electronic data may be broken down into three categories: documentation and care coordination, research applications, and safety and disease surveillance. In what follows, we describe each of these uses in detail.

## Documentation and Care Coordination

### Closed Electronic Health Records

An EHR is a longitudinal record of a patient's health information generated by one or more encounters in health care delivery settings. Many different types of information are included in this record, such as demographic information, progress notes, health problems, medications, vital signs, past medical history, immunizations, laboratory data, and radiology reports. At the core of the EHR lies the medical chart, or EMR, that provides a complete record of a clinical patient encounter, including evidence-based decision support, quality management, and outcomes reporting. As EHRs incorporate EMRs and because future electronic data sources will likely include much more than the medical chart, the term *EHR* will be used throughout this chapter to encompass both EMRs and EHRs.

The use of electronic means to complete medical charts, such as when a provider uses a handheld, laptop, or desktop computer to take notes during a patient encounter, the information captured is standardized for all patients. In cases in which different health care facilities employ the same EHR-S, medical charts may be standardized across them, enabling providers to document information and ensuring that the same information about a patient is available across facilities. Electronic medical information can be as simple as scanned versions of paper documents that are managed electronically to full systems in which data are directly entered, manipulated, and exchanged in the system.

Care coordination across facilities takes many forms, all of which are made easier when patient information is exchanged electronically. At a basic level, care coordination with EHRs allows medical histories, insurance information, prescription histories, and any lab or test information to be readily accessible wherever the patient is treated geographically. This enables providers to determine appropriate diagnoses and treatments based upon the patient's history.

More sophisticated EHR systems grant care providers electronic tools for making referrals, emailing prescriptions directly to pharmacies, ordering laboratory or radiology tests, providing decision support, and receiving data from other sources. By replacing a paper-based system with an electronic data management system, this information can be more easily stored, managed, communicated, and retrieved. The increased efficiency can result in care being allocated faster and more accurately.

## Open Electronic Health Records and Personal Health Records

Providers are not the sole beneficiaries of the advantages of EHRs. Patients themselves can access and manage their own electronic health data to improve the management of their health. For example, at the US Department of Veterans Affairs, which uses an EHR-S known as VistA (Veterans Health Information Systems and Technology Architecture), veterans enrolled in the VA health care system may access a portion of their EHR online and input some health information that can be reviewed and validated by their providers. This is one example of a patient portal into an EHR also known as an *open EHR*.

Through a website called My HealtheVet, veterans can view their own health information, such as blood pressure rates and cholesterol levels; access a list of locations where they received treatment and the health care providers they visited; view their prescription drug history; and record allergy and immunization information. In addition, users of My HealtheVet may refill prescriptions and print a personal health summary for any provider.

Personal health records (PHRs) enable patients to better manage their health information. Because all the potential data that a patient could store in a PHR is not necessarily relevant to their providers, whether or not PHRs should be integrated into EHRs is debatable because providers would have to validate all linked information. If a PHR were integrated with an EHR, the data included in the PHR would become part of the medical record and the provider would become responsible for that portion of the record as well. Proponents of integrating PHRs and EHRs believe that any health-related information should be relevant to the provider while critics feel that reviewing large volumes of information may be an inefficient use of providers' time.

For example, patients might use PHRs to track their daily diets. Patients who only visit providers occasionally would have a tremendous amount of information on diet and providers may review a sample of the daily logs to understand patients' diets for counseling and education purposes. However, if patients later have medical problems due to their diets, providers might be liable for potentially preventable problems. Consequentially, discussions are ongoing regarding how PHR information can be integrated into EHRs to maximize the benefit to providers and patients.

Many PHRs are available to patients in easily accessible forms. For example, Google has developed a PHR system called Google Health that allows anyone to build an online health profile. Google Health users can enter their medical conditions, medications, allergies, and lab results manually, or import their EHRs directly from their health insurance providers, and participating hospitals and pharmacies. This enables users to record a complete history of their medical conditions, medications, and test results in one easily accessible location. Google also plans to include tools that would enable users to schedule appointments, refill prescriptions, and use wellness programs.

More specific uses of PHRs are also being deployed across the United States. These targeted uses of PHRs have significant promise at improving patient self-management behaviors. For example, one study explored the use of an online PHR for the management of diabetes.[1] In this randomized controlled trial, both the treatment and control groups used PHRs, but the treatment group used a diabetes-specific PHR that incorporated clinical information on medications, provided decision support information to the patient, and enabled patients to create their own care plan that they would submit to their physicians. The control group only included family history and health maintenance information in their PHRs. Although this study did not find a statistically significant difference in risk factors between the 2 groups, it did find that treatment group members were more likely to adjust their diabetes-related medications than the control group.

## Telehealth and Telemedicine

Telemedicine involves the use of telecommunication and information technologies to provide clinical care to individuals at a distance. The advent of electronic health data and the Internet have had a profound effect on telemedicine as well as telehealth, which is similar in nature but encompasses a broader array of care, including health education, public health, research, and administrative functions. Both telemedicine and telehealth rely heavily on technology to deliver health care without requiring person-to-person contact. Most telemedicine systems have focused on 2-way interactive consultation capabilities, such as videoconferencing via telephone lines.

Newer telemedicine technologies allow clinical consultations between providers and patients to be communicated over the Internet. Recording these consultations allows them to be stored and reviewed at a later date as part of the patient's EHR and for research studies evaluating aspects of patient-provider interactions. This ability is particularly effective when, for example, a primary care provider seeks specialist consultation for a particular patient. The primary care provider may then forward the stored videoconference, along with any radiology images and other relevant data, to the specialist for review and analysis.

Telemedicine is most frequently used to provide health care to rural areas, where health care facilities or providers may be in short supply. It is also often used to provide care to patients with physical disabilities. In both instances, care may be literally brought into the patient's home. In cases in which patients in rural areas require mental health care, telemedicine may be used to conduct group therapy sessions. Providers can also monitor certain health indicators, such as pulse, weight, temperature, blood pressure, glucose levels, or heart irregularities of their patients over great distances by using remote monitoring devices. These devices may also include messaging services that can send reminders (for example, "Did you take your medicine today?") and health information (for example, "Egg yolks contain high amounts of cholesterol.") to patients.

Significant advances in telemedicine have been seen in cardiac care. In the case of heart monitoring, a wireless transmitter may be fitted to the patient's heart to communicate heart readings over the Internet to providers. Another example of an advance in telemedicine in cardiac care is weight monitoring following cardiac surgery for persons with chronic heart failure (CHF). Sudden weight gain for CHF patients is often an indicator of life-threatening fluid retention; these patients are at especially high risk of such complications following cardiothoracic surgery. Remote monitoring devices transmit frequent weight measurements along with telephone monitoring for these patients in the days following discharge when the patient is at the highest risk. Not only do monitoring technologies like this have the potential to help save lives and improve care, but they also might reduce hospital admissions, emergency room visits, and costs.[2]

As with other technological advances, telemedicine is not without opportunity costs as it reduces the face-to-face time between a patient and provider. Although this could be an advantage in some cases, it also has the potential to reduce the accuracy of providers' recommendations through missed information that would have been obtained through in-person examination. Additionally, there is the potential for miscommunication between the provider and the patient. Finally, as with any system, there are also financial costs for hardware and system maintenance. The benefits of telemedicine must be carefully weighed against the costs to determine the appropriateness of telemedicine for specific care and treatments.

### Administrative and Financial Data

While health care leaders are looking to EHRs as a mechanism for improving the quality and efficiency of health care delivery, providers often have different motivations for implementing EHRs. A study by the CommonwealthFund found that the tool was most routinely used by physicians for electronic billing—despite the purported benefits of other EHR applications.[3] EHRs may improve billing accuracy by ensuring the correct billing codes are associated with care delivered, and eliminate the need to enter charges or reimbursement information manually for each visit. Through EHR systems, provider orders and notes can be simply translated into administrative information for bills automatically and sent to insurers or patients for payments.

## Research Applications

### Data Abstraction and Preparation

EHRs provide many opportunities and advantages for advancing health research by making medical record data more accessible, improving data accuracy, and lowering the cost of using the data. Electronic data are much easier to locate and extract for statistical analyses than paper records that require the researcher to spend large quantities of time and money translating information into electronic form in preparation for analysis. Often, researchers need only be granted access to databases of health care information to make use of EHR data for studies.

An example of how EHR data can be used for data abstraction and preparation for research purposes is a 2008 study that used EHRs to locate clinical phenotype data for a genetic epidemiological study.[4] By filtering and extracting the information from EHRs, researchers were able to build a database of patient information for analysis that would have otherwise required vast amounts of time and money for recruitment and screening. In studies such as this, when data must be compiled from multiple sources, new database mapping and cleaning technologies may be employed to automate and expedite the process of compiling, abstracting, and preparing the data for research.

## Financial, Utilization, and Quality-of-Care Rates

Health care administrators and leaders increasingly rely on electronic data to improve the quality of care and reduce costs where possible. For example, electronic data may be used to evaluate the effectiveness and efficiency with which health care providers treat patients. Providers who have higher rates of patients returning for the same illness—taking into account specialty area and case-mix—may need to adjust their practices. Such a problem may go unnoticed without data to prove that a potential problem exists. Moreover, as quality improvement initiatives such as pay for performance proliferate and payers are not reimbursing for care such as *never* events or some readmissions, the stakes for being able to measure accurately the effectiveness of care delivery become higher for health care providers and organizations.

Electronic data may also be used to report, monitor, and calculate rates of patient safety errors including misdiagnosis, medication errors, and treatment or procedure errors. Electronic data and systems can be used to reduce errors and to detect them before they reach the patient. With the rate of medical misdiagnosis at 20%, there is much room for improvement. Data may be used to identify physicians more prone to error and work to prevent those errors from occurring.[5]

Another effective use for electronic data occurs in hospital emergency rooms, where managing patient flow and prioritizing patients by need may mean the difference between life and death. Electronic data systems can help perform these management tasks by tracking patient triage information and allowing administrators to organize the data either manually or automatically by patient need. In this way, an individual admitted to the emergency room for, say, heart failure or a communicable disease may be treated before a patient with a sprained ankle or similar ailment.

Using electronic data to analyze process and utilization can provide valuable information that can be used to improve the quality, cost, and efficiency of health care. For example, hospital administrators and leaders may be interested in analyzing trends in length of stay by diagnosis and procedure. When case-mix is adjusted for severity, differences in length of stay can signal possible quality issues, areas of inefficiency, or preventable complications. Additionally, outpatient providers may want to examine rates of hospitalization for ambulatory care sensitive conditions, which would be an indicator of inadequate outpatient care.

EHR data may also support HDM interventions conducted by health plans across multiple providers. Large-scale programs across the health plans' enrollee populations previously were not possible due to the resource intensity of clinical data collection from paper health records. Electronic data allow health insurance providers to monitor quality and performance measures, reducing the data reporting burden on providers.

## Clinical Research

Until recently, the use of EHRs for clinical research has been considered secondary, behind care coordination and documentation. But the full utility and benefits of EHRs for research applications are only beginning to emerge. Those benefits range from using electronic health data for disease prevalence and condition variance studies to identifying candidates for clinical trials and for conducting clinical outcomes research. In these studies, the entire patient population may be digitally transferred from one or a variety of databases for statistical analysis. This potentially reduces the time otherwise needed for recruitment, obtaining informed consent, entering information into a database, requesting health records from providers, and converting data from paper records into electronic form.

In some instances, the EHR may also include an indication of the patient's willingness to take part in research studies. EHR systems can automate the research recruitment step further by alerting attending physicians via electronic prompts of a patient's eligibility for ongoing clinical studies. Information about the trial may be linked to the prompt, so providers and patients can quickly learn more. To increase efficiency even more, informed consent procedures could be integrated into the EHR system as well as electronic record forms to collect additional data for the study. The technology seamlessly integrates research and clinical care—sectors of health care that often operate in isolation of one another.

## Safety and Disease Surveillance

### Safety

EHRs, if used properly, can be powerful tools for improving disease management by increasing care coordination and the availability of research data. But EHRs and EHR systems also can serve preventive roles, protecting the patient and public from misdiagnosis, drug interactions, and disease progressions or outbreaks. For instance, an EHR system that automatically identifies potentially harmful interactions between drugs prescribed to the patient alerts the provider to the possibility of a problem so that the physician has greater oversight of adverse reactions or altering the prescription regimen.

The simplest tools supply a pop-up reminder of potentially harmful interactions on the computer screen of a physician ordering drugs through the system. More sophisticated technologies monitor indicators of interactions in the body, alerting providers through pagers, text messages, and other automated means, if an adverse interaction could occur. These methods have been proven to cut down the number of unwanted interactions by up to 25%.[6] Similar tools alert health providers when abnormal lab test results are entered into the system either manually or automatically from the lab.[7] Highlighting these results ensures that nothing is overlooked and that the patient's problem is attended to promptly and properly.

EHR systems may also employ decision-making tools to ensure the safety of patients. Clinical decision support tools may be built into an EHR-S to aid the provider in determining accurate disease and illness etiologies. When physicians enter the chief complaints of the patient into the EHR-S, a list of potential causes of those symptoms is automatically produced. Such clinical decision support tools have been shown to be associated with improved health outcomes.[8] Additionally, these technologies may also link the clinician to protocols, care plans, critical paths, literature, pharmaceutical information, and other health care databases. Rapid access to the information can be extremely powerful, particularly in busy environments in which patient caseloads are high and providers are rushed for time.

## Disease Surveillance

EHRs can encompass a far greater spectrum of information than simply a digital copy of a patient's medical charts. Data incorporated into the EHR vary widely and may even include reports generated by computer systems that monitor real-time trends in diseases and illnesses within a population. Hospitals can deploy these automated epidemiological systems as an early detection tool to determine abnormal rates of a particular illness before a true disease outbreak occurs.

An example of the use of EHRs for disease surveillance was developed by Dr. Randall Moorman, who helped develop a bedside monitoring system to predict the likelihood that sepsis would occur in a newborn baby.[9] The system works by analyzing heartbeat signals obtained from a bedside heart rate monitor. The computer program records the heart signals and investigates them for patterns that provide an indication that the baby is developing signs of sepsis.

The Real-time Outbreak Detection System (RODS) is a disease surveillance system that takes a broader approach to analyzing EHR data. RODS prevents, detects, and responds to natural outbreaks of disease, as well as attacks with biological warfare agents such as anthrax. The system works like an Internet search engine by combing through and filtering electronic hospital admissions records around the country to locate where people become ill, how old they are, and what symptoms they have. A computer algorithm analyzes the data.

Johns Hopkins University's applied physics laboratory built a similar system, known as the Electronic Surveillance System for the Early Notification of Community-based Epidemics, that compiles data such as emergency room visits and over-the-counter drug sales to identify early recognition of patterns that could indicate the outbreak of a disease. The system was widely used in the Washington, DC, area immediately following the Sept. 11, 2001, terrorist attacks, and is now used to monitor irregularities in disease prevalence within the District of Columbia and its surrounding counties, Maryland, and Virginia.

## 2. Considerations for Using Data for Health and Disease Management

Users of EHR data include health care providers, administrators, health insurance providers, researchers, and policy makers. Each group of users may have unique motivations for utilizing electronic data, but limitations may exist that make data access or use more difficult. To ensure each user understands the strengths, weaknesses, and limitations of the electronic data, general considerations for evaluating how and whether or not to use electronic data are presented in the section.

Before using electronic data, the user must first identify his or her research question(s). Put plainly, the researcher must ask, "What do I want to do with the data?" and "What are my needs?" While these may seem like obvious questions, determining the specific need or application of the data is critical to understanding whether or not EHR data will help answer a specific research question, even if a question is exploratory in nature. HDM applications of EHR data can be categorized into whether the management occurs at the individual patient or population level. Table 1 lists common uses of EHR data by user and indicates whether the use is typically at the patient or population level. Additional considerations are listed below and categorized by the type of user.

## Considerations for Researchers

Many of the following considerations may have been investigated previously, so it is always important, and will save time, to look for past studies using the data source and validation by other researchers, which should highlight potential weaknesses and possible methodological solutions.

### Data Availability

Evaluating which data are available and whether or not the data meet your needs are critical to understanding the potential limitations of a study's results. To accomplish this, the researcher must consider:

- whether or not the data source, such as health plan, provider group, or integrated delivery systems (IDS) data, is appropriate for the study.
- if the types of services and settings represented in the data will enable the study's research questions to be addressed.
- if the types of services and settings excluded from the data are limitations that can be overcome.

- if the time period the data covers is sufficient.
- whether or not the appropriate outcomes to be examined are likely to have been recorded for all patients.
- if data were complete over that time period.
- if data were recorded consistently over time and across the dataset.

## Patient Representativeness

Determining whether or not the patient population available for a research study via EHR data is representative of a population that can adequately address all the study's research questions is paramount. To determine representativeness, researchers must identify if the number of patients in the data is adequate and if the population is appropriate to answer the study research questions. For example, if the EHR data comes from providers who mostly care for Medicare patients, researchers must determine how this will affect their results.

Researchers should also determine if there is a particular subgroup of the population represented in the data, such as those with a specific medical condition or particular socioeconomic status. Researchers must then determine how they will define that subgroup, and if the subgroup is appropriate to address their research questions. Although the appropriate variables and/or fields may be in the database, the completeness and accuracy of those variables must also be considered. For example, the presence of one diagnosis of a particular condition may not accurately represent a true diagnosis, such as in cases when the diagnosis code/value is also used to rule out a diagnosis.

## Supplemental Data

Given the data that are captured in the EHRs, researchers should consider whether or not other data are necessary to answer their research questions and if those data are accessible and can be linked with the EHR data. For example, perhaps the EHR does not have complete laboratory data for all patients, but electronic data from a national laboratory vendor are available. In order to be used for the analysis, the laboratory data must be able to be linked to the EHR data through a unique patient identifier that is either the same in both systems or available via a crosswalk to link the patients across systems. Without the same unique patient identifier or a crosswalk, the supplemental data cannot be linked to the EHR data at the patient level definitively.

## Temporal Access Issues

When data from a long period are included in an analysis, researchers must be aware that the science of medicine may have progressed and that the context in which the data were collected may have changed. Consider, for example, conducting a 30-year study about cancer outcomes. In the span of 30 years, medical treatments may have changed so rapidly that a patient with cancer—who 30 years ago had little chance of survival—might now be cured. Studying cancer outcomes, without adjusting for the evolution of medicine, might introduce considerable validity problems that must be accounted for in the analysis. Similarly, a surgical procedure that was once performed exclusively in a hospital may now be accomplished in an outpatient setting. This change in process affects the availability of the data in the hospital EHR. If the analysis of a specific research problem is limited to inpatient data, for example, important information from outpatient procedures is lost and a study may become underpowered or lead to biased conclusions.

Along with the progress of medicine, other external and internal factors will affect the reliability and validity of data over time. For example, medication formularies will change, new data items may be collected, or information might be recorded in more or less detail due to organizational or government policy changes. Also, the physical system itself will have changed over time with systems having the capacity to collect greater volumes of data and more complex data (such as digital images) as they evolve. Changes in computer and coding systems will also affect the use of the systems perhaps *forcing* users to record data in different ways; for example, a system change could ensure that meaningful diastolic and systolic blood pressure measurements were always collected for a hypertensive patient.

## Data Context

Understanding the context of the data is important for knowing how EHR data can be used appropriately. The context of the data may influence not only its clinical meaning, but also its analytic value. For example, creatine phosphokinase (CPK) lab values are compared to norms that may be set by the lab on the entire population of patients tested on the previous day. As patients' illnesses and patterns of utilization of health services change, the nature of an abnormal CPK finding also changes. A value abnormal for one population is not abnormal for another. Likewise, a value considered abnormal a year ago may be considered normal now. When patients' treatment shifts radically from the hospital to the outpatient clinic (as it has in recent years), many less severe values of tests are no longer available at the hospital lab and tests at the lab should be recalibrated.

## Standardized Data Organization

Before analysis can begin, there is a need to use standard query language to organize the data. EHR data are not always available in one place. Most data users are acquainted with a table of variables in the columns and patients as rows within the table. Unfortunately, in EHRs, data are dispersed in numerous tables. A visit table may include information about the visit and a link to a patient table that includes information about the patient, much like a relational database.

Another problem is that different types of information are collected from various patients. For example, for one patient, there may be a diagnosis of shock, but for another, a blood pressure of less than 90 may indicate that the patient has gone into shock. Consequently, statistical analysis of operational data is fraught with difficulties because there are multiple ways to measure the same variable. Before starting, the researcher must spend a great deal of time and effort to define variables of interest in redundant ways. For example, both *diagnosis of shock* and *blood pressure of less than 90* must be mapped to a third variable called report of shock.

Researchers must also keep in mind the interaction between the patient's treatment and conditions. A normal blood pressure may be a sign of effective treatment. A patient may go into shock and arrest but be stabilized by emergency medical workers on the way to the hospital. The EHR will indicate that the patient has a normal blood pressure but, in reality, if it were not for the treatment, the patient would be in crisis.

## Considerations for Providers

### Data Availability

Evaluating which data are available is critical for providers to understand the patient's complete health profile. While many universities and hospitals use EHRs, only 30% of office-based physicians in the United States use electronic health data.[10] Thus, electronic health data queried about the patient is likely to be incomplete, leaving the patient to fill in the gaps in documentation. It is important that providers not rely too heavily on electronic data without first inquiring if the patient has received care for problems that may have been documented in paper form.

### Data Errors

When using EHR systems, there is a danger of user error if, for instance, a health care professional accidentally checks the wrong field while documenting a problem. Such an error may result in an incorrect diagnosis and, consequently, incorrect treatment. Providers should take extra care to avoid input errors and ensure that the data they are reviewing are intuitive. Similarly, personal health records (PHRs) managed by patients are also prone to error. Often, the data are manually entered into these systems instead of imported, giving rise to the potential for improper documentation by the patient. Providers should ensure the etiologies, treatments prescribed, and prescriptions recorded make sense before relying on this type of data.

### Accessing All Information

Oftentimes, when using EHR-S, data is mapped to multiple databases. To the dismay of some physicians, some EHR systems do a better job at providing a one-page health summary for patients than others. As a result, additional navigation may be necessary to pull the information sought on the patient from the system. Providers should be careful not to overlook important data that may not be immediately visible within the system.

## Data Standardization

Given the fact that there are many different vendors of EHR systems, it is possible for 2 disparate systems not to be capable of communicating with each other. In these cases, providers may have access to outside electronic health data but be unable to import the data into their own EHR system. Third-party data mapping technologies are available to help disparate systems communicate, but such technologies may be expensive to implement. The easiest solution may be to create a hyperlink to an outside system or simply print out the information.

## 3. Conclusion

Electronic health data can be used for a wide variety of applications. From automating billing processes to disease surveillance, electronic health data has the ability to improve profoundly, if not revolutionize, health and disease management. As the overall adoption rate of EHR systems increases, additional uses for electronic health data will be discovered. But as the technology constantly evolves and improves, it is important to keep in mind which data are available, the quality and completeness of that data, and how it will be used.

**TABLE 1.** Common Uses of EHR Data by Type of User and Level

| | Health Care Provider | Administrator | Health Plan | Purchaser | Researchers and Policy Makers |
|---|---|---|---|---|---|
| Clinical decision support | patient | N/A | N/A | N/A | N/A |
| Evidence-based care | patient, population | population | population | population | population |
| Error prevention | patient, population | population | population | population | population |
| Practice management | N/A | patient, population | population | N/A | N/A |
| Utilization review | population | patient, population | patient, population | N/A | N/A |
| Provider profiling | N/A | population | population | population | population |
| Clinical registries | population | population | population | population | population |
| Clinical effectiveness | patient, population | patient, population | population | population | population |
| Health outcomes | patient, population | patient, population | population | population | population |

patient level / population level

# References

1. Grant RW, Wald JS, Schnipper JL, et al. Practice-linked online personal health records for type 2 diabetes mellitus: a randomized controlled trial. *Arch Intern Med*. 2008;168(16): 1717-1782.
2. Polisena J, Tran K, Cimon K, et al. Home telemonitoring for congestive heart failure: a systematic review and meta-analysis. *J Telemed Telecare*. 2010;16(2):68-76.
3. Audet AJ, Doty MM, Shamasdin J, Schoenbaum SC. *Physicians' Views on Quality of Care: Findings From the Commonwealth Fund National Survey of Physicians and Quality of Care*. New York, NY: The Commonwealth Fund; 2005.
4. Wood GC, Still CD, Chu X, et al. Association of chromosome 9p21 SNPs with cardiovascular phenotypes in morbid obesity using electronic health record data. *Genomic Med*. 2008;2(1-2):33-43.
5. Papier, A. Seeing is believing: visual diagnostic decision support. *Digital HealthCare & Productivity*. Available at: http://www.bio-itworld.com/2008/11/20/VDDS.html. Accessed November 20, 2008.
6. Fowles JB, Weiner JP, Chan KS, et al. *Performance Measures Using Electronic Health Records: Five Case Studies*. New York, NY: The Commonwealth Fund; 2008.
7. Koeller, Rodney L. IT Applications in Health Care: The Electronic Medical Record. University of Maryland; 2002. Retrieved May 12, 2003, from http://faculty.ed.umuc.edu/meinkej/inss690/koeller.pdf.
8. Sintchenko V, Coiera E, Iredell JR, Gilbert GL. Comparative impact of guidelines, clinical data, and decision support on prescribing decisions: an interactive web experiment with simulated cases. *J Am Med Inform Assoc*. 2004;11(1):71-77.
9. Moorman JR, Lake DE, Griffin MP. Heart rate characteristics monitoring for neonatal sepsis. *IEEE Trans Biomed Eng*. 2008;53(1):126-132.
10. Hing E, Burt CW, Woodwell DA. Electronic medical record use by office-based physicians and their practices: United States, 2006. Advance data from vital and health statistics; no. 393. Hyattsville, MD: US Department of Health and Human Services, CDC, National Center for Health Statistics; 2007. Available at: http:///www.cdc.gov/nchs/data/ad/ad393.pdf. Accessed September 23, 2012.

CHAPTER 8

# Strengths and Weaknesses of Using Electronic Health Records for Health and Disease Management

Carla Zema, PhD; Steven R. Simon, MD, MPH; Sam Ho, MD;
Edward Kim, MD, MBA; Jaspal Ahluwalia, MD, MPH; Andrew B. Einhorn, MS; Farrokh Alemi, PhD; and Brent Gibson, MD, MPH, FACPM

This chapter presents methodological issues related to the use of electronic health data by evaluating the benefits and limitations of electronic health records (EHRs), personal health records (PHRs), and EHR systems (EHR-Ss). Health and disease management (HDM) initiatives often rely on information and data from patients' medical records. However, the inability to access and exchange clinical information rapidly and accurately can be a barrier to operating effective HDM programs.[1]

An EHR-S is considered a key component in improving the effectiveness, efficiency, and safety of health care.[2] The deployment of an EHR-S, which significantly improves operating efficiencies and patient safety, is estimated to save the health care system $81 billion annually—a significant portion of which is derived from improved care for chronic conditions.[3] While the magnitude of such cost-savings is debated, the increase in efficiency, safety, and overall quality of patient care is widely accepted.[4-6]

The terms *EHR* and *electronic medical record (EMR)* are often used interchangeably, although they signify slight technological differences (see Chapter 6). An EMR incorporates only medical data from inside a single department or organization, such as a private practice, while an EHR includes all electronic health, financial, administrative, and other data about a patient across multiple departments and/or organizations. But given the direction of technology development and the push to incorporate many different health data points inside an EHR, we use the term *EHR* throughout this chapter and section.

## 1. Electronic Health Records

### Benefits of Using Electronic Health Records

Health care experts and policy makers view EHR adoption as essential to increasing the quality, safety, and efficiency of the health care system.[7] EHRs have significant advantages that enable effective HDM that is not possible with paper-based record keeping systems.

## General Benefits Compared to Paper Medical Records

EHRs eliminate or significantly reduce many of the limitations of paper medical records. With EHRs, medical record data are compiled into an electronic database, making the data more easily accessible and enabling users to review data for a larger number of patients than is possible with paper medical records. Because data entered at multiple locations may be included in one database and may be accessible by multiple providers all at once, the physical location of the data entry is typically irrelevant. Similarly, difficulties in data abstraction from paper records, along with resources needed to re-enter data from paper records, do not exist with EHRs. The elimination of these barriers to data exchange and consolidation lowers the administrative costs of using EHR data in lieu of paper medical records, once all stakeholders become familiar with the electronic system.

## Standardization of Data Categories

Differences in the type and level of documentation across health care providers oftentimes make it difficult to conduct research based on data collected via chart review. However, such variation in health care provider documentation can be reduced with EHRs through the standardization of data categories by using defined and categorical variables, enabling the identification of information across a patient population. For example, smoking history and smoking status are often inconsistently documented in medical records. Variables such as whether or not the patient currently smokes and how long the patient has been smoking could be required in the EHR.

## Data Quality and Completeness

EHRs have the potential to improve the quality and completeness of medical record data. Providers often receive electronic prompts and reminders via the EHR to provide documentation based on a particular standard established by condition-specific or procedure-based templates. Standardized data categories with range and logic checking, as well as electronic prompts and alerts, can improve providers' documentation of health care encounters. In primary care settings, where comprehensiveness and care coordination are essential to patient care, providers using an EHR were 4 times less likely to report missing clinical information compared with providers not using an EHR.[8]

## Technology-Driven Applications to Improve Health Care Delivery

In addition to capturing clinical encounter data in an electronic format, many EHRs have clinical applications that support the delivery of medical care. One example of such a clinical application includes clinical decision support (CDS) systems that aid the provider in making a diagnosis about the patient's problem. Others include computerized provider order entry (CPOE) forms that help avoid misinterpretation by enabling providers to order medical tests and procedures directly. Similar tools also issue automated medical alerts for patients being monitored.

While these applications do not change the underlying medical record data recorded, they do increase the quality, efficiency, and safety of the care delivered to the patient. Although several studies do not identify a link between EHR use and increased quality of care,[9,10] one study with a similar finding determined that the use of specific EHR features were associated with higher performance on some quality measures.[11] This suggests that the promise of EHRs may not be realized simply through the adoption of a basic system, but rather through the implementation of more comprehensive EHR features.

## Improvement in Diagnostic and Procedural Coding

An important attribute of EHRs includes automated, accurate, and complete coding of symptoms, diagnoses, procedures, and treatments provided to patients. Health care providers use medical codes to organize medical information rather than free text, making their record keeping and practice management more reliable, consistent, and simple. This also makes analysis and research of EHR data possible by eliminating the need for free text searching methodologies. Such coding captures comorbidities, symptoms, treatment, case-mix, and severity of illness so that appropriate identification and stratification of various cohort populations can be made for appropriate referrals and enrollment of eligible patients into HDM programs.

## Limitations of Electronic Health Records

Despite the promise of significant cost-savings while simultaneously realizing gains in quality and safety, EHRs have some limitations. For example, while EHRs may reduce some errors, others may arise.[12] Awareness of the limitations of EHRs is critical to realizing the full potential of EHR data for HDM.

## Reimbursement-Driven and Idiosyncratic Coding

Despite their organizational efficiency and cost advantages over paper medical records, EHRs are still plagued by limitations that have helped to prevent their widespread adoption. For instance, although the accuracy and completeness of diagnosis procedure and service coding may be improved with EHRs, they may still not capture the true underlying characteristics of the population. Consider a patient with multiple chronic conditions. In some instances when the EHR is linked to financial systems, the diagnostic code that generates the actual reimbursement is the only one that is used. Secondary and tertiary comorbidities may not be reported unless they justify reimbursement in claims data. Sometimes, clinical charts capture the greater complexity of comorbidities; however, practitioners may use idiosyncratic terms within the coding dictionaries that may not be readily abstracted or aggregated.

## Data Access

Accessing EHR data may also prove challenging depending on where the data are stored. If the data are in a central repository or data warehouse, advanced IT expertise or training may be needed to extract it. Moreover, data extraction is not standardized and is likely system specific, making access much more difficult. While many vendors offer a user friendly portal to access data, data queries are often limited to standardized reports and do not offer the ability to generate ad hoc reports. Systems utilizing predefined reports or data queries can prevent users from accessing and analyzing the data. Similarly, custom data queries may require sophisticated analytic skills, creating access barriers for average users.

## Interoperability

Another drawback to EHRs comes from the fact they, by definition, function within one type of organization or setting. Unless a patient visits multiple providers affiliated with the same organization, such as at a hospital, university, or government organization, a visit is typically recorded as a single encounter in the EHR, rather than a record covering multiple episodes of care. Few examples exist of electronic exchanges of clinical information between unaffiliated clinical providers. This stems partly from a decentralized health care system, wherein EHR-Ss differ from facility to facility and are thus unable to communicate information with one another. For example, applications like computerized provider order entry tools create a record of the order in the EHR, but a record of the results will likely not be present unless it is reported back to the ordering provider in a separate report. Even filing results with the ordering provider requires multiple systems to interface.

Despite significant technological advances, system interoperability presents challenges, especially if the systems were not purchased in tandem or as part of one entire unit. Standardization of record categories has helped to reduce some inoperability issues, but standardization of interfaces between systems is still required before EHRs can be used on a widespread basis to improve HDM for patients across episodes of care involving multiple providers and/or settings of care.

## Free Text Fields

By using menu-driven fields, EHRs were once thought to offer the potential to streamline care delivery by making it easier for providers to document their findings. However, there is little consensus on exactly which fields should be structured and which left for free text entry for the provider to adequately capture the richness of each individual clinical encounter. Although well-defined and categorical medical record form fields can improve the data available in the EHR, providers are often frustrated when an EHR requires the use of too many drop-down menus or checkboxes, restricting their ability to convey concisely and clearly in free text what they want. Until providers become more accustomed to using EHRs, using predefined checkboxes may increase the time it takes for a provider to record a patient encounter adequately. On the other hand, because reimbursement is often tied to using the prepopulated parts of the EHR (like drop-down menus or checkboxes), providers might be incented to enhance use of EHRs.

In using predefined fields, providers may end up with a record that can be difficult for them to read if the information is not contained in an intuitive way. Free text fields built into EHR systems offer a reprieve from potentially confounding checkboxes. An unfortunate drawback is that such free text fields—lacking any structure to the data—can be difficult to aggregate and analyze, even in electronic form. As with any electronic database, there are technologies to automate the extraction of data from free text fields, but those strategies, such as coding algorithms, are imperfect and can be expensive to implement.

### Data Quality and Completeness

EHR data-capture methods and data-input templates are often not designed to meet the needs of different providers, work styles, and patient care situations. Consequently, providers may not use the EHR consistently, resulting in incomplete data. This frequently occurs during the implementation phase, which can last from several months to several years. Moreover, implementation of an EHR requires changes in workflow and dedicated resources. Providers can underestimate these needs and, in an effort to reduce costs, make decisions that lead to inadequate hardware, insufficient training, or insufficient support. Additionally, providers often do not know which features to choose when selecting an EHR, because they often do not recognize the need for some features until after implementation begins. Thus, until providers are more accustomed to using EHRs, the data included in them might be incomplete and inconsistent.

## Cost-Benefit of Electronic Health Records

Despite the significant cost of adopting EHRs for medical practice, cost-benefit studies find that overall benefits outweigh the costs of implementation even for small practices.[3,5,8] However, the length of time over which it takes to recoup the investment made to implement EHRs is unknown. A review of EHR cost-benefit studies found that the time necessary to break even after adopting an EHR ranged from 3 to 13 years.[5] While the rate of adoption of EHRs is increasing,[13] progress has been slow in the United States, especially among small practices.[14] While small practices recouped the cost of the EHR in approximately 2.5 years on average, in another study some practices faced significant financial risk and could not recover as quickly.[15] However, the same study found that practices profited after they were able to pay for the EHR. Initial EHR costs in these small practices averaged $44,000 per full-time equivalent (FTE) provider with annual maintenance costs averaging $8,500 per FTE provider.

In 2007, the Medical Group Management Association (MGMA) conducted a survey of medical groups regarding their use of EHRs and identified the average EHR implementation cost was about $50,000 per physician (median $25,000) with annual maintenance costs of $1,295 per physician (median $500).[16] The MGMA survey found that most practices experienced increased costs, decreased productivity, and other challenges during the first 6 to 24 months following implementation. However, after this period, the benefits of EHR implementation increasingly exceeded its costs. In fact, over 40% of practices began to experience decreasing costs after 6 months and most wondered how they conducted business without an EHR.

## 2. Personal Health Records

Personal health records (PHR) typically include all aspects of a patient's health and are maintained by the patient, not the provider. With PHRs, patients can save a history of their medical conditions, list their medications, test results, schedule of appointments, and their vitals over time. The primary hub of the PHR is the patient portal where patients are primarily responsible for entering information, although various organizations are working to automate this process.[17]

### Benefits of Personal Health Records

Advantages of PHRs, especially in HDM programs, include the engagement and activation of patients by providing a mechanism for them to become involved in their own health care. Many aspects of health care are best measured from the patient's perspective, and PHRs provide a way for patients to provide information not available elsewhere, such as details on symptoms and qualitative assessments of health status. PHRs can also interface with equipment (for example, smartphones or personal computers) that could collect other information such as vital signs or dietary habits and exercise routines.

PHRs can also interface with EHRs to enhance information available to providers. Suppose, for example, a patient participates in an employer-based wellness program that interfaces with the PHR. As part of the program, the patient tracks physical activity—both type and duration. This information can be passed to the provider via the PHR as part of the EHR.

Another advantage of PHRs is their ability to be accessed from any computer with an Internet connection. This can be extremely useful if the patient cannot, for example, recall when speaking to a physician which medications he or she takes. If the provider is unfamiliar with the patient's history, the patient can simply access his or her records instantly and find out exactly which medications he has taken. In this way, PHRs may provide a bridge across EHR-S interoperability issues or simply substitute for an EHR when an EHR-S is unavailable.

### Limitations of Personal Health Records

Despite their promise, PHRs have drawbacks. First, patient-reported information can often be unreliable and incomplete as patients may not enter data into the system properly. Due to potential errors, providers may ask patients seemingly redundant questions in order to refine the information needed for diagnosis and/or assessment. Second, PHRs integrated into EHRs often transfer only a subset of information provided by the patient.[17] Given the large amount of information that a patient can potentially record in a PHR, this helps to limit the data transferred to that which is relevant for the provider. Third, although providers should validate information transferred from the PHR into the EHR, they may view data from PHRs embedded in EHRs as validated simply because they appear in the health record. It is possible that a physician could mistake PHR information for data entered by a clinician and make diagnosis and treatment decisions based on that information. Finally, interoperability is a drawback of PHRs. This is especially problematic for stand-alone PHRs (as opposed to those that are part of an EHR) that may not be built to communicate with EHRs or EHR-Ss.

## 3. Electronic Health Records Systems

Electronic Health Records Systems (EHR-Ss) may span multiple organizations, types, and health care settings. These networks rely on compatible software and hardware systems to facilitate electronic data exchanges. Interoperability eliminates electronic data silos, allowing multiple hospitals, clinics, pharmacies, laboratories, and other ancillary facilities within or among networks to share data seamlessly. Through these networks, medical records and other health data may be easily accessible to any health care provider. Consequently, episodes of care can be examined as opposed to only a single encounter. Providers may devise more accurate and effective treatment plans for their patients, improve patient monitoring and follow-up, and more readily consult with other health providers.

### Types of Electronic Health Record Systems

The most common sources of EHR-Ss are integrated delivery systems (IDSs), Regional Health Information Organizations (RHIOs), and health information exchanges (HIEs). IDSs are systems in which multiple types of care are provided within the system. One well-known and comprehensive IDS is the Veteran's Health Administration (VA). The VA EHR-S captures ambulatory, inpatient, ancillary, and long-term care services. Other examples of IDSs include many academic medical centers that have their own network of affiliated outpatient providers and other services.

RHIOs facilitate the exchange of health information within a specific geographic location. These collaborative networks face many challenges, including technical issues with linking and/or pulling data from multiple systems, as well as legal issues with data privacy and ownership. The Refugee Health Information Network (RHIN) represents another important foray into electronic health data management. An effort of the National Library of Medicine, RHIN is a national collaborative partnership whose purpose is to provide quality, multilingual health information resources for health care providers of refugees and asylees (asylum seekers).[18] Managed by refugee health professionals, the network serves as an electronic backstop to frontline health care providers working with these underserved populations. Currently, information from RHIN is provided on the following chronic diseases: diabetes, cardiovascular disease, hypertension, and cancer. All have implications for HDM programs among the refugee and asylee populations.

## Limitations of Electronic Health Record Systems

Since only 4% of physicians reported having an EHR-S in a national survey, very few patients have their care managed by providers that use an EHR-S. While the technical and logistical challenges of establishing an EHR-S are daunting, there are tangible benefits to all stakeholders. Although data from EHRs are useful for HDM, the data are also the least generalizable to the entire population.

In addition, data from EHRs may still be incomplete. Patients may receive care from outside the system, which may not be captured in the EHR unless reported back to a provider within the system. Even if reported back within the system, how the data are captured typically makes extraction more challenging. Examples include a patient who seeks medical care from a physician who is not part of the IDS or an ancillary service, such as a laboratory or radiology department that does not provide results electronically to the system. The likelihood of a patient seeking care outside of an IDS depends upon the size and market penetration of the IDS, as well as the comprehensiveness of the services offered within the IDS. Similarly, one of the critical success factors for RHIOs is the participation of providers, facilities, health systems and vendors in the region.

## 4. Conclusion

As with any data source, there are advantages and disadvantages to using EHR data for HDM. Understanding these characteristics will enable data users to choose the most appropriate data source as well as to design analyses using the data that account for these strengths and weaknesses. As new technologies, policies, and collaborations increase EHR adoption rates, these data will become even more valuable for HDM. Moreover, these data will also become more generalizable to the general population providers who use EHR.

## References

1. Hunt J, Siemienczuk J, Erstgaard P, et al. Use of an electronic medical record in disease management programs: a case study in hyperlipidemia. *Stud Health Technol Inform.* 2001;84: 825-829.
2. O'Toole MF, Kmetik KS, Bossley H, et al. Electronic health record systems: the vehicle for implementing performance measures. *Am Heart Hosp J.* 2005;3(2):88-93.
3. Hillestad R, Bigelow J, Bower A, et al. Can electronic medical record systems transform health care? Potential health benefits, savings and costs. *Health Aff.* 2005;24(5):1103-1117.
4. Chaudhry B, Wang J, Wu S, et al. Systematic review: impact of health information technology on quality, efficiency, and costs of medical care. *Ann Intern Med.* 2006;144(10):742-752.

## Part 2: Electronic Health Records

5. Shekelle PG, Morton SC, Keeler EB. *Costs and Benefits of Health Information Technology: Evidence Report/Technology Assessment No. 132*. (Prepared by the Southern California Evidence-based Practice Center under Contract No. 290-02-0003.) Rockville, MD: Agency for Healthcare Research and Quality; 2006. AHRQ Publication 06-E006.
6. Goodman C. Saving in electronic medical record systems? Do it for the quality. *Health Aff*. 2005;24(5):1124-1126.
7. Blumenthal D. Stimulating the adoption of health information technology. *NEJM*. 2009;360: 1477-1479.
8. Smith PC, Araya-Guerra R, Bublitz C, et al. Missing clinical information during primary care visits. *JAMA*. 2005;293:565-571.
9. Kayhani S, Hebert PL, Ross JS, Federman A, Zhu CW, Siu AL. Electronic health record components and the quality of care. *Med Care*. 2008;46(12):1267-1272.
10. Zhou L, Soran CS, Jenter CA, et al. The relationship between electronic health record use and quality of care over time. *J Am Med Inform Assoc*. 2009;16(4):457-464.
11. Poon EG, Wright A, Simon SR, et al. Relationship between use of electronic health record features and health care quality: results of a statewide survey. *Med Care*. 2010;48(3):203-209.
12. Koppel R, Metlay JP, Cohen A, et al. Role of computerized physician order entry systems in facilitating medication errors. *JAMA*. 2005;293:1197-1203.
13. Simon SR, Soran CS, Kaushal R, et al. Physicians' use of key functions in electronic health records from 2005 to 2007: a statewide survey. *J Am Med Inform Assoc*. 2009;16(4):465-470.
14. Gans D, Kralewski J, Hammons T, Dowd B. Medical groups' adoption of electronic health records and information systems. *Health Aff*. 2005;24(5):1323-1333.
15. Miller RH, West C, Brown TM, Sim I, Ganchoff C. The value of electronic health records in solo or small group practices. *Health Aff*. 2005;24(5):1127-1137.
16. Medical Group Management Association. Electronic health records: perspectives from the adopters. 2007. http://www.mgma.com/WorkArea/mgma_downloadasset.aspx?id=21086. October 2007. Accessed Sept 18, 2012.
17. Tang PC, Ash JS, Bates DW, Overhage JM, Sands DZ. Personal health records: definitions, benefits, and strategies for overcoming barriers to adoption. *JAMA*. 2006;13(2):121-126.
18. Refugee Health Information Network. *Welcome to the Refugee Health Information Network (RHIN)*. October 17, 2007. Retrieved November 28, 2008, from http://www.rhin.org/welcome.aspx.

CHAPTER 9

# Electronic Health Record Implementation Challenges at the Practice Level

Rachel Shapiro, MPP

As presented in the last chapter, there are advantages and disadvantages to the use of electronic health records (EHRs) for health and disease management (HDM). It is important to understand both how EHRs are expected to improve care coordination and the barriers to their effective use. This chapter examines the challenges of using EHRs in physician practices. Because a majority of US physicians are in practices of 8 physicians or fewer,[1] understanding the challenges these practices face will be essential to greater and more effective use of EHRs, as well as development of policies to further influence EHR use by providers.

First, this chapter examines barriers to adoption and use, including cost of the systems and training. Then, it describes the availability and provider use of EHR features, as well as EHR system limitations. Finally, it summarizes the policy implications of these challenges, specifically in light of the Health Information Technology for Economic and Clinical Health Act (HITECH) and its potential to further adoption and effective use of EHRs by primary care providers for care coordination. A full discussion of the use of EHR data for health and disease management from a policy perspective is presented in Chapter 11.

EHRs have the potential to transform health care and, specifically, to improve care coordination across providers through immediate electronic access to clinical information at the point of care.[2] It is widely believed that, through the effective use of EHRs and their multiple functions, providers will be able to offer their patients more comprehensive care, thereby improving care quality and efficiency. In light of this potential for care improvement, Congress passed HITECH as part of the American Recovery and Reinvestment Act of 2009 (ARRA) to promote the adoption of health IT.[3] Under HITECH, eligible providers can receive additional Medicare payments for adoption and meaningful use of certified EHRs. Three programs were established by the Office of the National Coordinator for Health Information Technology (ONC) to support implementation of the HITECH Act[4]—Regional Extension Centers to further adoption among small practices, health information exchanges to further development of infrastructure for providers, and training of a health IT workforce to sustain the infrastructure being built.

Although EHRs have great promise, there remain many hurdles to their adoption by providers and, in particular, those providers in small to mid-sized practices. One national study indicates that, as of 2008, only 17% of United States physicians had

Part 2: Electronic Health Records

implemented an EHR system and, of those, only 4% had a fully functional system. Furthermore, it found that when compared to physicians in small practices (with 3 or fewer physicians), those in large practices (with more than 50 physicians) were 3 times as likely to have a basic system and more than 4 times as likely to have a fully functional system.[5]* Fulfilling the promise of the use of EHR data is dependent upon the successful adoption and use of EHRs by provider practices.

# 1. Barriers to Provider Adoption of Electronic Health Records

## Cost of an Electronic Health Record System

Ideally, providers would like to be able to adopt an EHR system that does not require a large upfront cost and is easily maintained. If they do adopt a system, providers would like to be assured that it will conform to meaningful-use criteria, will provide a return on investment, and will have some interoperability with other systems with which providers interact, such as hospital, laboratory, and radiology systems.[5-7] However, EHRs are costly, both to implement and maintain, although this may change with modular and cloud systems. Estimates show total costs for ambulatory EHRs range between $25,000 and $45,000 per physician and annual ongoing costs at $3,000 to $9,000 per physician, due to software licensing fees, staff training, technical support, continued system maintenance, and decreased patient load during the transition period from paper to electronic records.[6,7]

There are also significant costs associated with connecting laboratories with EHRs.[8] Generally, operating costs are much more substantial for physicians in small, independent practices.[6] Several EHR vendors have recognized the upfront and continuing costs to providers, and have derived web-based solutions, which have lower initial and ongoing costs.[9,10] However, it is too early to determine whether or not these solutions will help further the adoption of EHRs by provider practices.

## Choosing a System

Providers also encounter multiple barriers in trying to find an optimal EHR system. Providers are concerned that they purchase the right system; that is, a system that will not become obsolete or discontinued, be certified to meet the meaningful-use incentives available under HITECH, and meet the practice's needs.[5,7,11]

In June 2010, ONC issued a final rule to establish a temporary certification program for EHRs, under which multiple organizations are providing certification of EHRs that meet the established meaningful-use incentives.[12,13] On July 13, 2010, the Centers for Medicare & Medicaid Services (CMS) and ONC issued a final rule on

---

* This study defined a basic system as having patient demographics, problem lists, medication lists, clinical notes, orders for prescriptions, and the capability to view laboratory and imaging results. A fully functional system was defined as having all of the basic system functionality, as well as medical history and follow-up notes, laboratory and imaging test orders, prescriptions and orders sent electronically, the capability to view electronic images, and clinical decision support.

what will constitute meaningful use of EHRs by eligible providers in the first 2 years (2011 and 2012) of the incentive program.[14] In January 2011, ONC issued a final rule to convert the temporary EHR certification program to permanent status by early 2012.[15] In August 2012, ONC released a final rule that requires providers to adopt and demonstrate meaningful use of EHR systems by October 2014 or face a 1% penalty to reimbursement from Medicare.

While ONC lists over 2,000 certified complete and modular ambulatory EHRs and their capabilities on its website,[16] it does not provide a meaningful way to assess which product is best for a practice. Physicians and other practice staff must invest time in testing products from several vendors to identify the system that is most effective for their practice workflow. Even after providers have acquired a certified system and are able to meet the first stage of meaningful use, they will face a number of hurdles related to their ability (1) to meet the definitions of meaningful use in 2 later stages, and (2) to expand the expected functions of EHRs, including uses for disease management, clinical decision support, medication management, and quality measurement and research.[17]

In addition to the overall cost of the EHR system and its ability to meet certification requirements, practices are faced with practice-specific barriers, including the time required for and cost of provider and staff training, and impacts on productivity.[1,6,18-20] During the transition from paper to electronic records, physicians are often unable to treat as many patients or expand their workday to see the same number of patients, thereby increasing the time investment in adjusting to the system, potentially reducing financial benefits of the system, and impacting time the physician can spend on quality improvement.[18] It takes more time to document patient visits in the EHR than on paper because of the numerous templates within EHRs that require providers to enter more information than they may have previously.[20] Hence, while the EHRs improve the amount that is documented from each visit, and potentially the accuracy of what is documented, additional time is required to enter patient notes. Several physicians found that this additional time did not decrease 2 years after the EHR was implemented in their practices.[20]

## 2. Availability, Use, and Limitations of Electronic Health Record Features in Practice Settings

### Availability and Use of Electronic Health Record Features

EHRs, as advertised by vendors to providers, should have the ability to operate smoothly, be used easily *out of the box*, and improve quality of care. Physicians and other practice staff should be able to enter, retrieve, and manage clinical information effortlessly on the templates within the EHR systems, thereby improving office workflow and efficiency. Perhaps most relevant to the provision of patient care, EHRs have multiple features that are meant to enhance care coordination, including clinical decision support features such as access to clinical guidelines and reminders, drug-drug interactions, and other alerts.

EHRs also enable providers to document clinical and demographic data electronically, prescribe electronically, and view and exchange results of laboratory tests and imaging. Fully functional systems can use all of these features, while basic systems lack certain order-entry and clinical decision support capabilities, and generally are limited to including patient demographics, patient problem lists, patient medication lists, clinical notes, orders for prescriptions, and electronic viewing of laboratory and imaging results.[5,21]

In addition to these features, if EHRs improve care coordination, they may ultimately improve quality of care and provider efficiency. As discussed in Chapter 6, moving to an electronic system would eliminate the need for paper records, thereby reducing the time spent pulling charts and perhaps improving provider productivity and enabling a better exchange of health care information across providers. The improved documentation available through an EHR could also help providers avoid duplicated or inappropriate diagnostic tests and adverse drug events, as well as promote appropriate prescribing of prescription medications.[5]

Although adoption rates remain low, among those with a basic system, providers are largely able to use all of the functions at least some of the time.[5] Part of the reason for this widespread use of functions in the basic system could be that providers find electronic notes more accessible, organized, and legible than their paper counterparts.[2,18,20] While physicians may use these basic functions, there is wide variation in terms of how they are used; some continue to dictate or use free text fields, rather than the templates (electronic forms) to enter clinical notes and other documentation.[18,20] Furthermore, although EHR vendors state that their products have care coordination functionalities, oftentimes physicians are unable to use these features and develop their own manual methods to extract the needed information from the EHRs.[2]

## Limitations in Use of Electronic Health Record Features

Most EHR systems require an extensive training period and considerable technical support to customize them to the practice for effective and efficient use by physicians. Moreover, more often than not physicians and their staff do not have adequate time or resources to devote to learning the systems. Even after the systems have been set up, providers and practice staff may not use the system confidently, reducing the system's effectiveness. At the same time, when physicians invest the time to learn how to use the system most effectively and redesign their workflow for this purpose, they are unable to devote time to quality improvement.[8,18,22] As with issues relating to cost, larger practices are better able to devote resources to customization and organization of the EHR than small practices; however, customization remains a time-consuming and burdensome issue even for the larger practices.[18]

Problems with usability are especially visible after practices have implemented the EHR systems. While providers find clinical information is easier to access and document through the EHR system, they also find that the systems do not work as effectively as advertised by vendors. Specifically, providers find that systems slow down workflow due to the numerous templates and actions (clicks) required to document clinical data, as well as software glitches and errors that require technical assistance to resolve.[11,20] In order to bypass the extra time it might take to enter clinical information into the various system templates, providers may instead use the free text entry allowed in the clinical notes field, burying information related to clinical quality (such as the receipt of tests and procedures) and leaving the system unable to process it because of a lack of standardized coding of data and inclusion of numeric results in the text. Such information would be useful to providers when reviewing patients' care, especially in the case of patients with chronic conditions, who require much more coordination of care.

Providers can be annoyed by some of the functions in the EHR that are supposed to increase efficiency, such as alerts and warnings of drug-drug interactions and other patient problems. Some providers reported that these alerts seemed to involve most of their practice's patients and were so numerous that they were likely to cause providers to have alert fatigue.[20] Although these alerts can be customized, physicians often do not have the adequate knowledge or resources to do so.[11]

An unintended consequence of the reliance on EHRs is the potential for information overload, which could hinder coordination of care. Physicians may enter repetitive information in several templates and may also not use the templates appropriately. For example, medication lists could be lengthy and out of date, resulting in medication errors, making it difficult to locate or verify the accuracy of information to help coordinate a patient's care.[20] While this information might be helpful within one practice in terms of real-time decision making for patients, it may prove to be less helpful in coordinating care across practices and settings, when providers spend more time searching for patient-specific data in the electronically stored information than communicating face-to-face.[2]

## 3. Policy Implications

There still remains much potential for the use of EHRs in small to medium-sized physician practices, even with the multiple challenges to their adoption and use. Given the importance placed on meaningful use of EHRs by Congress, providers should be offered assistance when choosing and adopting EHRs, including adequate training and assessment of practice needs. HITECH is a first step in this direction with the institution of the Health IT Extension program. It is possible that the extension program's Regional Extension Centers (RECs) will be able to address or mitigate these challenges by providing much-needed support to at least 100,000 primary care providers, through participating nonprofit organizations with the goal of helping the providers achieve meaningful use of EHRs and enabling nationwide health information exchange.[23]

The extension program established 60 regional centers in the first 2 rounds of awards in February and April 2010. In September 2010, 2 RECs were established, 2 existing RECs received additional funding to expand coverage areas, and 46 existing RECs received additional funding to support critical access and rural hospitals. Further funding was made available to existing RECs in January and February 2011.[24] Each REC cooperative agreement is for a 4-year project period with 2 separate 2-year budget periods. Renewals or extensions of the second 2-year budget period are dependent on performance and a determination by the US Department of Health and Human Services that a continued agreement with the REC is in the best interest of the program.

ONC's expectation is that the RECs awarded in the first 2 rounds will be fully functional by the middle of 2010 and self-sustaining by the middle of 2014. As required by the HITECH Act, the RECs must provide technical assistance to providers in: (1) selecting a certified EHR that offers the best value to meet their needs; (2) achieving implementation of an EHR system; (3) redesigning clinical and administrative workflow to achieve meaningful use of EHRs; and (4) complying with requirements to protect the integrity, privacy, and security of patients' health information.[25]

In addition to overseeing the RECs, the extension program established a Health IT Research Center that will support the RECs with information on effective practices. The resource center will also facilitate a peer-learning network through which the RECs will work with each other and relevant stakeholders to identify and share best practices in EHR adoption, effective use, and provider support.[25] The hope is that the RECs will be able to share learning experiences (for example, the more experienced providers will be able to offer ideas to assist practices as they implement both new EHRs and more complex features within the EHRs), leading to widespread meaningful use of EHRs by primary care providers.

It is not clear that the RECs alone will help practices adopt and implement EHRs effectively with a goal of quality improvement. Further funding will be necessary to help advance the adoption of EHRs by 2014 when the RECs are no longer funded by the federal government and must become self-sustaining. It is possible that these regional centers, in combination with the promise of a newly trained health IT workforce (though highly dependent on the availability of a faculty to train them), will provide enough of a jump-start to help practices embrace the adoption of EHRs, and start to use them more effectively for management and coordination of care.

Existing evidence points to the likelihood that providers will continue to be slow to adopt EHRs, even with incentive payments for meaningful use and technical assistance offered through the RECs and the resource center. The reasons for this reluctance to invest in EHR systems are both financial and cultural. On the financial side, providers may simply decide that it is not worth the time and effort to ensure that they have adopted a certified EHR and are using the system *meaningfully* in order to qualify for the incentive payments from CMS. Moreover, with continued threats of declining compensation from Medicare, including a 27% decrease in Medicare payment that could go into effect in 2013,[26] providers may choose to *jump ship* and refuse to see new Medicare and Medicaid patients. Ultimately, providers may find that the size of the incentive payment and offers of technical assistance through the RECs are not worth the cost of investment in an EHR, due to a potential negative impact on practice productivity, workflow, and finances.

On the cultural side, a number of necessary factors for the kind of practice transformation that EHRs will demand of physician practices are not addressed in HITECH or in its specific programs. These include the change of culture in practice data collection and use of information to make evidence-based decisions to serve their patients, as well as the redistributed workload among physicians and support staff that results from re-engineered practice workflows. Perhaps most significant to physicians is the likely loss of professional independence that EHRs may impose, as well as the preference and tastes of physicians and their staff for this kind of technology.

Ultimately, it remains unclear if financial incentives for well-paid and highly trained professionals are attractive enough to convince them to embark on an untested program that imposes multiple demands on their time and resources, particularly at a time when they are also being asked to change how they provide services to Medicare and Medicaid beneficiaries (through the Patient Protection and Affordable Care Act of 2010).

## References

1. Baron RJ, Fabens EL, Schiffman M, Wolf E. Electronic health records: just around the corner? Or over the cliff? *Ann Intern Med*. 2005;143(3):222-226.
2. O'Malley AS, Grossman JM, Cohen JR, et al. Are electronic medical records helpful for care coordination? Experiences of physician practices. *J Gen Intern Med*. 2009. Available at: http://www.hschange.org/CONTENT/1104/OMalley.pdf. Accessed September 18, 2012.
3. Congressional Budget Office. Letter to the Honorable Henry A. Waxman, chairman of the Committee on Energy and Commerce, U.S. House of Representatives. January 21, 2009. Available at: http://www.cbo.gov/sites/default/files/cbofiles/ftpdocs/99xx/doc9965/hitechwaxmanltr.pdf. Accessed September 18, 2012.
4. Blumenthal D. Launching HITECH. *N Engl J Med*. 2010;362(5):382-385.
5. DesRoches CM, Campbell EG, Rao SR, et al. Electronic records in ambulatory care: a national survey of physicians. *N Engl J Med*. 2008;359(1):50-60.
6. Congressional Budget Office. Evidence on the costs and benefits of health information technology. May 2008. Available at: http://www.cbo.gov/sites/default/files/cbofiles/ftpdocs/91xx/doc9168/05-20-healthit.pdf. Accessed September 18, 2012.
7. Moreno L, Peikes D, Krilla A. Necessary But Not Sufficient: The HITECH Act and Health Information Technology's Potential to Build Medical Homes. (Prepared by Mathematica Policy Research under Contract No. HHSA290200900019I TO2.) AHRQ Publication No. 10-0080-EF. Rockville, MD: Agency for Healthcare Research and Quality. June 2010. Available at: http://pcmh.ahrq.gov/portal/server.pt/gateway/PTARGS_0_11787_950288_0_0_18/HITECH%20White%20Paper--8.10.2010%20with%20new%20cover.pdf. Accessed September 18, 2012.
8. Baron RJ. Quality improvement with an electronic health record: achievable, but not automatic. *Ann Intern Med*. 2007;147(8):549-552.

Part 2: Electronic Health Records

9. iHealthBeat. GE Healthcare unveils online EHRs for small physician practices. June 16, 2010. Available at: http://www.ihealthbeat.org/articles/2010/6/16/ge-healthcare-unveils-online-ehrs-for-small-physician-practices.aspx. Accessed September 18, 2012.
10. eWeek. Dell, Practice Fusion to Offer Medical Records System. June 3, 2010. Available at: http://www.eweek.com/c/a/Health-Care-IT/Dell-Practice-Fusion-to-Offer-Medical-Records-System-805388/. Accessed September 18, 2012.
11. Felt-Lisk S, Johnson L, Fleming C, Shapiro R, Natzke B. Toward understanding EHR use in small physician practices. *Health Care Financ Rev*. 2009;31(1):11-22.
12. iHealthBeat. Final rule issued for temporary EHR certification program. June 18, 2010. Available at: http://www.ihealthbeat.org/articles/2010/6/18/final-rule-issued-for-temporary-ehr-certification-program.aspx. Accessed September 18, 2012.
13. Office of the National Coordinator for Health Information Technology (ONC). ONC-authorized testing and certification bodies. February 2011. Available at: http://healthit.hhs.gov/portal/server.pt?open=512&mode=2&objID=3120. Accessed September 18, 2012.
14. Blumenthal D, Tavenner M. The "meaningful use" regulation for electronic health records. N Engl J Med. 2010; 363:501-504. Available at: http://content.nejm.org/cgi/reprint/NEJMp1006114.pdf?ssource=hcrc. Accessed September 18, 2012.
15. Establishment of the permanent certification program for health information technology. 45 Federal Register 170. January 7, 2011;76(5):1262-1326. Available at: http://origin.www.gpo.gov/fdsys/pkg/FR-2011-01-07/pdf/2010-33174.pdf. Accessed September 18, 2012.
16. ONC. Certified Health IT product list. February 2011. Available at: http://onc-chpl.force.com/ehrcert/EHRProductSearch. Accessed September 18, 2012.
17. Buntin MB, Jain SH, Blumenthal D. Health information technology: laying the infrastructure for national health reform. *Health Aff*. 2010;29(6):1214-1219.
18. Miller RH, Sim I. Physicians' use of electronic medical records: barriers and solutions. *Health Aff*. 2004;23(2):116-126.
19. Miller RH, West CE. The value of electronic health records in community health centers: policy implications. *Health Aff*. 2007;26(1):206-214.
20. Fernandopulle R, Patel N. How the electronic health record did not measure up to the demands of our medical home practice. *Health Aff*. 2010;29(4):622-628.
21. Hogan SO, Kissam SM. Measuring meaningful use. *Health Aff*. 2010;29(4):601-606.
22. Linder JA, Ma J, Bates D, et al. Electronic health record use and the quality of ambulatory care in the United States. *Arch Intern Med*. 2007;167(13):1400-1405.
23. ONC. HITECH priority grants program: health information technology extension program. Facts-at-a-glance. September 2009. Available at: http://healthit.hhs.gov/portal/server.pt/community/extension_program_facts_at_a_glance/1331/home/16358. Accessed September 18, 2012.
24. ONC. Health information technology extension program. February 2011. Available at: http://healthit.hhs.gov/portal/server.pt/community/healthit_hhs_gov__rec_program/1495. Accessed September 18, 2012.
25. ONC. HIT extension program: frequently asked questions. May 2010. Available at: http://healthit.hhs.gov/portal/server.pt?open=512&objID=1329&parentname=CommunityPage&parentid=15&mode=2&in_hi_userid=11113&cached=true#. Accessed September 18, 2012.
26. Barr S. CBO Says Medicare Spending Growth Slower than Expected. Kaiser *Health News*, August 22, 2012. http://capsules.kaiserhealthnews.org/index.php/2012/08/cbo-says-medicare-spending-growth-slower-than-expected/?referrer=search. Accessed September 18, 2012.

CHAPTER 10

# Real-Time Applications of Electronic Health Record Data

Farrokh Alemi, PhD; Brent Gibson, MD, MPH, FACPM; and Carla Zema, PhD

The use of the electronic health record (EHR) in medical practice has brought with it many challenges but also many advantages, including that EHRs are designed to store information about every patient encounter. When a patient appears for treatment, the information from previous visits can be retrieved easily and made available to guide decision making. When the EHR is used actively to guide clinical practice and other decision making at the time the data are identified and stored, the data are referred to as *having real-time application*.

The use of real-time data in clinical settings is an area of interest for all health professionals. Real-time data linked to, or originating from, the EHR have the potential to assist with clinical decision making and the detection of safety signals, other adverse events, and sentinel events of public health importance. Beyond this, data gathered for real time or near-real time may be used in rapid turnaround research and evaluations. This chapter will introduce statistical process control charts and outline some specific examples of the use of real-time and near-real-time electronic health information.

## 1. Statistical Process Control

A common tool of real-time data monitoring is the statistical process control chart that is used to monitor a particular process continuously by sampling from electronic data and reporting when the process parameters have changed. In one example of a control chart, time is plotted on the X-axis while the Y-axis identifies the outcome. Another example of a control chart has the occurrence of each incidence of an event on the X-axis and the time to the event on the Y-axis. To decide if outcomes are different from expected patterns, a user can calculate the upper control limits (UCL) and lower control limits (LCL). These limits will differ depending on the type of control chart being used.

A typical process control chart might compare a clinician's performance in the denial of claims to his or her peers (Figure 1). If data from the relevant peer organizations, providers, or similar entities are used to construct upper and lower limits of expected outcome, identifying these limits can be interpreted as the best and worst performers. Typically, researchers organize these limits in such a way as to ensure that 99% of expected values fall within them. In this control chart, the points that fall outside the upper and lower limits identify the need for process change. For example, in the 10th incident of a denial, the organization was performing a great deal better than its peers. Over time, however, the performance deteriorated and eventually fell, at the 18th incident reaching a performance level lower than its worst performing peer.

**FIGURE 1.** Components of a control chart

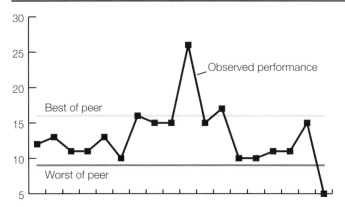

In real-time analysis, the time interval used for estimating the control limit is held constant. Figure 1 shows data over 4 months as the solid red line. These limits are extrapolated forward to see if the new data point is within the control limits. As time progresses, if the data used for calculating the control limits change, the distance between the limits changes and the extrapolated portion of the limits changes. The newest data point is compared to the control limit calculated from a previous time, in this case the last 4 months. If the data are outside the control limit, then there is a statistically significant probability that the process has changed.

## 2. Real-Time Applications of Electronic Health Record Data

### Real-Time Monitoring of Health Outcomes

While many consider the EHR simply to be a digital copy of the patient medical chart, in reality, it encompasses a far greater spectrum of medical reports. One such report is generated by computer systems that monitor, in real time, trends in disease and illness within a population. Hospitals often deploy these automated epidemiological systems as an early detection tool. Reports on population health outcomes may be monitored to determine abnormal rates of a particular illness before a true disease outbreak occurs.

For example, several syndromic surveillance systems monitor frequency of diseases in emergency departments. These systems operate by pooling data across EHRs in different hospitals. One study finds that these systems can identify the emergence of influenza 1 to 4 weeks before actual isolation of influenza virus in the community through other means.[1] Such decision aids rely on predetermined sets of encoded rules that tell the system to monitor health outcomes and report variations in those outcomes when specific numeric targets are met.

## Detection of Rare Sentinel Events

Another important use of real-time data from EHRs is the identification of rare sentinel events or safety signals. The Joint Commission defines a *sentinel event* as an unexpected occurrence involving death or serious physical or psychological injury, or the risk thereof. The prevention of sentinel events is dependent upon the ability to identify risks and recognize safety signals prior to the event occurring. Researchers have identified signals and risks of sentinel events in medical records as early as 1990 using retrospective chart reviews of paper medical records.[2] Implementation of EHRs makes it feasible to monitor patient care for such safety signals and risks in real time, and to alert health care professionals to potential risks in order to reduce the likelihood of a sentinel event.

Once an EHR is in use within a medical system, designers can develop methods for identifying and transmitting specified data to clinic or physician displays. Such *dashboards* are widely in use in hospital emergency department information systems (EDIS) where they display either clinical or administrative data being collected in real time. The Microsoft Amalga Unified Intelligence System, for example, is an EMR-S that is able to gather, integrate, and analyze information from disparate clinical data sources. Researchers have used the system to develop a query tool to detect temporal patterns in patient histories.[3] Such a tool would be useful not only for clinical medicine and research but also to help clinicians and administrators detect sentinel events.

Another method uses algorithms to identify rare or sentinel events in administrative claims data that can be modified for real-time monitoring using EHRs. Quality indicators (QIs) developed by the Agency for Healthcare Research and Quality (AHRQ) are calculated using hospital administrative discharge claims data. One of the 4 QI modules is patient safety indicators (PSIs), which focus on potentially avoidable complications and iatrogenic events. Miller and colleagues calculated the 12 adverse event rates in this module and their association with patient- and hospital-level characteristics.[4] The indicators could be identified using EHRs in order to identify rare sentinel events or potentially detect increased risk of adverse events in real time, enabling physicians and staff to take preventive measures. The PSIs have also been tested with regard to evaluating the US Veterans Administration's health care services.[5]

## Monitoring Rare Events for Quality Improvement

Quality indicators developed by AHRQ and other entities measure rare events of clinical importance. Although these measures accurately identify and consistently monitor sentinel events and adverse effects, statistical analysis can be limited due to the rare occurrence of such events. Beyond this, early in the experience of using a new drug, device, or other treatment, rare events may be early indications of a serious issue—potentially revealing what will eventually be understood to be more common events.

An alternative to measuring the rates of these events is to monitor the time to a sentinel event or adverse effect using the statistical process control described earlier. Such measures are best calculated using real-time EHR data rather than administrative data. Instead of calculating the rate of occurrence of such rare events, the time between rare events is measured. This alternative eliminates the statistical issues that arise when trying to compare the rates of rare events.

An example of a specific measure used in these automated epidemiological systems includes the incidence of central line-associated bloodstream infections (CLABs). Each year, according to CDC estimates, 250,000 CLAB cases occur in United States hospitals with an estimated attributable mortality of 12 to 25%.[6] Quality improvement efforts in this area have shown that significant reductions in CLAB rates to nearly zero are possible using surveillance to monitor hospital-acquired infection data in real time. Information obtained from such surveillance can then be used to identify and mitigate the causes of these infections.[7,8] Continuous data monitoring provides valuable feedback to the staff on the progress of their improvement efforts. Statistical process control charting of the measure offers a simple and visual feedback tool to drive further improvement. This data can be calculated easily using EHR data in real time.

## Evidenced-Based Medicine Using Real-Time Data

Delays in care can jeopardize health outcomes and often arise from the inability to obtain physician input quickly in response to rapid changes in patients' conditions. Data-driven decision algorithms and protocols based on evidence-based standards enable providers to manage patients in many instances without delays.

One example of such an algorithm would be an insulin infusion protocol to manage blood glucose. Traditionally, a physician order would be necessary to change infusion rates. However, evidence-based algorithms allow nurses to adjust the infusion rate according to immediate blood glucose levels readings. Nursing decision making plays an important role in managing the hour-to-hour treatment of hospitalized patients, especially those in intensive care units. Kim and colleagues conducted an analysis of using a rule-based system as compared to actual nursing decisions made based on data extracted from medical records.[9] Data collected included readily available measures such as the number of activity assistants and basic neurological assessment scores, including the Glasgow Coma Scale and the Ramsey Sedation Scale. While the results of this particular trial did not consistently show agreement with human decision making, poor alignment was likely due to low-quality source data and incomplete decision rules. Analogous limitations are encountered on a daily basis in clinical practice.

Expanding upon the idea of an electronic real-time decision tool geared toward nursing practice, the Knowledge-Based Nursing Initiative (KBNI) of Aurora Health Care, Cerner (an EHR vendor), and the University of Wisconsin-Milwaukee College of Nursing have operationalized the concept of a continuously updated, web-based clinical decision-making tool.[10] Based on the multidirectional flow of clinical information among a data repository and specific areas of clinical activity (such as patient assessment, diagnoses, intervention, and clinical outcomes), the KBNI provides users with up-to-date and evidence-based recommendations for clinical care. In addition to informing clinical decisions, information from clinical practice adds to and integrates with the data repository to assist other users moving forward.

The application to clinical, translational, health economic, and other research is evident as current peer-reviewed knowledge can be applied to patients quickly, without the delay of traditional dissemination through journal clubs, scientific conferences, formal training programs, or other means. Likewise, ongoing or planned research projects will have access to a wide variety of up-to-date patient data.

EHRs may also improve patient care by interfacing with registries and generating real-time reports and information. One example is a multidisciplinary surgical outcomes database described by Newcomb.[11] This system relies on inputs from clinical staff, hospital billing information, and the patients themselves. This particular database currently manages data from 14 specific surgical procedures with the potential to expand to others. Some reports are available in real time and information gathered in the outcomes database may be rapidly analyzed and made available to clinicians in a matter of hours.

A final example of an innovative, real-time monitoring initiative geared specifically toward patient safety is that undertaken by the Massachusetts General Hospital with respect to anesthesia care and patient allergies.[12] In a study by Sandberg, facility-specific software designed to scan the EHR for discrepancies or errors that would affect reimbursement was redesigned to scan the record for other user-defined data such as patient allergies. Prior to implementation of the monitoring software, as many as 30% of patient charts were missing information on allergies—a potentially life-threatening documentation error. The system reduced the prevalence of missing allergy information to about 8% within a few days. The specific mechanism of notifying providers of the missing information was a message sent via pager.

## Practice Management Using Real-Time Data

In addition to applications related to patient care, real-time data applications are also relevant to practice management processes. Real-time monitoring may be used to monitor billing and claims denial. For instance, real-time analysis of data for the time to the next claims denial can help organizational decision makers focus their quality improvement efforts and understand whether or not the organization is receiving payment for services rendered. If there are problems in specific clinics, with specific providers, or with specific services, management can target these areas before significant reimbursement losses occur.

Several organizations have introduced real-time analysis of patient feedback.[13] Patients provide comments on the web, through a comment card, through a postcard, by e-mail or by phone. These comments are analyzed using sentiment analysis and classified into complaints or praise. Time to complaint is then used to provide a numerical measure of patient satisfaction in real time.

## 3. Challenges to Real-Time Analysis

Despite the benefits of using EHR data in real-time applications, several challenges exist. Before analysis begins, standard query language must be used to organize the data. One problem with operational data is that different types of information are collected from various patients for whom the data have very different clinical meanings. For example, for one patient, there may be a diagnosis of shock and, for another patient, a systolic blood pressure reading of less than 90 may indicate the patient is in shock. In the first case, a clinician has made a determination; whereas, in the second case, clinical data indicate the diagnosis. Statistical analysis of operational data is fraught with similar difficulties because there are multiple ways to measure the same variable. Before starting, the researcher must define variables of interest in redundant ways.

The context of the data may also influence its clinical meaning and analytic value. As patients' illnesses and patterns of utilization of health services change, the normal ranges for a particular laboratory test may also change. A value abnormal for one population may not be abnormal for another and a value considered abnormal a year ago may not be considered abnormal today. When patients' health care setting shifts from a hospital to an outpatient clinic, then critical values must also be adjusted as patients who are not admitted will be potentially more difficult to manage. When analyzing real-time data, all of these considerations must be built into the analytic algorithms so that the clinician or researcher has meaningful information.

## 4. Conclusion

The examples above demonstrate how specific, innovative applications using EHR information can have an important impact on health and disease management. Interventions may be simple and involve modifications of existing software or may be more complex and involve multiple collaborating systems, databases, and interactions. The common theme in these systems is cooperation among different functional areas within the health system. Providers, information technology experts, administrative professionals, and other staff play important roles in maximizing meaningful information exchange and build-out of innovative quality and safety initiatives.

The relevance of real-time interpretation is largely designed to improve clinical care at or around the time of treatment. However, there are important public health, research, and administrative applications of real-time data as well. The health researcher is accustomed to looking across populations and seeing and acting on trends in the data with little or no input directly from patients. The clinician, on the other hand, gathers information from the current or recent personal encounters with the patient and makes decisions accordingly.

While the researcher may rely on computers to analyze data, the clinician relies on his or her training, experience, and some clinical references to decide on a course of action. This professional judgment, while difficult to quantify, is needed for clinical encounters. There is no other way to diagnose and treat based on the many subtle and personal cues and exam findings that inform treatment. Although individuals have the capacity to process much information, a well-designed interface is necessary in order for health care professionals to use EHR data effectively in the care of their patients. Well-designed, clinically oriented, real-time EHR applications will become a truly indispensable adjunct to the research, policy, and clinical communities.

## References

1. Lemay R, Mawudeku A, Shi Y, Ruben M, Achonu C. Syndromic surveillance for influenza-like illness. *Biosecur Bioterror*. 2008;6(2):161-170.
2. Brennan TA, Localio AR, Leape LL, et al. Identification of adverse events occurring during hospitalization. *Ann Intern Med*. 1990;112:221-226.
3. Plaisant C, Lam S, Shneiderman B, et al. Searching electronic health records for temporal patterns in patient histories: a case study with Microsoft Amalga. *AMIA Annu Symp Proc*. 2008;601-605.
4. Miller MR, Elixhauser A, Zhan C, Meyer GS. Patient safety indicators: using administrative data to identify potential patient safety concerns. *Health Serv Res*. 2001;36(6 pt 2):110-132.
5. Rosen AK, Rivard P, Zhao S, et al. Evaluating the patient safety indicators: how well do they perform on Veterans Health Administration data? *Med Care*. 2005;43(9):873-884.
6. Centers for Disease Control and Prevention. Reduction in central line-associated bloodstream infections among patients in intensive care units: Pennsylvania, April 2001-March 2005. *MMWR*. 2005;54:1013-1016.
7. Shannon RP, Frndak D, Grunden N, et al. Using real-time problem solving to eliminate central line infections. *Jt Comm J Qual Patient Safety*. 2006;32(9):479-487.
8. Zack J. Zeroing in on zero tolerance for central line-associated bacteremia. *Am J Infect Control*. 2008;36(10):S176.e1- S176.e2.
9. Kim H, Harris M, Savova G, Speedie S, Chute C. Toward near real-time acuity estimation: a feasibility study. *Nurs Res*. 2007;56:288-294.
10. Lang N. The promise of simultaneous transformation of practice and research with the use of clinical information systems. *Nurs Outlook*. 2008;56:232-236.
11. Newcomb WL, Lincourt AE, Gersin K, et al. Development of a functional, internet-accessible department of surgery outcomes database. *Am Surg*. 2008;74:548-554.
12. Sandberg WS, Sandberg EH, Seim AR, et al. Real-time checking of electronic anesthesia records for documentation errors and automatically text messaging clinicians improves quality of documentation. *Anesth Analg*. 2008;106:192-201.
13. Alemi F, Torii M, Clementz L, Aron DC. Feasibility of real-time satisfaction surveys through automated analysis of patients' unstructured comments and sentiments. *Qual Manag Health Care*. 2012;21(1):9-19.

CHAPTER 11

# Policy Maker Perspectives on Electronic Health Records

Ryung Suh, MD, MPP, MBA, MPH; Jason Ormsby, PhD, MBA, MHSA; Sarah Johnson Katz, MS; and Brent Gibson, MD, MPH, FACPM

Across diverse health care settings, many different agents, including physicians, hospitals, health care provider networks, and select government agencies, have created and implemented successful electronic health record systems (EHR-Ss). However, the entities implementing these systems are relatively isolated from one another and often encounter cultural, political, economic, and technological barriers to full EHR adoption. With sound input from patients, providers, health care administrators, technology specialists, and others—coupled with a clear vision for system functionality, architecture, confidentiality, and cost-benefit—policy makers can avoid these barriers and encourage the meaningful use of health care information technology (HIT) tools. This chapter examines the role of policy making in establishing effective, large-scale, and interoperable EHR systems. By analyzing recent public and private EHR initiatives for strengths and weaknesses with respect to the policies used to create and redefine them, a clear roadmap for implementing EHR systems may emerge.

## 1. Government Electronic Health Record Expansion Policies and Initiatives

### The First Electronic Health Record Systems

As early as the late 1960s, some forward-thinking hospitals developed early EHRs, primarily to reduce paperwork and overhead by linking clinical and administrative functions. The most successful of these EHR prototypes include the Help Evaluation through Logical Processing (HELP) system at LDS Hospital in Utah, the Computer Stored Ambulatory Record System (COSTAR) at Massachusetts General Hospital, The Medical Record (TMR) system at Duke, and the Regenstrief Medical Record System (RMS) in Indiana.[1] By the 1980s, the designers of these and other EHR systems shifted their focus away from maintaining electronic patient records and reducing administrative overhead to developing clinical decision support systems that would improve outcomes and reduce medical errors.

These clinical decision support systems perform different functions, but they generally assist physicians by presenting focused treatment options for likely diagnoses given the specific data available at baseline and gathered during the encounter. Clinical decision-making support may run the gamut from merely providing commonly used dosing regimens for medications to aiding in the diagnosis to providing comprehensive and specific treatment guidelines for certain conditions.

## The US Department of Veterans Affairs

Federal policy makers built upon clinical decision support and other ideas learned from these early EHR experiments to design and implement systems on a larger scale. By the mid-1980s, federal interest in EHRs had grown considerably, particularly in the US Department of Veterans Affairs (VA). Using the same computer language as the COSTAR system, the VA adopted the Decentralized Hospital Computer Program (DHCP) that was designed to use health care software applications within a complete hospital information system. This system evolved into the Veterans Health Information Systems and Technology Architecture (VistA) that is still in use today.

The VA has harnessed the power of VistA by adding components, such as a comprehensive suite of clinical applications called the Computerized Patient Record System (CPRS) in 1997. CPRS offers comprehensive clinical decision-making aids such as a real-time order checking system, notification system, patient posting system, clinical reminder system, and a remote data view, as well as other innovations.[2] The positive experiences of VistA and a few other EHR systems were successfully disseminated to the broader health care community in several Institute of Medicine (IOM) reports beginning with *The Computer-Based Patient Record: An Essential Technology for Health Care in 1991.*[3] The reports greatly increased interest in EHR within the health care sector but particularly within certain federal agencies.

## The US Department of Health and Human Services

EHR system initiatives from the US Department of Health and Human Services (HHS) targeted 2 main areas. First, federal funds supported the adoption and implementation of EHRs through its quality improvement organization (QIO) program within the Centers for Medicare & Medicaid Services (CMS). QIOs have helped providers to implement EHR solutions, encouraged the use of EHRs for quality improvement with a focus on health and disease management (HDM), and educated providers on how to use their EHR capabilities to improve screening and immunization rates.[4]

The Office of the National Coordinator for HIT (ONC) was created in 2004 and has since directed national EHR research and demonstration programs to provide the secretary of the US Department of Health and Human Services with recommendations on how best to promote uptake of EHRs and other HIT technologies, and to improve interoperability and security of the national health information infrastructure. Of particular note, in 2004 alone, HHS provided $228 million for

EHR-related initiatives ranging from support for development of standard terminologies to funding geographically linked health information exchanges.

## Recovery and Health Reform Legislation

Building upon both public and private experimentation, as well as input from stakeholders, Congress offered unprecedented opportunities for nationwide EHR advancement through the American Recovery and Reinvestment Act of 2009 (ARRA). With an estimated $48 billion in HIT-related funding across all areas of the federal government, the overall national strategy is to improve health care quality, safety, outcomes, and efficiency by stimulating the widespread adoption of EHR systems, establishing a standards-based, secure nationwide health care data exchange, and offering providers financial incentives to encourage the proper use of HIT.

By far, the most extensive new funding opportunity from ARRA involves the direct subsidization of EHR systems for providers. Beginning in 2011, CMS was responsible for distributing $29 billion in Medicare and Medicaid incentives to encourage physicians, hospitals, and other providers to have *meaningful use* of EHR systems to address various issues including improving care coordination, reducing health care disparities, engaging patients and families, improving population health, and maintaining data privacy and security. Physicians could have received up to $44,000 over 5 years and hospitals could have received up to $11 million. For providers who fail to adopt EHRs, ARRA cuts their Medicare payment rates by 1% in 2015, and up to 5% thereafter. Due to these incentives, and other factors, Congress predicts that approximately 90% of doctors and 70% of hospitals will adopt certified EHRs within the next decade. In turn, that could save the federal government more than $12 billion (through reduced spending on Medicare and Medicaid, and other programs) and generate additional savings in the health care sector through improvements in quality, care coordination, and reductions in medical errors and duplicative care.

ONC is also directing over $600 million in grants for the establishment of up to 70 HIT regional extension centers (RECs) that will offer technical assistance, guidance, and information on best practices to support and accelerate health care providers' efforts to become meaningful users of EHR. Sixty RECs were established by December 2010. ARRA funding also supports a national Health Information Technology Research Center (HITRC) that will gather relevant information on effective practices and help the RECs collaborate to identify and share EHR adoption, effective use, and provider support.

The Patient Protection and Affordable Care Act of 2010 (ACA) was an unprecedented expansion of US health care and heavily promotes the use of HIT systems and tools, particularly EHR. Although ACA does not provide the level of funding for HIT implementation contained in ARRA, it views HIT as way to connect the wide array of new public and private coverage and care expansions. Specifically, ACA builds upon ARRA funding to further promote the use of EHR for quality measurement, quality improvement, HDM, patient-centered care and medical home care models, and comparative effectiveness research. Of note are references to the promotion of open-source VistA for public and private providers, and its proven capabilities with HDM and other care management systems and tools.[5]

## State and Local Efforts

Since a 2004 Executive Order encouraging HIT interoperability and EHR adoption, every state has some type of program to promote EHR adoption underway.[6] For example, Texas and Wisconsin initiated innovative EHR programs. The Texas Statewide Healthcare Coordinating Council directs state health care workforce policy and, with the help of a Health Information Technology Advisory Committee (HITAC), develops ways to use EHRs to improve quality and lower costs. The state of Wisconsin has also analyzed HIT adoption with attention to integration with patient safety systems and found that there is significant HIT in use even in rural areas and in smaller hospitals, often with an impact on patient safety.[7]

At the regional and local levels, various stakeholders are working to encourage the adoption and implementation of EHR systems. Several insurers offer financial incentives to providers that adopt EHRs intended to offset the capital cost of initial EHR investment. Regional efforts, including regional collaborations and purchasing coalitions, also support adoption and implementation by offering technical assistance and consulting to educate providers. Foundations and other philanthropic organizations have also supported such efforts. These initiatives often bring multiple stakeholders together to achieve common quality and safety goals.

## 2. Policy Barriers to Electronic Health Record Adoption and Implementation

### Data Security and Privacy

Of the many challenges facing the uptake of EHRs, the one that generates the most publicity—and, perhaps consequently, creates the greatest implementation barrier—is data security. For a number of reasons, privacy advocates, patients, health care providers, and health care administrators are concerned with the security of electronic data. A major concern is that others will seek to take advantage of patients by stealing their identities and gaining access to electronic data. Another concern is that the data will be lost, corrupted, deleted, or altered more easily than what occurs with paper records.

Anyone who has used a computer understands the risk of files being misplaced, accidentally mislabeled or deleted, or not updated properly. Furthermore, while few would argue against the utility of using EHRs to enhance HDM programs, the potential threat posed by identity thieves, viruses, and user error is enough to delay widespread EHR adoption. Public and private users of EHRs must demonstrate that advances in technology can securely guard against data intrusions, system failures, and human errors in order to diminish the opposition to widespread adoption.

## Data Validity

HDM and other EHR-enhanced health care maintenance and improvement programs potentially offer an attractive environment in which to field EHR systems; however, their usefulness depends on the data not only being secure but also valid and presented in a way that enhances understanding of the clinical encounter. Many HDM programs require monitoring patient prescription drug usage, but some may be more comprehensive and monitor for rare adverse events and potentially assist providers with understanding causal relationships.

To further complicate matters, there may be concern about how collected data accurately reflect patient experience. For example, without adequate notes, a patient's experience with unusual and/or unnecessary pain following a procedure would not be noted even if a procedure were a success. Additionally, if the electronic system depends directly on patient input, as in the case of a personal health record (potentially prone to inaccuracy) rather than objectively obtained data such as laboratory values (that can be invalid), then decision making for that patient may be inappropriate. This, in turn, erodes the effectiveness of the program and user confidence.

## Cost

While a comprehensive cost analysis for implementing EHRs is beyond the scope of this chapter, a few comments are worth noting. As noted in Chapter 9, the federal government has estimated the capital investment needed for equipment, software, training, and support when implementing EHRs. For example, the Congressional Budget Office determined that for a physician office, start-up costs for installing a basic EHR system range from $25,000 to $45,000 per physician, while annual operating costs range from $3,000 to $9,000.[8] Although ARRA and other legislation have addressed some of these investment costs by providing practices up to $44,000 per year, practices also incur opportunity costs as physicians and others must devote time to learning the system instead of generating revenue through patient care activities.

Although the total costs for some practices and other providers (such as hospitals) might be prohibitive for some, researchers and policy makers have identified a financial benefit of EHR adoption within a modest timeframe. Using data from a hypothetical primary care panel generated from the Partners Healthcare System at the Brigham and Women's Hospital and Massachusetts General Hospital, researchers found that implementation of an EHR reaches a financial break-even point between the second and third years after adoption.[9]

## 3. Private Sector Policy Trends and Industry Developments

At the forefront of the health informatics sector are the American Medical Informatics Association (AMIA) and the American Health Information Management Association (AHIMA). These organizations formed a Joint Workforce Task Force to address the skills needed by people who use or work with EHRs.[10] This task force identified care competencies in 5 domains: health information literacy and skills, health informatics skills using the EHR, privacy and confidentiality of health information, health information/data technical security, and basic computer literacy skills.

The AMIA published a white paper addressing the use of HIT and EHRs as they relate to HDM and wellness programs, with an emphasis on changing from institutional to patient-centric applications. This would represent an important shift from designing programs around the requirements and needs of hospitals, clinics, and other institutions to those of patients. For HDM programs, this is especially important as the patient's role in maintaining health and wellness, especially over the long-term, is critical to the program's success. Innovations such as Internet applications, mobile devices, and home telehealth programs facilitate the patient's central role in HDM. Previously, care was unidirectional, flowing from provider to patient. It has evolved to be interactive and bidirectional, flowing from patient to provider back to patient in multiple iterations. Systems capable of capturing these iterations will aid in improving case management and ultimately disease management.

## 4. Policy Issues Regarding Electronic Health Record Utilization in Health and Disease Management Evaluation

Despite the many perceived advantages to using EHRs in HDM programs, some of the general concerns present when fielding HIT in general—such as access, quality, safety, efficacy, funding, and maintaining confidentiality—are likely also to be present in HDM applications. Along the lines of access, one area of concern is that increasing the use of EHRs may have the unintended consequence of reducing access to certain services. This would potentially occur through economic barriers brought on by more expensive electronic HDM programs that increase the overall cost of care.

In addition, for those programs requiring access to a digital central support system via the Internet, some families or entire communities may be locked out owing to a lack of high-speed communications where they live or work. The growing digital divide between the telecommunication and information haves and have-nots is a possible harbinger with regard to health care.[11] Other concerns regarding EHR utilization in HDM evaluation include the safety and efficacy of health care devices and the potential need for FDA review of new technologies, as well as the interoperability of patient-centered technologies requiring data transfer across multiple physical and technological settings. Awareness of these potential problem areas will assist policy makers as they introduce new programs and technologies.

## 5. Perceptions of Data Source Reliability and Validity among Federal Agencies

Federal agencies such as HHS, AHRQ, and CMS are key players in standardizing and supporting interoperability of EHRs and other aspects of HIT that make HDM programs possible. In addition to having extensive experience with EHRs and being a major purchaser of health care services, federal agencies also have visibility across large jurisdictional areas, such as states, and large-practice environments, such as integrated health systems. Efforts at standardizing and bolstering data reliability and validity may indeed originate at the federal level.

Thus, it is useful to review recent federal efforts designed to advance the general HIT and EHR agenda. AHRQ has launched several projects potentially related to EHR interoperability, including HDM evaluation and EHR/HDM integration. While beyond the scope of this chapter, these projects deployed HIT in rural settings to bridge gaps in coverage, and in urban areas to create an EHR/HDM system for community health centers. CMS is also active at the federal level in implementing both HDM and HIT. In the past decade, over 20 state Medicaid agencies have instituted HDM programs and the agency has also fielded an EHR demonstration project. How data from these programs are stored, exchanged, and utilized across clinics and providers will provide a valuable blueprint for nationwide HIT and EHR efforts.

For other agencies, complementary EHR system interoperability is a longstanding issue. The VA and the US Department of Defense (DOD) share many patients who also may seek care outside of either system. This presents an enormous challenge for providers who have limited or no knowledge of treatments outside of their systems. The VA has several ongoing research projects related to HDM (under the VA's Office of Research and Development's Health Services Research and Development Service), and the VA and DOD have worked on mechanisms to share EHRs and patient data under the Joint Electronic Records Interoperability (JEHRI) strategy.[12]

## 6. Conclusion

Building a secure, interoperable nationwide EHR system will likely allow for the comprehensive exchange of health care data between many providers. As a result, the enhanced use of health care management programs may improve access, quality, safety, outcomes, and efficiency. So, as the implementation of both HDM programs and EHRs moves forward, understanding their interaction should be a priority research area. Their full potential will be realized with proper stewardship and guidance at the national, state, and community levels. EHR research and implementation programs sponsored by DHHS, AHRQ, CMS, VA, and DoD will help build the foundation of a complicated and incongruous HIT infrastructure.

# References

1. Reel SF, Mandell SF. History. In: Lehmann HP. *Aspects of Electronic Health Systems*. New York: Springer; 2006:chap 2.
2. Office of Enterprise Development, Department of Veterans Affairs. *VistA-HealtheVet Monograph*. Washington, DC: Department of Veterans Affairs; July 2008.
3. Institute of Medicine. *The Computer-Based Patient Record: An Essential Technology for Health Care*. Washington, DC: National Academy Press; 1997.
4. Institute of Medicine. *Medicare's Quality Improvement Organization Program*. Washington, DC: National Academy Press; 2006.
5. 111th Congress. Public Law 111-148. Patient Protection and Affordable Care Act. Washington, DC: Government Printing Office. http://www.gpo.gov/fdsys/pkg/PLAW-111publ148/pdf/PLAW-111publ148.pdf. Published March 23, 2010. Accessed November 26, 2010.
6. National Association of State Chief Information Officers (NASCIO). *Profiles of Progress: State Health IT Initiatives*. Lexington, KY: NASCIO; 2006.
7. Rural Wisconsin Health Cooperative. *Density of HIT Adoption in RWHC Member Hospitals*. Sauk City, WI: Rural Wisconsin Health Cooperative; 2006.
8. Congressional Budget Office. *Evidence on the Costs and Benefits of Health Information Technology*. Washington, DC: Congressional Budget Office; 2008.
9. Wang SJ, Middleton B, Prosser LA, et al. A cost-benefit analysis of electronic medical records in primary care. *Am J Med*. 2003;114(5):397-403.
10. American Health Information Management Association and the American Medical Informatics Association. *Joint Work Force Task Force: Health Information Management and Informatics Core Competencies for Individuals Working with Electronic Health Records*. Bethesda, MD: American Medical Informatics Association; 2008.
11. Cooper R, Kimmelman G. *The Digital Divide Confronts the Telecommunications Act of 1996: Economic Reality Versus Public Policy*. Yonkers, NY: Consumer Union; 1999.
12. US Department of Veterans Affairs. VA/DoD health IT sharing program. May 2008. Retrieved November 30, 2008, from http://www1.va.gov/VADoDHealthITSharing/.

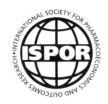

# PART 3

## Patient-Reported Outcomes

CHAPTER 12  Introduction to Patient-Reported Outcomes ............................ 133

CHAPTER 13  Patient-Reported Outcomes Instrument Design
and Development ................................................................................. 141

CHAPTER 14  Psychometric Methods for Patient-Reported
Outcomes Assessment .......................................................... 151

CHAPTER 15  Health-Related Quality of Life/Functional Status
and Health and Disease Management ..................................... 172

CHAPTER 16  Work Outcomes in Health and Disease Management ............... 188

CHAPTER 17  Patient Satisfaction and Health and Disease Management ....... 206

## CHAPTER 12

# Introduction to Patient-Reported Outcomes

Robin S. Turpin, PhD; and Heidi C. Waters, MS, MBA

This chapter defines patient-reported outcomes and their uses in health and disease management. It also discusses the potential biases introduced as a result of low- or differential-response rates, difficulties with recall or social desirability, issues of trust and confidentiality, and the influence of incentives on data quality. The chapter then concludes with a brief description of the other chapters in this section.

## 1. Defining Patient-Reported Outcomes

Ernest Codman[1] called for careful scrutiny of patient-reported outcomes (PROs) in his seminal 1914 publication, *The Product of a Hospital*, but it was not until the 1980s that the patient point of view became a focus of health care providers, payers, policy makers, and researchers. In what is perhaps the largest series of validation studies of a data collection instrument, the Medical Outcomes Study (MOS) was launched in 1986 to develop a practical tool for the routine monitoring of patient outcomes.[2] This research resulted in the 36-item Short Form Health Survey (SF-36) that includes an 8-scale profile of functional health and well-being scores, as well as psychometrically based physical and mental health summary measures and a preference-based health utility index. Subsequent validation studies resulted in shortened versions used most often for population studies, including the SF-20, SF-12, SF-8, and SF-6D. PROs increased in importance in health services and drug effectiveness research over the ensuing 3 to 4 decades, but were utilized less often in health and disease management.

### Definition

A PRO is any direct report from patients about how they function or feel in relation to a health condition and/or its therapy, without interpretation, comment, or revision by physicians or others.[3] *PRO* is a broadly defined umbrella term that includes physical functioning and pain; symptom reporting and global health perception; psychological well-being and happiness; and treatment adherence and satisfaction.[4] PRO data collection instruments can be either generic or disease-specific. Generic instruments, such as the SF-36, allow researchers to compare outcomes across a wide range of conditions and populations.

In health and disease management, generic instruments are particularly useful at assessing the overall health of an employed population, and evaluating general changes in health perception and physical functioning. Disease-specific instruments have a more narrow scope, focus on the symptoms associated with specific conditions (such as asthma or arthritis) and are more sensitive to changes in health perception than generic measures.[5,6] Examples of disease-specific instruments include the Beck Depression Inventory that measures the depth or intensity of depression[7] and the Back Pain Classification Scale that is used to distinguish low back pain due to psychological disturbance from that due to organic disease.[8]

Regardless of the generic or specific nature of the patient-reported measure, evaluators should develop data collection instruments with extensive patient input to ensure all health issues pertinent to a particular patient group are captured. For example, for a new instrument to assess health-related quality of life (HRQOL) in patients with endometriosis, researchers should interview patients about their condition and its impact on their HRQOL before finalizing the content.[3] The measure should be well grounded in psychometric or preference-based theories, with appropriate validation before use, and as necessary, appropriate language and cultural translation.[9,10] Given the increasing use of PROs in both clinical and population studies, there exists a wide array of generic and disease-specific instruments, generally eliminating the need for health and disease management program planners and evaluators to create their own.

## Uses of Patient-Reported Outcomes

There are many uses for patient-reported outcomes in health and disease management, including:

- a screen for particular conditions (for example, depression in chronic obstructive pulmonary disease (COPD) or heart failure).[11,12]
- an assessment of clinical improvement (for example, migraine pain).[13]
- an end point for conditions with little hope of cure (for example, anxiety levels in end-stage renal disease).[14,15]
- an indicator of program success (such as treatment satisfaction).[16]

For some conditions, PROs are strongly related to long-term treatment outcomes. For example, for persons with diabetes, positive well-being and self-management are linked to overall treatment success,[17,18] while for persons with psoriasis, negative well-being is associated with depression and suicidal ideation.[19]

## 2. Impact of Response Rates

The reliability of PROs is directly related to response rates. Low-response rates, for either an entire instrument (total nonresponse) or individual questions on that instrument (item nonresponse), may bias findings, making them difficult to generalize.[20] This is particularly true if nonresponders and responders differ systematically. However, if the characteristics of the nonresponders and responders are similar, a low-response rate may not be indicative of bias.

Response rates can vary between types of studies and instrument administration methods. An analysis of published patient satisfaction studies found that those that used an in-person interview methodology in either subject recruitment or data collection have higher response rates than those that utilized mail methods.[21] Another study showed that sending written or telephonic reminders for mail-based surveys increases response rates.[22] The number of contacts made with participants and the provision of monetary incentives also increases the likelihood of response.[23] Health and disease management programs that utilize face-to-face contact or telephonic follow-up may reduce the impact of nonresponse bias on PROs. Other disease management programs that utilize Internet-based methods of administration, which may improve follow-up for some, might introduce bias as not all participants may have equal access to the Internet. However, the US Census Bureau estimates that approximately 70% of the US population has some access to the Internet, so this bias may not be as large as it was in the past.[24]

There are various methods to control for the effects of nonresponse bias, including the comparison of research results to similar results from the population under study and assessing these similarities,[25] or weighting techniques based on currently available data and using regression estimation.[26] Each of these methods has potential pitfalls. Small biases typically can be corrected by weighting procedures, but the larger the population of nonresponders, the more difficult bias correction becomes.

## 3. Response Biases

Several sources of response bias can be introduced in the collection of PRO data, including problems with recall, response sets, and the response shift phenomenon.

### Recall

Potential biases associated with recall difficulties are well documented,[27] and most PRO instruments have been developed and validated to minimize their impact. Nonetheless, certain types of recall bias can have an impact on the evaluation of health and disease management programs and should be identified in advance. For example, a placebo response has been identified in fibromyalgia patients, who report higher levels of pain when asked to recall incidences over the past month than when they record their current pain level.[28] The same phenomenon has been reported in a broad range of conditions.[29,30]

Many PRO instruments for dementia embed a mini mental status exam to help limit potential recall bias. For PROs outside of a dementia study, where cognitive status is an issue, there may be additional difficulties in collecting reliable data. Generally recall bias tends to result in exaggerated positive effects of health and disease programs. The best approach to limit the impact of recall bias is to collect data in the shortest timeframe possible depending on the condition of interest, preferably in real time via participant diaries and/or electronic devices.

## Response Sets

Another challenge to the validity of PRO instruments is that respondents might answer questions systematically in a manner unrelated to the questions being asked, but strongly associated to their own individual characteristics, a phenomenon known as *response sets*.[31,32] There are several well-known response sets, including social desirability, extremity of responses, and acquiescence.

*Social desirability* is the tendency to respond in the most socially acceptable manner. Researchers have demonstrated that this has an effect on such areas as underestimating the difficulties associated with cancer,[33,34] inaccurately reporting height, weight, and body mass index (BMI),[35] and exaggerating adherence to medical treatment.[36] There are several approaches to minimizing the impact of social desirability, including requiring a forced choice between 2 equally desirable responses, selecting items about which social desirability is not an issue, assuring respondents of anonymity or that there are no right or wrong answers, and minimizing personal contact when the desire to respond appropriately is compounded. In health research, the potential measurement error created by social desirability may be mitigated by comparison to a control or placebo group, but this is not always possible in health or disease management.

*Extremity of responses* is the tendency to respond in the most positive (the optimist) or negative (the pessimist) manner available. This is generally an inherent characteristic of individual respondents. One approach to minimize this impact is to utilize dichotomous questions (for example, true-false), or items with a Likert scale for response categories with multiple response choices. However, during the instrument development process, researchers must test for floor and ceiling effects (when most respondents report positive outcomes and there is no variability) and remove items to mitigate these effects when present.

The *acquiescence response* set is the tendency for a respondent either to agree or disagree consistently with any question, and is related to the acceptance response set (the tendency to accept all positively worded items and reject all negatively worded items). Utilizing a balanced data collection instrument, with equal numbers of positive and negative responses, can help minimize the impact of these response sets. Validated PRO instruments will be structured to minimize the impact of each of these response sets, but these issues must be addressed if health and disease management evaluations utilize "home-grown" instruments or adapt validated instruments.

## Response Shift

*Response shift* refers to the tendency for respondents to recalibrate their perspective of their health status over time.[37,38] Response shifts can be negative (over time, participants believe their health was worse than they originally reported) or positive (participants believe their health was better than they originally reported). The phenomenon has been demonstrated across a wide range of conditions including arthritis, cancer, and diabetes, and results in difficulties in interpreting change over time, often leading investigators to wonder whether changes were due to a health care intervention or disease management program or merely response shift. Response shift is different from recall bias as respondents actually experience a shift or a redefinition of their internal standards, values, or concepts about their health condition or quality of life. Since response shifts can be either negative or positive, they can either overestimate or underestimate the impact of a disease management program.

The standard approach to assessing whether or not a response shift has occurred is to use a *then-test*. This consists of 2 measurements of the same item: first, in real time at baseline and second, at a later point of the program. For example, patients with chronic pain may be assessed for their baseline pain levels at program initiation, and then asked about their baseline pain level several months later. A response shift occurs if respondents report different baseline pain levels. The best approach to minimizing impact is to measure outcomes in real time or to incorporate a comparison group in which one would assume a similar level of response shift so that any incremental change shown in the treatment group can be assumed to be real. But if these are not possible, it is important to assess and understand the impact that response shift can have on program results.

## 4. Confidentiality

With the growing need for research to support health and disease management programs, patient confidentiality is critical. The Health Insurance Portability and Accountability Act of 1996 (HIPAA) was originally established to ensure that employees who changed jobs would be able to obtain insurance at their new place of employment regardless of health conditions reported under previous insurance carriers.[39] As such, HIPAA mandated the protection and privacy of individually identifiable health information but provided little guidance on how this applied to research. The result was a variety of interpretations of HIPAA and much confusion for those conducting research.

Wolf and Bennett found that the enactment of HIPAA initially increased the financial and time resources needed for research recruitment threefold, but once a HIPAA-compliant recruitment policy was enacted, the resource constraints fell by approximately 70%. Another study found that consent for follow-up in patient registries dropped by two-thirds following the enactment of HIPAA, and that heterogeneity among those who did consent also decreased. The decline in the number of patients willing to participate in research has introduced selection bias into studies.

When planning disease management programs, researchers must be aware of the impact of patient confidentiality provisions and build extra resources into the budget to account for reduced enrollment rates. Also, when analyzing findings, the effects of potential selection bias as a result of confidentiality concerns should be thoroughly explored and analyzed.

## 5. Impact of Incentives on Data Quality

Recruitment in research is often enhanced by providing something of value to the research participants. Providing cash as an incentive for participation has a greater effect on participation than other forms of rewards.[40,41] One study found that when a monetary incentive was promised to survey participants, contingent on the return of a questionnaire, the average increase in the response rate was 7%. The larger the incentive offered, the more the response rate increased, regardless of the survey population.[42] Several studies have demonstrated that providing financial incentives or other material incentives to study participants did not affect the quality of data[42,43] or the study outcome.[44] Many employer-based wellness programs offer monetary incentives for participation, including health insurance rebates, cash bonuses, and paid vacation days.

Literature is mixed regarding whether or not monetary incentives lead to desired behavior. Studies assessing the effectiveness of incentives on smoking cessation programs indicated that incentives generally increase participation rates[45,46] and have initial impact on smoking cessation, but this impact tends to decrease over time.[44-46] However, other research indicates that appropriately structured incentives can have a long-term impact on employee behavior[47,48] and that relative effectiveness and participation in the programs is directly correlated with the dollar value of the incentive.[49] When designing a disease management program, consideration should be given to providing incentives for participation and achievement of results, but at a level considered sufficient for effort in participating and nothing more.

## 6. Organization of this Part of the Book

This chapter provides only a sample of the issues associated with measuring very complex human phenomena through PROs. In Chapter 13, we describe PRO instrument design and validation, with particular attention on administration methods, linguistic validation, and approaches to standardization. Chapter 14 provides a primer on psychometric methods, detailing the issues that must be addressed when developing a new instrument. Chapter 15 examines health-related quality of life and functional status instruments, and the differences between them. Chapter 16 describes the use of PROs to measure work outcomes, absenteeism, presenteeism, and productivity. Finally, Chapter 17 discusses the role of patient satisfaction in health and disease management, especially the relationship of patient, provider, or caregiver satisfaction to health-related quality of life.

## References

1. Codman EA. The product of a hospital. *Surg Gynecol Obstet.* 1914;18:491-496.
2. Ware JE. *SF-36 Health Survey: Manual and Interpretation Guide.* Boston, MA: The Health Institute, New England Medical Center; 1993.
3. Patrick DL, Burke LB, Powers JH, et al. Patient-reported outcomes to support medical product

labeling claims: FDA perspective. *Value Health.* 2007;10(suppl 2):125-137.
4. Arpinelli F, Bamfi F. The FDA guidance for industry on PROs: the point of view of a pharmaceutical company. *Health Qual Life Out.* 2006;4(85):1-5.
5. Marquis P, Arnould B, Acquadro C, Roberts WM. Patient-reported outcomes and health-related quality of life in effectiveness studies: pros and cons. *Drug Develop Res.* 2006;67:193-201.
6. Guyatt GH, Feeny DH, Patrick DL. Measuring health-related quality of life. *Ann Intern Med.* 1993;118:622-629.
7. Beck AT, Steer RA, Garbin MG. Psychometric properties of the Beck Depression Inventory: twenty-five years of evaluation. *Clin Psychol Rev.* 1988;8:77-100.
8. Leavitt F. Comparison of three measures for detecting psychological disturbance in patients with low back pain. *Pain.* 1982;13:299-305.
9. Revicki DA, Ehreth JL. Health-related quality-of-life assessment and planning for the pharmaceutical industry. *Clin Ther.* 1997;19(5):1101-1115.
10. US Department of Health and Human Services FDA Centers for Drug Evaluation and Research; Biologics Evaluation and Research; and Devices and Radiological Health. Guidance for industry: patient-reported outcome measures: use in medical product development to support labeling claims: draft guidance. *Health Qual Life Out.* 2006;4(79):1-20.
11. Oga R, Nishimura K, Tsukino S, Sato S, Hajiro T, Mishia M. Longitudinal deteriorations in patient reported outcomes in patients with COPD. *Respir Med.* 2007;101(1):146-153.
12. Smith B, Forkner E, Zaslow B, et al. Disease management produces limited quality-of-life improvements in patients with congestive heart failure: evidence from a randomized trial in community-dwelling patients. *Am J Manag Care.* 2005;11:701-713.
13. Campinha-Bacote DL, Kendle JB, Jones C, et al. Impact of migraine management program on improving health outcomes. *Dis Manag.* 2005;8(6):382-391.
14. Sands JJ. Disease management improves end-stage renal disease outcomes. *Blood Purif.* 2006;24(4):394-399.
15. Anand S, Nissenson AR. Utilizing a disease management approach to improve ESRD patient outcomes. *Semin Dial.* 2002;15(1):38-40.
16. Sen S, Fawson P, Cherrington G, et al. Patient satisfaction measurement in the disease management industry. *Dis Manag.* 2005;8(5):288-300.
17. Krumholtz HM, Currie PM, Riegel B, et al. A taxonomy for disease management. Circulation [serial online]. 2006: 114(13):1432-45. http://www.circulationaha.org. Accessed August 15, 2008.
18. Rubin RR, Peyrot M, Siminerio LM. Health care and patient-reported outcomes: results of the cross-national Diabetes Attitudes, Wishes and Needs (DAWN) study. *Diabetes Care.* 2006;29(6):1249-1255.
19. Bhosle MJ, Kulkarni A, Feldman SR, Balkrishnan R. Quality of life in patients with psoriasis. *Health Qual Life Outcomes.* 2006;4(35):1-7.
20. Sax LJ, Gilmartin SK, Bryant AN. Assessing response rates and nonresponse bias in web and paper surveys. *Res High Educ.* 2003;44(4):409-432.
21. Sitzia J, Wood N. Response rate in patient satisfaction research: an analysis of 210 published studies. *J Qual Health Care.* 1998;10(4):311-317.
22. Asch DA, Jedrziewski K, Christakis NA. Response rates to mail surveys published in medical journals. *J Clin Epidemiol.* 1997;50(10):1129-1136.
23. McColl E, Jacoby A, Thomas L, et al. Design and use of questionnaires: a review of best practice applicable to surveys of health service staff and patients. *Health Technolo Assess.* 2001;5(31):1-6.
24. Bureau of the Census. Adult computer and adult internet users by selected characteristics 1995 to 2006. In: *Statistical Abstracts of the United States: 2008.* 127th ed. Table 1128. Washington, DC: US GPO; 2008.
25. Armstrong JS, Overton TS. Evaluating nonresponse bias in mail surveys. *J Marketing Res.* 1977;14:396-402.
26. Bethlehem JG. Reduction of nonresponse bias through regression estimation. *J Official Stat.* 1988;4(3):251-260.

**Part 3: Patient-Reported Outcomes**

27. Aday LA. *Designing and conducting health surveys: A comprehensive guide.* 2nd ed. San Francisco, CA: Jossey-Bass; 1996.
28. Williams DA, Gendreau M, Hufford MR, Groner K, Gracely RH, Clauw DJ. Pain assessment in patients with fibromyalgia syndrome: a consideration of methods for clinical trials. *Clin J Pain.* 2004;20(5):348-356.
29. Broderick JE, Stone AA, Calvanese P, Schwartz JE, Turk DC. Recalled pain ratings: a complex and poorly defined task. *J Pain.* 2006;7(2);142-149.
30. Asimakopoulou KG, Hampson SE. Biases in self-reports of self-care behaviors in type 2 diabetes. *Psychol Health Med.* 2005;10(3):305-314.
31. Oskamp S. *Attitudes and Opinions.* Englewood Cliffs, NJ: Prentice-Hall; 1977.
32. Rust J, Golombok S. *Modern Psychometrics: The Science of Psychological Assessment.* 2nd ed. New York, NY: Routledge; 1999.
33. O'Leary TE, Diller L, Recklitis CJ. The effects of response bias on self-reported quality of life among childhood cancer survivors. *Qual Life Res.* 2007;16(7):1211-1220.
34. Johnson TP, O'Rourke DP, Burris JE, Warnecke RB. An investigation of the effects of social desirability on the validity of self-reports of cancer screening behaviors. *Med Care.* 2005; 43(6):565-573.
35. Craig TW. Assessing motivational response bias: the influence of individual, item, and situational characteristics on the measurement of self-reported health indicators. *Dissertation Abstracts International.* 2007;68(4-B):2707.
36. Balkrishnan R, Jayawant SS. Medication adherence research in populations: measurement issues and other challenges. *Clin Ther.* 2007;29(6):1180-1183.
37. Osborne RH, Hawkins M, Sprangers MAG. Change of perspective: a measurable and desired outcome of chronic disease self-management intervention programs that violates the premise of preintervention/postintervention assessment. *Arthritis Rheum.* 2006;55(3):458-465.
38. Rapkin BD, Schwartz CE. Toward a theoretical model of quality-of-life appraisal: implications of findings from studies of response shift. *Health Qual Life Out.* 2004;2(14):1-12.
39. Wolf MS, Bennett CL. Local perspective of the impact of the HIPAA privacy rule on research. *Cancer.* 2006;106:474-479.
40. Deehan A, Templeton L, Taylor C, Drummond C, Strang J. The effect of cash and other financial inducements on response rate of general practitioners in a national postal study. *Br J Gen Prac.* 1997;47:87-90.
41. Perneger TV, Etter JF, Rougemont A. Randomized trial of use of a monetary incentive and reminder card to increase the response rate to a mailed health survey. *Am J Epidemiol.* 1993;138(9):714-722.
42. Hopkins KD. Response rates in survey research: a meta-analysis of the effects of monetary gratuities. *J Exp Ed.* 1992;61:52.
43. Shaw MJ, Beebe TJ, Adlis SA, Jensen H. The use of monetary incentives in a community survey: impact on response rates, data quality, and cost. *Health Serv Res.* 2001;35(6):1339-1346.
44. Goritz AS. The impact of material incentives on response quantity, response quality, sample composition, survey outcomes, and cost in online access panels. *Int J Market Res.* 2004;46: 327-345.
45. Matson DM, Lee JW, Hopp JW. The impact of incentives and competitions on participation and quit rates in worksite smoking cessation programs. *Am J Health Promotion.* 1993;7(4): 270-280.
46. Hey K, Perera R. Competitions and incentives for smoking cessation. *Cochrane Database Syst Rev.* April 2005. 18:(2):CD004307.
47. Bains N, Pickett W, Hoey J. The use and impact of incentives in population-based smoking cessation programs: a review. *Am J Health Promot.* 1998;12(5):307-320.
48. Finkelstein EA, Hossa KM. Use of incentives to motivate healthy behaviors among employees. *Gender Issues.* 2003;21(3):50-59.
49. Chapman L. Employee participation in workplace health promotion and wellness programs: how important are incentives and which ones work best? *NC Med J.* 2006;67(6):431-432.

CHAPTER 13

# Patient-Reported Outcomes Instrument Design and Development

Gergana Zlateva, PhD; Anandi V. Law, BPharm, PhD, FAACP, FAPhA; and Elizabeth Molsen, RN

---

This chapter describes the design and development of patient-reported outcomes (PRO) instruments. We provide a brief background on the history of PRO instrument development, followed by an overview of constructing a new PRO instrument and issues related to use of existing instruments. The Food and Drug Administration's (FDA) PRO guidelines are discussed as the standard document in outlining steps in the creation of new instrument. This chapter also discusses differences between validated and nonvalidated PRO instruments, administration methods, translation into other languages, and other issues.

## 1. Introduction

With the increasing significance of PROs to both drug development and clinical practice, there are a number of agencies and consortia that have provided information on the use of PROs. For example, 2 of the largest regulatory bodies in the world—the FDA and the European Medicines Agency (EMA)—have developed guidelines regarding the use of PROs. PROMIS (Patient-Reported Outcomes Measurement Information System), which is funded by the National Institutes of Health (NIH), was formed by a group of outcomes scientists from various research organizations, academia, and the NIH.[1] The goals of this ongoing project are to standardize measurement properties of PRO instruments, provide guidance on the selection and implementation of the measures, and serve as a resource on PROs.

Organizations such as the International Society for Quality of Life (ISOQOL) and the International Society for Pharmacoeconomics and Outcomes Research (ISPOR) have established their own working groups and task forces to address various aspects of PRO development, evaluation, and utilization. For example, in 2002, ISOQOL's Good Practices Working Group explored the availability of health-related quality-of-life (HRQOL) instruments and a more formal review of quality-of-life (QOL) instruments use in clinical trials.[2]

Since 1999, ISPOR has had a series of initiatives in this area starting with a paper on the primary principles and standards for use of QOL data to support label claims, eventually resulting in a number of PRO articles published in *Value in Health* as well as consensus ISPOR PRO Task Force Reports.[2,3] ISPOR reports have focused on topics such as evaluating and documenting content validity,[4-6] good research practices for translation and linguistic validation[7] as well as the adaptation and equivalence of electronic PROs.[8] In addition, ISPOR has provided recommendations on approaches to using the same language in different countries and also pooling data from different countries.[4,7]

The result of the activities described above has been the ready availability of information on PROs development and guidance on how to use them. Yet, although much information is available, a gold standard for PRO development and use does not exist. The FDA and EMA guidelines are a recommended starting point for health care research as they were constructed by obtaining input from researchers in academia, government agencies, pharmaceutical companies, and scientific associations. The focus of the guidelines was the development and use of PROs in the context of assessing therapeutic interventions and potential label claims.

The EMA guideline process was initiated when the Committee for Human and Medicinal Products (CHMP) of the EMA published a white paper entitled *Reflection Paper on the Regulatory Guidance for the Use of Health-related Quality of Life Measures in the Evaluation of Medicinal Products*.[5,9] This document was the first step in presenting a European regulatory perspective on PRO use in interventional clinical trials for product registration. The FDA followed in February 2006 with a more detailed and in-depth draft guidance to industry, *Patient Reported Outcome Measures: Use in Medical Product Development to Support Labeling Claims* in December 2009.[6,10] Unlike its European counterpart, the FDA focused this guidance on the appropriate development and psychometric testing of PRO instruments, such that they eventually can be used by researchers or manufacturers if a label claim about a PRO is an objective of the clinical trial program.

## 2. Developing an Instrument to Assess Patient-Reported Outcomes

### Definition and Value of Patient-Reported Outcomes

Although the definition of a PRO can differ by type of health care service or disease being studied, one place to start would be the definition set forth by the FDA:

> A PRO is "any report of the status of a patient's health condition that comes directly from the patient, without interpretation of the patient's response by a clinician or anyone else. The outcome can be measured in absolute terms (eg, severity of a symptom, sign, or state of a disease) or as a change from a previous measure."[8]

PROs are valuable to evaluations of Health and Disease Management (HDM) initiatives because they are designed to enable patients (or their proxies) to assess their treatment. In contrast, clinical measures or formal clinical assessments cannot always identify treatment effects experienced by a patient. For example, pain intensity and pain relief are symptomatic measures reported by a patient and used in the development of analgesic products. PRO pain measures include pain visual analogue scales (VAS) or numeric rating scales (NRS). A multidimensional scale, such as the Brief Pain Inventory, includes questions that allow the assessment of both pain severity (average, worst, least) and pain interference (with sleep, mood, function, or other issues.)[7,11] However, clinical assessments of pain by providers fall short when they do not incorporate patients' perspectives.

Evaluations of HDM programs can be enhanced in many ways through the use of PROs. For instance, some PROs identify treatment satisfaction or preference for one type of intervention versus another (for example, the Pain Treatment Satisfaction Scale).[8,12] PRO measures can also augment clinical and psychological evaluations by providing evidence for patient improvement or decline that is not necessarily associated with clinical measures.[13] Finally, the significance of PROs in capturing changes in patient functioning and quality of life deserves attention as they are often used as an indirect preference-based measure in health economic modeling.

## Framework Used to Design Instruments Measuring Patient-Reported Outcomes

PRO instruments are challenging to design because they incorporate patients' perspectives on how they feel and/or function, and are therefore open to subjective interpretation. Outcome measures can range from a simple symptom measure (for example, an incontinence diary) to more complex measurements such as quality of life (QOL), which is a multidimensional concept that often captures physical, psychological, and social components. Further complicating this issue is that the outcomes could be observable and nonobservable events, behaviors, and/or feelings experienced by patients. However, it is the ability of PROs to capture the patient's interpretation of disease or the impact of treatment that makes them particularly valuable in HDM programs.

The general framework recommended by the FDA to develop and validate an instrument has included a mixed methods approach of both qualitative (outcomes are evaluated via text/sentences response) and quantitative (outcomes are evaluated via numerical response) methods. The PRO instrument development process has been outlined best by the FDA PRO guidance.[8,10]

A patient reported outcome (PRO) instrument measures a concept relevant and important to the patient's condition and its treatment. Generally, the first step in PRO instrument development is to define the conceptual framework for the instrument that identifies the outcomes to be measured. For PRO instruments, items and domains as reflected in the scores of an instrument should be important to the target population of patients and comprehensive with respect to patient concerns concerning the concept being assessed. Developers of new PRO instruments are encouraged to start by mapping the concepts or target areas to be evaluated with the new instrument.

A simple example is the assessment of patients with asthma, where creation of a conceptual framework for a new asthma PRO would involve selecting the outcomes to be evaluated (such as daily activities, physical exertion, asthma-related sleep interference, productivity impact, quality of life or other concepts); prioritizing the outcomes; and identifying the expected relationship of the treatment on all outcomes. The conceptual framework should also include the expected relationship between the items to be measured, including hypotheses on the effect of the treatment or intervention. At this stage, the developer should also consider whether or not the proposed instrument is appropriate for the population by considering the average age, average education level, and ethnicity profile of its members.

## Construction of a New Patient-Reported Outcome

PRO instrument development is a multistep process. The first step involves item generation—deciding what specific questions to include through a review of peer-reviewed literature, to identify outcomes of the disease and intervention, and any PROs that already exist. Although literature reviews help identify important aspects that should be included, they are dependent on the quality of data collected; the interpretation of findings from each manuscript; and the settings or patient groups on which the research was conducted. Moreover, even if a PRO that is found is not suitable in its entirety, there may be individual items within it that can be used in a new instrument.

In addition to a literature review, researchers might use other approaches for item generation, including focus groups or interviews, which have their own advantages and disadvantages.[9,14] Focus groups and/or face-to-face interviews are other important steps in item generation. These are conducted with patients (or their proxies), and/or health care providers, when applicable. The primary advantage of focus groups is that they provide insights into important outcomes from the patients themselves. These can often include outcomes that have not yet been measured in the existing literature. However, focus groups and face-to-face contact can be costly and time-consuming, and require trained moderators to direct the group discussion effectively. An alternative to face-to-face interviews is to contact patients via telephone or Internet surveys. Regardless of the method chosen to contact patients, these interviews are key to item generation.

After conducting the literature review and/or making contact with patients or providers, the PRO developer should have a pool of potential items to be included in the proposed instrument. The next step is to narrow down this pool to include only those items that will measure the outcome(s) of interest. This involves a number of processes such as *factor analysis*, in which items are grouped according to the concepts to be measured. This can be readily accomplished using a number of statistical software packages. Expert opinion can also be used to choose the items. Sometimes researchers use the *Delphi Method*, in which a group of experts repeatedly chooses the items of interest until consensus is reached.

Making the decision on the format of the responses is a process that can be completed in parallel with item generation. This involves, for example, whether to include a simple yes/no response or to have the potential responses presented in the form of a scale. Consideration must be given to respondents' ability to understand the response scale and differentiate between its components, skip patterns based on responses to some items (that is, "If you answered 'yes' to question 5, go to question 10, if 'no' continue to question 6."), and the direction of the responses (circling number 5 means 'highest' for one question, but 'lowest' for the next question). There are a number of scales and options available for responses (Table 1).

**TABLE 1.** PRO response options*[8,10]

| Type | Description |
| --- | --- |
| Visual Analog Scale (VAS) | A line of fixed length with words that anchor the scale at the extreme ends and no words describing intermediate positions. Patients are instructed to place a mark on the line corresponding to their perceived state. |
| Likert Scale | An ordered set of discrete terms or statements from which patients are asked to choose the response that best describes their state or experience. |
| Rating Scale | A set of numerical categories from which patients are asked to choose the category that best describes their state or experience. The ends of rating scales are anchored with words but the categories do not have labels. |
| Checklist | A simple choice between a limited set of options, such as 'yes,' 'no,' and 'don't know.' Some checklists ask patients to place a mark in a space if the statement in the item is true. |

* Adapted from the original version.

In addition to the scale that is used to measure the outcomes, when designing the final questions, researchers should consider the time span the respondent will be asked to consider. Recall bias, part of which is the inability of the respondent to remember what happened in the past (for example, asking about concomitant drug utilization in the previous year), can affect the quality of the data collected. To minimize the potential for bias, the respondent should be asked to consider the question in context of a reasonable time period. Oftentimes, the selection of the best time period depends on the nature of the disease (acute versus chronic) or type of outcome being measured.

After the potential items are selected and the format chosen, the new instrument should be assessed for face and content validity. Face validity is a subjective measure, wherein the new instrument is assessed by a patient and expert panel to examine if the instrument *on the face of it* appears to measure that which it intends. This is often done by testing the instrument with a small number of people from the target population prior to implementation. The purpose of this step is to determine patients' ability to understand the questions and interpret them appropriately. Content validity can be assessed by an expert panel to determine if the items in the instrument appear meaningful, useful, or essential, given the domains they are expected to cover.

The instrument must also be tested for reliability. This involves patients filling out the instrument and then conducting further statistical tests on the items such as reliability assessment, which measures the ability of the instrument to measure consistently that which it intends. Reliability and validity tests can sometimes be accomplished in parallel. The results of these processes will allow inclusion of only those items that pass all the tests, resulting in a list of final items for the new instrument.

ISPOR published a 2-part PRO task force report on the specific process of establishing and reporting the evidence of content validity in newly developed patient-reported outcomes (PRO) instruments for medical product evaluation. The report details the process for eliciting concepts for a new PRO instrument and then assessing respondent understanding.[5,6]

## Patient-Reported Outcome Administration

There are a number of ways to administer a PRO instrument, including via a trained interviewer or by self-administration (where the patient/respondent completes the instrument without assistance). Both interviewer- or self-administered instruments can be completed with paper and pencil or electronic devices (such as a mobile phone, over the telephone using a live operator, through an interactive voice response system, or on the Internet.

When choosing a form of administration, researchers should consider how the characteristics of patients in the study population might affect PRO administration and comprehension. Some of the characteristics to take into account are the average literacy levels of the subjects (note that the interviewer-administered version is preferred for those with lower levels of literacy), access to telephone or Internet, and the presence of many extended family members who may bias the patient's response if the questionnaire is completed at home. Researchers should also consider the frequency with which the PRO instrument will be administered. If it is to be administered daily, then an electronic device will be more reliable; if a lengthier period such as every 6 months is desired, a paper format would be better.

If the instrument will be administered multiple times or to several different groups, it is preferable that the same administration method is used unless the equivalency of different modes can be demonstrated. For an existing instrument, such equivalency can customarily be found in the published literature. If there is no published research on equivalency, ISPOR has published an overview of the evidence necessary to demonstrate equivalence between electronic PROs (ePROs) and the paper-based PRO measures from which they were adapted.[8] If a research study spans several sites or countries, training study site staff members in the patient interview process will enable consistent PRO instrument administration over multiple visits.

PRO instruments should be accompanied by a set of instructions to ensure the best possible comprehension and completion rate. For example, an instrument administered over the telephone would require instructions for both the administrator and the respondent. Instructions for respondents should be concise and written at the appropriate level for optimal comprehension. Instructions designed for the study staff who conducts the interview can include greater detail.

When completing a self-administered PRO instrument, the patient should be instructed to respond to the questions to the best of their ability without concern about giving a right or wrong answer. Typical guidance for administration also recommends that the subject should be in a quiet, comfortable environment, where friends or relatives will not influence the response. Similarly, the presence of a physician in the room or as an interviewer may bias the patient's response.

If the PRO instrument is administered by an interviewer, a brief training of the interviewer is recommended. Some instruments that are more complex may require more formal training; also, many computer-based tools will require formal administration and rater training. Interviewers should receive specific instructions on explaining the purpose of the instrument and how to obtain assistance with any administrative questions. Uniform administration of PRO instrument (via the same interviewer or consistent instructions) over different assessment periods is critical for the reliability of the collected data.

Respondent burden is an important consideration in PRO administration. This includes, but is not limited to, practical issues such as instrument length, font size, and possible use of different recall periods. For example, a font size that is too small may lead to an inability of the respondent to answer the questions accurately. There may also be administration burden such as a complicated set of instructions on how to administer the instrument. Both patient and administrator burden can compromise data quality and subsequent completion rates.

## Scoring a Patient-Reported Outcome Instrument

An instrument with questions that yield quantitative (that is, numerical) responses might be used to calculate a score to proxy for outcomes. For example, an instrument with questions that yields a score ranging from 0 to 100 might indicate unfavorable outcomes (0) or favorable outcomes (100). Scoring of a new instrument is driven by a number of considerations. Most importantly, the response choices should reflect a relevant numerical value. Compiling the final score can be as simple as summing the number of specific responses for a total score, or as complex as an elaborate scoring algorithm that weights various items and domains based on their relative impact on the overall measure.

## 3. Use of Existing Patient-Reported Outcomes

The development of a new, validated, and well-documented PRO instrument may be expensive and associated with a long development cycle. Researchers and practitioners working with disease management and patient health management programs that do not have such resources can consider alternative solutions to instrument development. In particular, they can choose to use an existing validated instrument or a nonvalidated one.

Sometimes there are existing tools that are not specific to the research question of interest but measure health care or some other outcomes from an overall perspective. The benefit of using one of these is that they are often validated and thus have predictable measurement abilities. For example, a commonly used global instrument is the Short Form Health Status-36 questions (SF-36).[15] The primary drawback of this approach, however, is that the instrument may be too broad and miss small, but important, changes in patients' function or quality of life. Adding exploratory questions to supplement a validated scale is a possibility; however, these questions must themselves be validated, which may be possible by using data from the study.

For example, if a disease management program for restless leg syndrome (RLS) wants to involve the spouse or partner of the RLS patient, a question might be included in a program questionnaire regarding disturbance from the perspective of the partner and would be a candidate to be added to a current instrument such as the International Restless Legs Syndrome Study Group (IRLS) rating scale; however, if items are added or altered to allow a partner to also complete, then instrument revalidation would be required.[16] ISPOR details the process of validating existing or modified PRO instruments for medical label claims in a PRO task force report published in *Value in Health*.[4]

When no existing validated instrument is available, researchers may decide to use an instrument that is not validated. A number of such examples exist on health-related websites where visitors are invited to complete a questionnaire that can either result in a predicative score indicating the chance of a certain pathologic condition or simply invite one to bring along the survey results to their health care provider for further evaluation. Such use of nonvalidated tools may be acceptable for certain purposes. The primary disadvantage of a nonvalidated tool is the lack of information on its measurement properties and its relevance of its untested attributes to the patient population, which may impact its ability to detect meaningful change experienced through the disease management program.

## 4. Translation of Patient-Reported Outcomes for International Studies

PROs are often developed in English and must be translated and adapted to other languages, dialects, and cultures before they are used in countries or regions where English is not the primary language. The following steps for instrument translation are provided by ISPOR's PRO Good Research Practices Task Force on translation and linguistic validation:[7]

1. Forward Translation: Two translations to the target language are completed by native speakers of the target language who are also fluent in English. A consensus version is then produced from these 2 forward translations, referred to as *reconciliation*.

2. Back Translation: Two translations of the consensus version are translated back to English by native English speakers and compared to the original version.

3. Back Translation Review: Comparison of the back-translated versions of the instrument with the original is conducted to identify discrepancies between the original and the back-translated versions.

4. Harmonization: Any discrepancies between the original and back-translated versions are resolved to a single version.

5. Cognitive Debriefing: The harmonized version is administered to a small group of respondents who are not involved in the study and are native speakers of the target language.

6. Final Version: The final version is produced after reconciliation of feedback from the cognitive debriefing to address any issues surrounding respondents' understanding of questions.

Research conducted in an area with a small patient population whose members speak an uncommon language would require a longer lead time to prepare the necessary linguistic validations. Identifying the appropriate language for a PRO instrument will depend on site location and an assessment of the feasibility of using specific translations at the site (that is, using a language that is comprehended by both staff and patients). It is important to start planning early to prevent an instance in which linguistic experts may not be readily available. Given the wide use of PROs in clinical trials, some broadly used instruments have translations in many languages available on specialized websites.

## 5. Conclusions

There are a number of steps that are involved in development of a new PRO instrument. This chapter has only provided an overview; some of the individual steps can involve even more complex processes, particularly in the statistical methods used to generate instrument items. There are many organizations that exist to assist in or complete the development process. Whether researchers construct a new PRO instrument alone or in tandem with a study partner often depends on available resources. Alternatively, existing instruments can be utilized with the strengths and areas of improvement associated with this method. Whether developing a new PRO instrument or using an existing instrument, when evaluating outcomes outside of the clinical realm, PROs can be valuable to determining effects of health and disease management programs.

## References

1. Patient Reported Outcomes Measurement Information System (PROMIS). Available at: http://www.nihpromis.org/. Accessed September 21, 2012.
2. ISPOR. Patient Reported Outcomes and Quality of Life Initiative. Available at: http://www.ispor.org/research_initiatives/qol_initiatives.asp. Accessed November 19, 2012
3. Leidy K, Revicki D, Geneste B. Recommendations for evaluating the validity of quality of life claims for labeling and promotion. *Value Health*. 1999;2(2):113-127.
4. Rothman M, Burke L, Erickson P, et al. Use of existing patient-reported outcome (PRO) instruments and their modification: the ISPOR good research practices for evaluating and documenting content validity for the use of existing instruments and their modification PRO task force report. *Value Health*. 2009;12;1075-83.
5. Patrick DL, Burke LB, Gwaltney CJ, et al. Content validity: establishing and reporting the evidence in newly-developed patient-reported outcomes (PRO) instruments for medical product evaluation: ISPOR PRO good research practices task force report: Part 1—eliciting concepts for a new PRO instrument. *Value Health*. 2011;14;967-977.
6. Patrick DL, Burke LB, Gwaltney CJ, et al. Content validity: establishing and reporting the evidence in newly-developed patient-reported outcomes (PRO) Instruments for medical product evaluation: ISPOR PRO good research practices task force report: Part 2—assessing respondent understanding. *Value Health*. 2011;14; 978-988.
7. Wild D, Eremenco S, Mear I, et al. Multinational trials: recommendations on the translations required, approaches to using the same language in different countries, and the approaches to support pooling the data: the ISPOR patient reported outcomes translation & linguistic validation good research practices task force report. *Value Health*. 2009;12:430-440.
8. Coons S, Gwaltney C, Hays R, et al. Recommendations on evidence needed to support measurement equivalence between electronic and paper-based patient-reported outcomes (PRO) measures: ISPOR ePRO good research practices task force report. *Value Health*. 2009;12: 419-429.
9. European Medicines Agency, Reflection Paper on the Regulatory Guidance for the Use of Health-related Quality of Life Measures in the Evaluation of Medicinal Products; paper # EMEA/CHMP/EWP/139391/2004. http://www.emea.europa.eu/docs/en_GB/document_library/Scientific_guideline/2009/09/WC500003637.pdf. Published July 2005. Accessed September 21, 2012.
10. U.S. Department of Health and Human Services, Food and Drug Administration. Patient-reported outcome measures: use in medical product development to support labeling claims. Federal Register 2009;74(35):65132-133. http://www.fda.gov/downloads/Drugs/GuidanceComplianceRegulatoryInformation/Guidances/UCM193282.pdf. Published December 2009. Accessed April 24, 2013.
11. Cleeland CS, Ryan KM. Pain assessment: global use of the Brief Pain Inventory. *Ann Acad Med Singap*. 1994;23(2):129-138.
12. Evans C, Trudeau E, Mertzanis P, et al. Development and validation of the pain treatment satisfaction scale. *Pain*. 2004;112:254-266.
13. Brown G, Sharma S, Brown M, Kistler J. Utility values in age-related macular degeneration. *Arch Ophthalmol*. 2000;119:47-51.
14. Salant P, Dillman DA. Deciding what information you need. In: *How to Conduct Your Own Survey*. 1st ed. New York, NY: John Wiley & Sons; 1994:chap 3.
15. SF-36.org. Community for Measuring Health Outcomes Using SF tools. Available at: http://www.sf-36.org/. Accessed September 21, 2012.
16. Hening Abetz L, Arbuckle R, Allen RP, et al. The reliability, validity and responsiveness of the international restless legs syndrome study group rating scale and subscales in a clinical-trial setting. *Sleep Med*. 2006;7:340-349.

CHAPTER 14

# Psychometric Methods for Patient-Reported Outcomes Assessment

I-Chan Huang, PhD, MSc; and Jane Speight, MSc, CPsychol, PhD, AFBPsS

Outcomes reported from the patient's perspective provide unique insight into various domains of health beyond traditional laboratory and clinical indicators. Measuring outcomes from the patient's perspective (or patient-reported outcomes (PROs)) is especially salient for patients with long-term or chronic conditions, who may have impaired functional status, or who require maintenance medications that may negatively impact their lifestyles. Several professional organizations (for example, the Disease Management Association of America[1] and the American College of Cardiology[2]) have identified the importance of measuring PROs in patients with chronic conditions.

In the context of health and disease management, measuring PROs can be useful in promoting patients' involvement in the treatment decision-making process, improving effective patient-doctor communication, and increasing patients' satisfaction with care.[3,4] Clinicians can use PROs to monitor patients' disease progression and to identify unexpected problems (especially psychosocial functioning) and other issues as a direct or indirect result of a condition or treatment.[1,5] Pharmaceutical companies and regulatory agencies are interested in the use of PROs to assess the effects of new drugs, medical devices, or health and disease management programs.[6] Evidence derived from valid and reliable PRO assessments may be used to support labeling and promotional claims for medical products.[7,8]

The purpose of this chapter is to describe the measurement properties of PRO instruments[9-12] Readers can apply this knowledge to help select and use appropriate PRO instruments for health and disease management. The remainder of this section will cover the topics of basic measurement theory and types of psychometric methods recommended by professional organizations. Methods of evaluating psychometric properties for PRO instruments will be explored in the following 2 sections, while the last part of this chapter focuses on the use of modern test theory.

## 1. The Value of Psychometric Evidence for PROs

Although clinicians and researchers express enthusiasm for investigating PROs in clinical practice and clinical trials, their application is challenging. This reflects the fact that PROs are:

- subjective, relying on the personal experience, interpretation, and self-report of the patient;

- complex, involving the measurement of abstract concepts from simple (for example, symptoms, pain, or fatigue) to more complex concepts (for example, satisfaction, well-being, or health-related quality of life), for which there is less consensus;[13,14] and

- costly to administer, requiring resources to collect and analyze data routinely.

Generic and condition- or disease-specific instruments capture various aspects of a patient's experience.[15] However, the ability of a PRO instrument to provide evidence of the impact of a disease or treatment, as well as to facilitate clinical decision making and health or disease management depends on the psychometric merits of the instrument. Essential psychometric properties of PRO instruments include reliability (the extent to which a measure yields the same results on repeated applications), validity (the extent to which an instrument measures what is intended), responsiveness (the extent to which an instrument distinguishes true change from random error), and interpretability (the extent to which results are unambiguous).

## Theories Underpinning Psychometric Methods

This section introduces the philosophy of psychometric methods for instrument development, which is important because the use of different measurement theories to develop or validate PRO instruments may lead to different psychometric evidence and potentially different conclusions. Readers should take these fundamental issues into account when evaluating and adopting PRO instruments.

Item response theory (IRT) and classical test theory (CTT) are 2 measurement theories used in the development and refinement of PRO instruments. IRT investigates the relationship between individuals' responses to items and their levels of the underlying construct. Compared to CTT, PRO scores estimated by IRT are sample- and scale-independent because IRT accounts for both instrument properties and respondent characteristics in PRO modeling simultaneously. Theoretically, item parameters (for example, item difficulty and discrimination) estimated by IRT are invariant; that is, the psychometric properties of items will not differ by respondent characteristics. In addition, IRT is characterized by subject invariance; that is, estimation of a respondent's underlying construct will not rely on the use of specific items.

The most widely used approach, CTT (also known as true score theory), assumes that the observed scores are composed of the true scores (that is, reflecting the exact values of respondents' underlying construct) plus random errors (for example, variability resulting from guesswork or fatigue), which are expected to be consistent over repeated measurements. The unique feature of CTT is that instrument properties (for example, item difficulty and discrimination) depend on the characteristics of the respondents. Therefore, the true score is both sample- and scale-dependent. The use of CTT for the development and validation of PRO instruments is relatively easy to understand for clinicians compared with IRT because the latter is technically complex and requires specific software to perform the analysis.

## Professional and Regulatory Guidance for Instrument Development and Validation

As a result of great interest in measuring PROs in clinical trials and clinical practice, as well as the subjectivity, complexity, and lack of consensus in this field, there has been a call by researchers, clinicians, and policy makers for practical guidance on the development and validation of PRO instruments. Several guidance documents and working groups have been established by research groups, such as the Medical Outcomes Trust (MOT)[16,17] and the European Regulatory Issues on Quality of Life Assessment (ERIQA) Group;[18] professional associations such as the International Society for Pharmacoeconomics and Outcomes Research (ISPOR);[19] and regulatory agencies such as the United States Food and Drug Administration (FDA)[8] and the European Medicines Agency (EMA).[7] Although there is not full consensus between these groups about key principles and criteria that should be used, all recognize that PRO instruments should focus on the properties of reliability, validity, responsiveness, and interpretability. In their guidance, research groups make recommendations detailing psychometric methods, principles, and criteria for determining quality of measurement properties. By contrast, regulatory agencies suggest the types of psychometric methods to be used rather than the principles and criteria. Table 1 compares the types and criteria of psychometric methods recommended for validating PRO instruments.

## 2. Reliability and Validity

### The Relationship between Validity and Reliability

The assessment of validity and reliability is concerned with the extent to which a measure is accurate (measures what it claims to measure) and consistent (repeatedly measures the same concept). Because a test cannot be valid unless it is reliable, but a reliable test is not necessarily valid, reliability is a necessary but not sufficient condition for validity.[9] It is important to note the variability of these issues between characteristically different samples and that even IRT does not presume invariance when the samples are different. Whereas reliability, at least in the form of internally consistent reliability, can and should be reported early in the life of a measure, full validation is an ongoing process and validity can take many years to demonstrate and may vary by context.

## Part 3: Patient-Reported Outcomes

**TABLE 1.** Professional and regulatory guidance regarding the types and criteria of psychometric methods recommended for PRO instrument validation

| Measurement Property | Type | Proposed by | Definition: The extent to which: | Method and Criteria |
|---|---|---|---|---|
| Reliability | Internal consistency | EMA, ERIQA, FDA, MOT | items in the same domain are intercorrelated. | 1. CTT: A single value in a domain based on Cronbach's coefficient (≥0.7 for group comparisons and =0.9-0.95 for individual comparisons)[7,17]<br>2. IRT: A range of values across different levels of latent trait in a domain using error variance, standard error of measurement and test information[17] |
|  | Test-retest reliability | EMA, ERIQA, FDA, MOT | the domain scores are reproducible or stable over time given no change has occurred in the concepts that the instrument is designed to measure. | Intraclass correlation coefficient or kappa coefficient (r≥0.7 for group comparisons and r=0.9-0.95 for individual comparisons)[7] |
|  | Inter-rater reliability | EMA, ERIQA, FDA, MOT | the domain scores are reproducible by different raters at one point in time. | Intraclass correlation coefficient or kappa coefficient (r≥0.8)[7] |
| Validity | Content validity | EMA, ERIQA, FDA, MOT | a specific domain of interest within a construct is fully captured by designed items and to which a construct of interest (health-related quality of life) is fully covered by the designed domains of the instrument. | Qualitative methods using patient and expert panels to judge the important themes of the domain and construct of interest, clarity, comprehensiveness, and redundancy of items and domains[7,17] |
|  | Structural validity[†] | EMA, ERIQA, FDA | the observed relationships between designed items support the hypothesized construct of the instrument. | 1. CTT: Exploratory factor analysis (factor loading ≥0.4) or correlation for the item-domain ≥0.4)[7]<br>2. IRT: Rasch analysis or confirmatory factor analysis to test the dimensionality in the construct of the instrument[7] |
|  | Convergent/ Divergent validity[†] | FDA | observed relationships between domains of one instrument and domains of other instruments confirm the hypotheses in the conceptual framework. | Moderate correlation (r=0.4-0.7) for similar domains and weak correlation (r<0.4) for heterogeneous domains |

[†] In various guidance, the terms are used interchangeably with and come under the broader heading of "construct validity."

**TABLE 1.** Professional and regulatory guidance regarding the types and criteria of psychometric methods recommended for PRO instrument validation

| Measurement Property | Type | Proposed by | Definition: The extent to which: | Method and Criteria |
|---|---|---|---|---|
| | Known-groups validity (known as clinical | EMA, ERIQA, FDA, MOT | the domain scores of an instrument discriminate between different groups of patients who differ by clinical conditions that are relevant to the construct of interest. | |
| | Criterion validity (known as concurrent validity) | EMA, ERIQA, FDA, MOT | domain scores are correlated to relevant domain of an acceptable gold standard. | Moderate correlation (r=0.4-0.7) for similar domains of the target instrument and gold standard, and weak correlation (r<0.4) for heterogeneous domains[7] |
| | Predictive validity | EMA, ERIQA, FDA, MOT | the current domain scores or the change of domain scores for an instrument are related future events or outcomes. | Area under the curve approach to refer the domain scores to dichotomous outcomes such as death (0.7 or higher) and Pearson's correlation coefficient for continuous outcomes (r≥0.4)[20] |
| Responsive-ness | Longitudinal validity (known as sensitivity to change) | EMA, ERIQA, FDA, MOT | the measured scores are stable when there is no change in patients' health conditions, and the scores change when there is a true change in patients' health conditions even if the magnitude of change is very small. | Distribution-based approach such as effect size (low=0.2-0.5; medium=0.5-0.7; large≥0.7), standard error of measurement, or standardized response means |
| Interpretability | Meaningful important difference (MID) and responder | EMA, ERIQA, FDA, MOT | the change in domain scores is clinically meaningful or interpretable. | Distribution-based or anchor-based approaches, or a combination of both |

## Reliability

Reliability is the extent to which an instrument yields the same score each time it is administered when the construct being measured has not changed. In CTT, reliability is based on scale-level analysis and is assumed to be constant across people who have different levels of a PRO domain. In contrast, IRT enables explicit demonstration of item- and scale-level reliability (also known as precision) that varies across people who have different levels of a PRO domain. The 3 methods recommended by CTT for evaluating the reliability of PRO instruments include internal consistency, test-retest, and inter-rater reliability.

### Internal Consistency

Internal consistency is an indication of the homogeneity of items within the domain or scale; that is, that they all measure a particular attribute. Internal consistency reliability is the average of all possible split-half correlations among all scale items.[11] Reliability coefficient values range from 0 to 1, with higher values indicating higher internal consistency. The most widely reported coefficient is Cronbach's alpha ($\alpha$).[21]

Although there is some disagreement among experts, most agree that $\alpha=0.7$-$0.9$ is sufficient to demonstrate reliability.[9] However, an $\alpha>0.95$ may indicate some redundancy among items and an unnecessary increase in respondent burden. Disagreement is fueled by the fact that Cronbach's alpha is dependent on the number of items in the scale; the brevity of the scale needs to be borne in mind when assessing its reliability.

For example, an $\alpha=0.7$ may be considered reliable for a 6-item scale but may be unsatisfactory for a 20-item scale. This is because items in a short scale may cover different aspects of the concept and therefore are not expected to be internally consistent. Some consider 10 homogeneous items to be the minimum number of items for a reliable test.[9] However, shorter scales or subscales may be reliable even when Cronbach's alpha is below 0.7, and perhaps as low as 0.5 for a 3-item scale.[22] Some recommend using a Spearman-Brown adjustment to a 10-item scale for scales of all lengths.[23] Comparing that to one's minimum criterion makes for easier interpretation. Item-total correlations may also be reported in a description of a scale's development: These are the correlations of individual items with the whole scale total omitting that item. The minimum acceptable item-total correlation for any item ranges from 0.2[24] to 0.3,[10] though higher thresholds are often adopted.

To demonstrate internal consistency, a large number of individuals must complete the PRO instrument. Expert opinion varies on the minimum sample size necessary to obtain a Cronbach's alpha of 0.7 (from 130 respondents[11] to at least 300[10]), and be confident that future replication of the coefficient alpha will remain above the minimum criterion. This needs to be borne in mind when assessing a reported reliability coefficient. In some research, large sample sizes are not always practical or obtainable.

## Test-Retest Reliability

Test-retest reliability (also known as stability), indicates the degree to which an instrument yields similar results on 2 or more administrations, assuming no actual change in respondents on the attribute being measured during the intervening period. A major challenge with this form of reliability is judging the appropriate timing of the second assessment—to ensure that sufficient time has passed so that respondents do not simply remember their previous responses and repeat them at second administration (artificially increasing the correlation between the 2 administrations), but not so much time that changes may have occurred in the respondent's condition or circumstances. There is no agreement among experts on the appropriate time interval between the first and second assessments: it varies from 2 to 14 days,[11] 2 weeks,[10] 3 months,[9] to 6 months for a more enduring attribute[10]). Practical problems include ensuring that there was no actual change in the attribute being measured and that the time interval is longer than the recall period of the survey so that responses do not overlap.

Test-retest reliability is generally measured with a Pearson correlation coefficient, with $r>0.70$ generally considered acceptable. ICCs, Bland-Altman, and repeated measures t-tests are also acceptable measures. Emotional states (for example, anxiety) can be transient and may only have coefficients of this magnitude when re-administered within 2 to 14 days.[11] A minimum of 100 respondents has been suggested as necessary for assessing test-retest reliability.[9]

## Inter-rater Reliability

Inter-rater reliability assesses the extent to which 2 observers or interviewers agree in their assessment of the underlying construct. As suggested, this type of reliability is required only when the PRO instrument is not completed by the patient and, as such, this type of reliability is not central to the aims of this chapter.

# Validity

Validity is the extent to which an instrument measures what it is intended to measure. The 4 aspects that are commonly recommended for evaluating the validity of instruments include face validity, content validity, construct validity, and known-groups validity.

## Face and Content Validity

Face validity pertains to whether or not the test *looks valid* to those who will use it (including clinicians and patients), while content validity is the extent to which the instrument actually measures the concept of interest. That is, the latter is an indication of the degree to which the PRO concept is comprehensively represented by the items in the instrument.[25] Both are entirely subjective judgments. Content validity is established based on evidence from literature reviews and focus groups or interviews with patients to inform the design of the instrument. This is followed by pilot testing and *cognitive debriefing* of the instrument with patients[26,27] to confirm ease of use and comprehension, as well as comprehensiveness without redundancy.

Content validity is, therefore, nonquantitative and best determined during the initial development of an instrument[10] or when used in a new condition or population. Arguably, it is the most fundamental aspect of scale selection[8] and it is essential that the researcher inspects the content of a scale to ascertain its suitability for a given study. The instrument should be an acceptable measure of the intended construct, without which the suitability of other measurement properties is irrelevant; evidence of other types of validity or reliability "will not overcome problems with content validity."[8]

Face validity is a qualitative assessment of whether or not the items *on the face of it* appear reasonable; that is, to determine if the items and scales conclusively capture all aspects of the construct and any additions.[25] Although it is often assessed by researchers or experts themselves once a scale has been developed, some believe that the respondent, not the expert, should be the judge.[28] A measure is likely to have higher face validity if respondents are involved in the development of the measure (opinions sought via interviews and/or focus groups), generating items, and then confirming the subject matter.[29] Thus, face and content validity, although assessed in different ways, are linked to each other.

## Construct Validity

An instrument has construct validity when there is evidence that supports the existence of the hypothetical construct that the instrument purports to measure (for example, satisfaction), but which cannot be directly observed. Construct validation involves testing hypotheses about the relationship of the construct with specific variables that can be measured. Thus, no single set of results will indicate that a measure has construct validity. Construct validation is an ongoing process in which hypotheses are tested about the construct as understanding of the construct increases.

## Structural Validity

Structural validity refers to the appropriate dimensionality of the PRO being measured. Factor analysis is a statistical method usually used to determine if a scale's items load (or cluster) together on factors in an expected or readily interpretable pattern to form scale (or subscale) scores. The analysis aims to simplify complex sets of data and any resulting factor is "a dimension or construct which is a condensed statement of the relationship between a set of variables."[30] Factor analysis can be either exploratory or confirmatory.

Exploratory factor analysis (EFA) is conducted when there are no particular expectations of the data or no clear hypothesis about the structure of the PRO.

Principal components analysis, a frequently used EFA method, simplifies a dataset by finding clusters of related items that correlate more highly with each other than with other variables in the set. Thus, it identifies *any* underlying dimensions, domains, or constructs in a PRO instrument. Where there are 2 or more distinct clusters of factors, this indicates the presence of subscales.

Confirmatory factor analysis (CFA) is used when researchers wish to test their model to confirm the expected number of factors in the scale and to test how a particular set of items should load on a specific scale. Traditionally, CFA is performed less often than EFA due, in part, to the need for large sample sizes, an appropriate fit index, and the difficulty of learning and operating specialty software. However, the use of CFA over the EFA is encouraged because, before conducting validation tests, researchers should hold *a priori* assumptions or propose a conceptual framework for the PRO measure.[8] Furthermore, compared to the EFA, the CFA has greater capability to handle ordinal data, has strength in the stability of the findings, and is able to compare multiple groups for invariance with relative ease.[10,30]

## Convergent or Discriminant Validity

As part of the construct validation process, a measure might be hypothesized to have stronger relationships with variables that are thought to be related to the construct (convergent validity), and weaker relationships (or ideally no relationship at all) with variables that bear little relation to the construct (discriminant or divergent validity). This validity is assessed by correlating one instrument (or subscale) with another to test predefined hypotheses about the relationship between the variables. For example, to test convergent/discriminant validity for the WHO-QOL-100,[31] one would correlate its scores with those of the SF-36.[32] We expect to observe a stronger correlation between the physical health domain of the WHO-QOL-100 and the physical functioning domain of the SF-36. In contrast, we expect to observe weaker correlation between the physical health domain of the WHO-QOL-100 and the mental health domain of the SF-36.

## Criterion Validity

The concept of criterion validity is similar to convergent/discriminant validity. Criterion validity is concerned with the comparison of the PRO measure with a gold standard instrument or criterion score, whereas convergent/discriminant validity is concerned with the relationship with measurable variables or instruments that are not necessarily accepted as the gold standard. Criterion validity applies only where a gold standard (or criterion), previously validated instrument measuring an attribute already exists and can be used to compare a new scale measuring that attribute. However, there are few gold standards in the PRO field and there are disagreements about appropriate criterion measures. There are 2 types of criterion validity: concurrent and predictive.

## Part 3: Patient-Reported Outcomes

*Concurrent Validity*

Where a gold standard instrument does exist, both instruments are administered at the same time to the same set of respondents and scores are correlated. Concurrent validity is confirmed if the correlation between the 2 instruments falls in the range of r=0.4-0.7.[7] Lower correlation indicates that either the reliability of one of the instruments is unacceptably low or that they are measuring different attributes.[20,33] As with construct validity, correlations can be positive or negative.

*Predictive Validity*

A test has predictive validity if it is able to predict a future criterion score, such as whether or not perceived stress measured in childhood predicts cardiovascular disease in adulthood. However, it is often difficult to find a clear criterion for prediction[8] and the results of the prediction may not be known for some time, possibly years later. The common example of predictive validity is whether or not a PRO can predict a future event such as death. The indicators commonly used to determine predictive validity are sensitivity, specificity, and C-statistics, which can be calculated through the receiver operating characteristic (ROC) approach. A value of 0.7 or greater is considered an indication of acceptable predictive validity.[20]

## Known-Groups Validity

Another version of discriminant validity (sometimes called extreme groups validity) is where different groups are hypothesized to have significantly different scores on a variable, and this is then shown to be the case. For example, patients with lower Eastern Cooperative Oncology Group (ECOG) performance scale scores from fully active (0) to completely disabled (4) are hypothesized to have greater physical functioning than people with higher ECOG scores. This type of validity is assessed by examining PRO scores between groups to test predefined hypotheses about the differences between 2 (or more) groups.[17,34-36,8]

## 3. Responsiveness and Interpretability

The principles and criteria for reliability and validity testing are well defined. Unfortunately, despite their relevance in clinical practice and trials, less attention has been paid to the assessment of responsiveness and interpretability. Responsiveness refers to the extent to which instrument scores: (a) are stable when there is no change in patients' condition, and (b) detect change when there is a true change in patients' condition or treatment. Interpretability is the extent to which the change in PRO domain scores is clinically meaningful or interpretable. In other words, responsiveness focuses on capability or performance of the instrument; by contrast, interpretability focuses on the meanings of the views (and changes in views) of respondents about the domains of interest.[17]

Conventionally, tests of statistical significance are often used to determine the extent of change of PRO scores over time. However, use of statistical tests alone can be misleading because a trivial numerical difference can become statistically significant given a sufficiently large sample. Providing transparent and intuitive guidance to interpret the meaning of PRO scores is critical to facilitating use of PROs in health and disease management.[34-36]

Focusing on the meaning attached to a change in score, interpretability is especially relevant to clinical practice, due to clinicians' and policy makers' lack of familiarity with PRO scores.[8] This is also known as the minimal important difference (MID), which can be described as the smallest change in a PRO score that is perceived by patients as beneficial or that would mandate a change in treatment.[37,38] In health and disease management, establishing the MID is especially useful for interpreting the progress of PROs in different conditions (for example, dementia based on the Alzheimer's Disease Assessment Scale-Cognitive Subscale (ADAS-Cog)[39] or diabetes based on the Diabetes Quality of Life (DQOL) questionnaire).[40]

Two methods are frequently used to measure responsiveness and MID. A *distribution-based approach* expresses observed change in a standardized metric by referring to statistical characteristics of a sample. FDA and MOT guidance recommend the use of distribution-based approaches because they provide insights about the magnitude of change and enable comparisons of responsiveness of PROs across different treatment groups and/or PRO instruments.[8,17] An *anchor-based approach* provides alternative information, referring the score change to external factors that have known meanings to patients or clinicians. Thus, anchor-based approaches examine whether observed change is important from the patients' or clinicians' perspectives. FDA, ERIQA, and MOT guidance recommend using anchor-based approaches to establish MID because they directly relate the PRO score change to interpretable anchors such as health status or life events.[8,18] Of note, the FDA suggests that the distribution-based methods for determining clinical significance of particular score changes should be considered as supportive and are not appropriate as the sole basis for determining MID.[8]

## Distribution-Based Approaches

A simple and frequently used distribution-based approach is Cohen's effect size (ES), which is defined as the discrepancy in mean scores between baseline and follow-up divided by the pooled standard deviation (SD) of the baseline and follow-up scores.[41] Opinions on the criteria to determine responsiveness vary. For example, researchers often cite Cohen's effect sizes: 0.2 SD as small and 0.5 SD as medium.[41] However, Cohen's cutoff scores were not empirically driven from clinical observations and were never intended to be used to assess responsiveness. Using data of patients with lung cancer, Cella and colleagues suggest that the use of 0.33-0.5 SD seems appropriate to capture clinically meaningful change on the Functional Assessment of Cancer Therapy-Lung (FACT-L) questionnaire.[42,43] Revicki and colleagues proposed 0.2-0.3 SD,[44] while Norman and colleagues suggest that 0.5 SD seems to be the most reasonable value to determine clinically meaningful change.[45]

An alternative distribution-based approach for establishing responsiveness and MID is based on the measurement precision of the instruments, such as standard error of measurement (SEM) and Reliable Change Index (RCI).[45] The SEM and RCI approaches are promising because they can quantify the amount of random variation that appears in repeated measures of PRO outcomes and the amount of error inherent in the measurement or the unreliability of the measurement. If a change in PRO score is smaller than the SEM or RCI cutoff, responsiveness can be interpreted as a result of measurement error rather than a true change in scores. Theoretical evidence suggests that the values of SEM and RCI are relatively stable across different populations. Therefore, compared to ES, the SEM and RCI approaches are recommended as a standard by which to evaluate an individual respondent's change in PRO scores. Several studies have proposed different criterion to determine responsiveness or MID, but no consensus has been reached.[45]

## Anchor-Based Approaches

Anchor-based interpretations are considered to be more understandable by clinicians than distribution-based approaches.[46] Several anchors have been recommended to estimate an MID given their high level of content validity. These anchors include clinically recognized end points (for example, laboratory measures, physiological measures, or clinical ratings); interventions with known effectiveness; subjective ratings for global assessments of change in health or symptoms by patients, their significant others, or their providers; a combination of clinical and patient-based end points; and socially recognized life events such as loss of job or significant others.[43,47,48]

Among anchor-based approaches, global assessments of change in health are frequently used. This method defines responsiveness or an MID as the mean score change across specific categories by which patients have experienced what they themselves considered to be minimally important change in their health.[49] For example, a global rating of change (GRC) approach has been recommended in which patients use a 14-point scale to rate magnitude of change.[49] Use of multiple independent anchors is recommended to examine and confirm responsiveness across multiple samples.[43] Jaeschke and colleagues found that when response options are presented on a 7-point Likert scale, an average score change of 0.5 per item in each PRO domain can be used as a sufficient and straightforward criterion to indicate an MID,[49] although this is dependent on the number of response options available.

In addition, the selection of anchors depends on the extent to which they are associated with changes in PRO scores. It is important to ensure that the anchors demonstrate acceptable quantitative properties, especially a moderate association with the PRO. For example, anchoring a PRO score on certain biomedical indicators may not be appropriate if the PRO is not expected to be well correlated with them.[50] It is recommended that the strength of the association of the anchor measure with the PRO should be between 0.30 and 0.50.[43,51] Understanding of the trajectory of health outcomes in the target disease is also helpful in correctly evaluating responsiveness or an MID.

## 4. Item Response Theory

### Limitations of Classic Psychometric Methods

Many PRO instruments have been developed based largely on CTT, but this approach has various disadvantages that may limit the use of PROs in clinical practice.[12,52] First, CTT is test or scale driven rather than item driven, meaning that the entire set of items must be administered to ensure the scale's reliability even though some items may not fit well with the respondent's underlying characteristics. For example, an item about capability to walk one block may be too difficult for someone with impaired mobility but must be included because of the way the instrument is designed. Administering items that are too easy or too difficult may threaten measurement precision. To make PRO instruments more practical, developers often compromise the range of content in the instrument, leading to large amounts of measurement noise and floor or ceiling effects.[53]

Second, in CTT, the measurement precision of a PRO is determined by internal consistency reliability. However, this is sample dependent and the precision of a PRO measure is assumed to be constant for all score levels. For example, in CTT, a physical functioning scale with a Cronbach's alpha equal to 0.8 would be applied to people of a group regardless of their level of underlying physical functioning. In reality, the precision of PRO measurement should rely on whether or not the content of the item and the patient's underlying PRO are matched.

Third, CTT cannot differentiate between a respondent's underlying outcome and the measurement properties of the instrument. For example, if 2 different instruments are used to measure an individual's physical functioning and result in scores of 50 and 70, we may not know the individual's true level of physical functioning because these scores may represent the instruments' measurement properties rather than the respondent's true physical functioning, or a combination thereof.

To better address psychometric issues encountered by CTT, several groups have devoted their efforts to IRT methodology. For example, the National Institutes of Health (NIH) launched a project of Patient-Reported Outcomes Measurement Information System (PROMIS) in 2004 that is dedicated to improve the reliability, validity, and precision of patient outcomes and PRO measurement using IRT.[54] One of the goals is to develop PRO item banks using IRT and technology of computerized adaptive tests.

### Item Response Theory Concept

Two types of IRT models are frequently used to design or refine instruments for PRO measurement. These models explicitly account for the properties of item difficulty alone (1-parameter model) and item difficulty together with item discrimination (2-parameter model). Item difficulty is defined as how easy or difficult it is for a respondent to endorse items. An easy item refers to one where almost everyone can endorse the attribute (for example, raising a hand). By contrast, a difficult item refers to one where only a few people can endorse the attribute (for example, running 1 mile). Mathematically, the item difficulty parameter is defined as the location of items on the continuum of the underlying PRO at which individuals endorse items with a probability of 50%. Item discrimination is defined as the magnitude of an item related to the underlying PRO domain (for example, physical functioning) measured by the scale.

A fundamental feature of IRT is that the item location on the latent continuum of a PRO domain is related to the estimated amount of a respondent's underlying PRO domain. In the IRT framework, an Item Characteristic Curve (ICC) is used to describe the probability of endorsing a dichotomous item (yes/no) associated with the level of underlying PRO domain (for example, running a mile). As the level of an underlying ability increases, the probability of item endorsement increases. For multiple overlapping, or polytomous, response items (such as Likert-type scale items), category response curves (CRCs) are used to describe the probability of endorsing a response category of an item associated with the level of the underlying PRO domain.

## Measurement Precision

In IRT, the precision of a PRO instrument is measured through an item and test information function. In contrast to CTT, which fixes measurement precision (reliability) to a certain value, IRT allows measurement precision of a PRO instrument to vary by levels of the underlying PRO domain on a latent continuum as a function of item difficulty and discrimination. For a particular item, the item information function is maximized around the *value of difficulty* parameter of this item if we place all items on a latent continuum. Items with a higher level of discrimination parameters tend to provide more information than items with lower discrimination parameters.

Test information function is the summation of a set of item information function. If we want to measure PROs across patients who have different levels of a PRO domain, use of item and test information can identify the gap in the latent continuum where the level of measurement precision is lower compared to other areas because the instrument does not include appropriate items. If the instrument is imprecise, it may be revised by adding items that provide additional information at a particular level of latent continuum. Item and test information function provide a useful message to suggest whether the use of some specific items rather than the entire set of items will be sufficient for measuring a respondent's PRO.

## Differential Item Functioning

In PRO measurement, it is assumed that individuals in different groups defined by, for example, age, race or ethnicity, disease severity, or languages that have the same underlying PRO domain will have the same probability of choosing a response category for an item. If this assumption is violated, this is termed *differential item functioning (DIF)*, which threatens measurement validity because items may measure different attributes that the instrument was not intended to measure.

DIF occurs when parameters for an item differ in a uniform or nonuniform way between groups. *Uniform DIF* is defined as the difference between the groups if the probability of endorsing an item is constant across all levels of the underlying PRO domain on the latent continuum. For example, given the same level of physical functioning (latent trait), we may find cancer patients undergoing chemotherapy more likely to respond that walking more than a mile is a problem than those in remission.

By contrast, *nonuniform DIF* refers to the difference between the groups if the probability of endorsing an item differs by the levels of underlying PRO domain. Using the aforementioned example, we may find that for a lower level of physical functioning, cancer patients undergoing chemotherapy are more likely to respond a problem than those in remission, whereas for a higher level, cancer patients and those in remission may equally respond a problem for walking more than a mile. From a visual perspective, uniform DIF means that the ICCs or CRCs for the 2 groups do not cross at any level of underlying PRO domain, while nonuniform DIF means that the item characteristics curves for the 2 groups cross.[55]

## Equating or Linking

Another useful aspect of IRT methodology is to link items from multiple instruments through the calibration process. Linking various items enables the generation of item banks that contain items with desired psychometric properties. Because the calibration process places all items on the same measurement metric, the estimated PRO scores are comparable among respondents across different ages, health conditions, and disease stages, irrespective of which items in the item bank are endorsed. For example, linking is helpful in addressing the issue of pediatric PRO measurement where the same items may not be equally applied to all cohorts of children because their cognitive maturity and perception of illness may differ.

Using IRT methodology, we can identify some items that are universally important for all developmental stages and others that are unique for specific developmental stages. Much easier items (for example, riding a bicycle) can be administered for younger children and more difficult items can be administered for adolescents (for example, mountaineering). We can use common items to link and calibrate developmental-specific items, allowing comparisons of PRO across entire developmental stages.

## Computerized Adaptive Tests

The use of computerized adaptive test (CAT) technology incorporated with IRT methodology (CAT/IRT) to measure PRO domains provides some practical advantages for health and disease management programs, especially those that focus on the elderly or people with chronic illness. CAT/IRT technology offers a feasible method of selecting some, but not all, items from item banks and administers the PRO survey in a systematic way. The result will better target a respondent's underlying PRO domain with the use of fewest items.

By design, CAT/IRT uses information from items already answered to select the next appropriate item, making it possible to present fewer items and achieve greater measurement precision. For example, if a patient reports difficulty in walking or moving around, he/she is less likely to report ease in running and playing sports. This is because the latter item offers no additional information. CAT/IRT can reduce the burden on patients during instrument administration and decrease data collection costs in clinical and research settings. Previous studies suggest that the use of only 10 items selected from a simulated CAT module for physical functioning may provide reliable and precise responses that are comparable to a much longer static questionnaire measuring physical functioning.[56] In these studies, the resulting correlation coefficients between the short and long versions were $r \geq 0.9$.[57-66]

## Limitations of Item Response Theory

Although the use of IRT in PRO measurement has many advantages, it is not without limitations that influence the slow adoption of this methodology. A primary limitation is the sample size requirements, with the simplest model (1 parameter) requiring sample sizes in excess of 200 respondents[67] and more complex models (2 or more parameters) requiring 2 to 5 times as many respondents.[68,69]

A second limitation is the additional assumptions of the IRT models, which are not required by CTT. The confidence of IRT results will greatly depend on the degree to which the assumptions are met and explicit tests of these assumptions are required. A third limitation is the complexity of performing IRT analyses, which generally are not supported by the standard statistical packages and require special analytic software and several different programs to implement the tests of the assumptions and estimate parameters.[70]

## 5. Conclusions

In summary, although the use of PROs can be advantageous for health and disease management, their measurement and application are challenging. Appropriate use of PRO instruments requires stakeholders to have a rudimentary understanding of the measurement theory upon which the instrument is based and to be confident in evaluating whether or not the instrument's psychometric properties are appropriate for the target population. Otherwise, stakeholders risk misinterpretation of the PRO assessment that may jeopardize clinical or policy decisions. The ability of a PRO instrument to provide unequivocal evidence of the impact of a disease and/or its treatment depends on its measurement properties. Reliability, validity, responsiveness, and interpretability are the essential psychometric properties of PRO instruments. The principles and criteria of reliability and validity for developing PRO instruments are largely well defined.

However, there is less consensus for the concepts of responsiveness and interpretability, which may be argued to be more clinically relevant. The use of CTT for development, refinement, and validation of PRO instruments is relatively easy and understandable by stakeholders. However, the use of CTT is sample- and scale-dependent, leading to confusion between a respondent's underlying PRO domain and the measurement properties of the instrument. Validation of PRO instruments is an expensive and time-consuming process. Various study designs, populations and availability of external anchors may require the use of different psychometric methods and establishment of new psychometric evidence for the PRO specific to the study criteria.

Part 3: Patient-Reported Outcomes

**APPENDIX.** Terminology and Definitions Used in this Chapter

| Terminology (alphabetical) | Definition |
|---|---|
| Common items | A subset of the same items which is universally used in different group (eg, disease group). Common items can be used to link and calibrate noncommon items from different groups on the same metric. |
| Differential item functioning (DIF) | Persons of different groups (eg, gender, race, etc.) have the same latent trait, but do not have the same probability of response to a category of an item. |
| Dimension | A component of the PRO measure. (eg, physical functioning) |
| Gap in latent continuum | A position where the latent continuum of a PRO scale does not have appropriate items. Ideally, a scale should cover items that represent corresponding latent traits the scale intends to measure. |
| Item Characteristic Curve (ICC) | A curve describing the probabilistic relationship between a person's response to each category of an item and his or her level of the latent trait. |
| Item difficulty | Describing how easy or difficult it is for people to endorse an item for the attribute the item intends to measure. Mathematically, it is the location of items on the latent continuum where individuals need to endorse items with a probability of 50%. |
| Item discrimination | Describing how strongly an item is related to the latent trait measured by the scale. Mathematically, it is the slope where individuals need to endorse items with a probability of 50%. |
| Item/Test information function | A curve describes the reliability of an item/scale across different levels of the latent trait. |
| Item pool | A collection of items from multiple instruments into a single source, which captures the best quality items. |
| Latent continuum | A display of different levels of latent traits along a specific axis. |
| Latent trait | Unobserved PRO construct (eg, physical functioning), which can be measured by a scale. |
| Multidimensionality | Multiple underlying PRO domains within an instrument. |
| Polytomous response category | An item having 2 or more response categories. (eg, a 5-point Likert type scale) |
| Scale | A component of an instrument, which consists of multiple items that measure a single domain. |
| Unidimensionality | One underlying PRO domain within an instrument. |

# References

1. Fitzner K, Sidorov J, Fetterolf D, et al. Principles for assessing disease management outcomes. *Dis Manag.* 2004;7(3):191-201.
2. Krumholz H, Baker D, Ashton C, et al. Evaluating quality of care for patients with heart failure. *Circulation.* 2000;101(12):E122-E140.
3. Detmar SB, Aaronson NK, Wever LDV, Muller M, Schornagel JH. How are you feeling? Who wants to know? Patients' and oncologists' preferences for discussing health-related quality-of-life issues. *J Clin Oncol.* 2000;18(18):3295-3301.
4. Detmar SB, Muller MJ, Wever LD, Schornagel JH, Aaronson NK. The patient-physician relationship: patient-physician communication during outpatient palliative treatment visits: an observational study. *JAMA.* 2001;285(10):1351-1357.
5. Walker D, McKinney B, Cannon-Wagner M, Vance R. Evaluating disease management programs. *Dis Manage Health Outcomes.* 2002;10(10):613-619.
6. McAlister F, Lawson F, Teo K, Armstrong P. A systematic review of randomized trials of disease management programs in heart failure. *Am J Med.* 2001;110(5):378-384.
7. European Medicines Agency (EMEA). Reflection paper on the regulatory guidance for the use of heath-related quality of life (HRQL) measures in the evaluation of medicinal products. http://www.emea.europa.eu/docs/en_GB/document_library/Scientific_guideline/2009/09/WC500003637.pdf. Published July 2005. Accessed September 21, 2012.
8. US Department of Health and Human Services FDA Centers for Drug Evaluation and Research, Biologics Evaluation and Research, and Devices and Radiological Health. Guidance for industry: patient-reported outcome measures: use in medical product development to support labeling claims. 2009. Accessed September 21, 2012. http://www.fda.gov/downloads/Drugs/GuidanceComplianceRegulatoryInformation/Guidances/UCM193282.pdf
9. Kline P. *The Handbook of Psychological Testing.* London, UK: Routledge; 1993.
10. Nunnally J, Bernstein I. *Psychometric Theory.* 3rd ed. New York, NY: McGraw-Hill; 1994.
11. Streiner DL, Norman GR. *Health Measurement Scales: A Practical Guide to Their Development and Use.* 3rd ed. Oxford,UK: Oxford University Press; 2003.
12. Chang CH, Reeve BB. Item response theory and its applications to patient-reported outcomes measurement. *Eval Health Prof.* 2005;28(3):264-282.
13. Gill TM, Feinstein AR. A critical appraisal of the quality of quality-of-life measurements. *JAMA.* 1994;272(8):619-626.
14. Naughton MJ, Shumaker SA. The case for domains of function in quality of life assessment. *Qual Life Res.* 2003;12 (suppl 1):73-80.
15. Garratt A, Schmidt L, Mackintosh A, Fitzpatrick R. Quality of life measurement: bibliographic study of patient assessed health outcome measures. *BMJ.* 2002;324(7351):1417.
16. Lohr KN, Aaronson NK, Alonso J, Audrey BM, et al. Evaluating quality-of-life and health status instruments: development of scientific review criteria. *Clin Ther.* 1996;18:979-992.
17. Scientific Advisory Committee. Assessing health status and quality-of-life instruments: attributes and review criteria. *Qual Life Res.* 2002;11(3):193-205.
18. Chassany O, Sagnier P, Marquis P, Fullerton S, Aaronson N, for the European Regulatory Issues on Quality of Life Assessment Group. Patient-reported outcomes: the example of health-related quality of life: a European guidance document for the improved integration of health-related quality of life assessment in the drug regulatory process. *Drug Inf J.* 2002;36(1):209-238.
19. ISPOR. ISPOR patient reported outcomes quality of life initiatives. http://www.ispor.org/research_initiatives/qol_initiatives.asp. Accessed July 14, 2009.
20. Iezzoni LI. *Risk Adjustment for Measuring Health Care Outcomes.* Chicago, IL: Health Administration Press; 2003.
21. Cronbach LJ. Coefficient alpha and the internal structure of tests. *Psychometrika.* 1951;16:297-334.
22. Todd C, Bradley C. Evaluating the design and development of psychological scales. In: Bradley C, ed. *Handbook of Psychology and Diabetes.* Chur, Switzerland: Harwood Academic Publishers; 1994:15-42.

### Part 3: Patient-Reported Outcomes

23. Pedhazur EJ, Schmelkin LP. *Measurement, Design and Analysis: An Integrated Approach*. New York, NY: Psychology Press;1991:81-117.
24. Kline P. *A Handbook of Test Construction*. London, UK: Methuen; 1986.
25. Guyatt GH, Feeny DH, Patrick DL. Measuring health-related quality of life. *Ann Intern Med*. 1993;118(8):622-629.
26. Bowling A. *Measuring Health: A Review of Quality of Life Measurement Scales*. 3rd ed. New York, NY: Open University Press; 2005.
27. Willis GB. *Cognitive Interviewing: A Toll for Improving Questionnaire Design*. Thousand Oaks, CA: Sage Publications; 2005.
28. Nevo B. Face validity revisited. *Journal of Educational Measurement*. 1985;22:287-293.
29. Fitzpatrick R, Davey C, Buxton MJ, Jones DR. Evaluating patient-based outcome measures for use in clinical trials. *Health Technol Assess*. 1998; 2(14).
30. Kline P. *An Easy Guide to Factor Analysis*. London, UK: Routledge; 1994.
31. The WHOQOL Group. The World Health Organization Quality of Life Assessment (WHOQOL): development and general psychometric properties. *Soc Sci Med*. 1998;46(12):1569-1585.
32. Ware JE, Sherbourne CD. The MOS 36-Item Short-Form Health Survey (SF-36): conceptual framework and item selection. *Med Care*. 1992;30(6):473-483.
33. Juniper EF, Guyatt GH, Willan A, Griffith LE. Determining a minimal important change in a disease-specific quality of life questionnaire. *J Clin Epidemiol*. 1994;47(1):81-87.
34. Kelleher CJ, Pleil AM, Reese PR, Burgess SM, Brodish PH. How much is enough and who says so? *BJOG*. 2004;111(6):605-612.
35. Osoba D, Rodrigues G, Myles J, Zee B, Pater J. Interpreting the significance of changes in health-related quality-of-life scores. *J Clin Oncol*. 1998;16(1):139-144.
36. Guyatt G, Walter S, Norman G. Measuring change over time: assessing the usefulness of evaluative instruments. *J Chronic Dis*. 1987;40(2):171-178.
37. Guyatt GH, Osoba D, Wu AW, Wyrwich KW, Norman GR. Methods to explain the clinical significance of health status measures. *Mayo Clin Proc*. 2002;77(4):371-383.
38. Molnar F, Man-Son-Hing M, Fergusson D. Systematic review of measures of clinical significance employed in randomized controlled trials of drugs for dementia. *J Am Geriatr Soc*. 2009;57(3): 536-546.
39. Huang I, Liu J, Wu A, Wu M, Leite W, Hwang C. Evaluating the reliability, validity and minimally important difference of the Taiwanese version of the diabetes quality of life (DQOL) measurement. *Health Qual Life Outcomes*. 2008;6:87.
40. Cohen J. *Statistical Power Analysis for the Behavioral Sciences*. 2nd ed. Hillsdale, NJ: Lawrence Erlbaum Associates; 1988.
41. Cella D, Eton DT, Lai JS, Peterman AH, Merkel DE. Combining anchor and distribution-based methods to derive minimal clinically important differences on the functional assessment of cancer therapy (FACT) anemia and fatigue scales. *J Pain Symptom Manage*. 2002;24(6): 547-561.
42. Cella D, Eton DT, Fairclough DL, et al. What is a clinically meaningful change on the Functional Assessment of Cancer Therapy-Lung (FACT-L) questionnaire? Results from Eastern Cooperative Oncology Group (ECOG) Study 5592. *J Clin Epidemiol*. 2002;55(3):285-295.
43. Revicki DA, Cella D, Hays RD, Sloan JA, Lenderking WR, Aaronson NK. Responsiveness and minimal important differences for patient reported outcomes. *Health Qual Life Outcomes*. 2006;4:70.
44. Norman GR, Sloan JA, Wyrwich KW. Interpretation of changes in health-related quality of life: the remarkable universality of half a standard deviation. *Med Care*. 2003;41(5):582-592.
45. Crosby RD, Kolotkin RL, Williams GR. Defining clinically meaningful change in health-related quality of life. *J Clin Epidemiol*. 2003;56(5):395-407.
46. Lydick E, Epstein RS. Interpretation of quality of life changes. *Qual Life Res*. 1993;2(3): 221-226.
47. Guyatt GH, Osoba D, Wu AW, Wyrwich KW, Norman GR; Clinical Significance Consensus Meeting Group. Methods to explain the clinical significance of health status measures. *Mayo Clin Proc*. 2002;77(4):371-383.
48. Marquis P, Chassany O, Abetz L. A comprehensive strategy for the interpretation of quality-of-life data based on existing methods. *Value Health*. 2004;7(1):93-104.

49. Jaeschke R, Singer J, Guyatt GH. Measurement of health status: ascertaining the minimal clinically important difference. *Control Clin Trials*. 1989;10(4):407-415.
50. Bradley C. Feedback on the FDA's February 2006 draft guidance on patient reported outcome (PRO) measures from a developer of PRO measures. *Health Qual Life Outcomes*. 2006;4(1):78.
51. Revicki DA, Hays RD, Cella D, Sloan J. Recommended methods for determining responsiveness and minimally important differences for patient-reported outcomes. *J Clin Epidemiol*. 2008;61(2):102-109.
52. Hays RD, Morales LS, Reise SP. Item response theory and health outcomes measurement in the 21st century. *Med Care*. 2000;38(9 suppl):II28-II42.
53. Ware JE Jr. Conceptualization and measurement of health-related quality of life: comments on an evolving field. *Arch Phys Med Rehabil*. 2003;84(4 suppl 2):S43-S51.
54. Cella D, Yount S, Rothrock N, et al. The Patient-Reported Outcomes Measurement Information System (PROMIS): progress of an NIH roadmap cooperative group during its first two years. *Med Care*. 2007;45(5 suppl 1):S3-S11.
55. Teresi JA. Different approaches to differential item functioning in health applications: advantages, disadvantages and some neglected topics. *Med Care*. 2006;44(11 suppl 3):S152-S170.
56. Siebens H, Andres PL, Pengsheng N, Coster WJ, Haley SM. Measuring physical function in patients with complex medical and postsurgical conditions: a computer adaptive approach. *Am J Phys Med Rehabil*. 2005;84(10):741-748.
57. Adams RJ, Wilson M, Wu M. Multilevel item response models: an approach to errors in variables regression. *J Educ Behav Stat*. 1997;22(1):47-76.
58. Bock RD, Gibbons R, Muraki E. Full-information item factor analysis. *Appl Psychol Meas*. 1988;12(3):261-280.
59. Haley SM, Coster WJ, Andres PL, Kosinski M, Ni P. Score comparability of short forms and computerized adaptive testing: simulation study with the activity measure for post-acute care. *Arch Phys Med Rehabil*. 2004;85(4):661-666.
60. Haley SM, Ni P, Ludlow LH, Fragala-Pinkham MA. Measurement precision and efficiency of multidimensional computer adaptive testing of physical functioning using the pediatric evaluation of disability inventory. *Arch Phys Med Rehabil*. 2006;87(9):1223-1229.
61. Hoijtink H, Rooks G, Wilmink FW. Confirmatory factor analysis of items with a dichotomous response format using the multidimensional Rasch model. *Psychol Methods*. 1999;4(3):300-314.
62. Muthen B. A general structural equation model with dichotomous, ordered, categorical and latent variable indicators. *Psychometrika*. 1984;49(1):115-132.
63. Petersen MA, Groenvold M, Aaronson N, Fayers P, Sprangers M, Bjorner JB. Multidimensional computerized adaptive testing of the EORTC QLQ-C30: basic developments and evaluations. *Qual Life Res*. 2006;15(3):315-329.
64. Takane Y, de Leeu WJ. On the relationship between item response theory and factor analysis of discretized variables. *Psychometrika*. 1987;52(33):393-408.
65. Wang WC, Chen PH, Cheng YY. Improving measurement precision of test batteries using multidimensional item response models. *Psychol Methods*. 2004;9(1):116-136.
66. Wang WC, Yao G, Tsai YJ, Wang JD, Hsieh CL. Validating, improving reliability, and estimating correlation of the four subscales in the WHOQOL-BREF using multidimensional Rasch analysis. *Qual Life Res*. 2006;15(4):607-620.
67. Linacre JM. Sample size and item calibration stability. *Rasch Measurement Transactions*. 1994;7(4):328.
68. Bjorner JB, Kosinski M, Ware JE Jr. Using item response theory to calibrate the headache impact test (HIT) to the metric of traditional headache scales. *Qual Life Res*. 2003;12(8):981-1002.
69. Tsutakawa RK, Johnson JC. The effect of uncertainty of item parameter-estimation on ability estimates. *Psychometrika*. 1990;55(2):371-390.
70. Deng N. References on non-commercial software for IRT analyses. Available at: http://www.umass.edu/remp/main_software.html. Accessed March 1, 2010.

CHAPTER 15

# Health-Related Quality of Life/Functional Status and Health and Disease Management

Anandi V. Law, BPharm, PhD, FAACP, FAPhA; I-Chan Huang, PhD, MSc; and Jayashri Sankaranarayanan, MPharm, PhD

This chapter provides a brief historical perspective and conceptual underpinnings of health-related quality of life (HRQOL) as well as a description of functional status as an aspect of HRQOL. Further, the chapter describes HRQOL measurement via different approaches, including health index versus health profile and generic versus disease-specific instruments. Measurement of HRQOL is described with a focus on health and disease management. Finally, the chapter presents issues specific to the use of HRQOL measures, including standardization, cross-cultural translation, response shift, personality, and proxy issues.

The World Health Organization defines a *healthy state* as one of complete physical, mental, and social well-being and not merely the absence of disease or infirmity.[1] *Health-related quality of life (HRQOL)* has been defined as the "value assigned to duration of life as modified by the impairments, physical, social and psychological functional states, perceptions and opportunities that are influenced by disease, injury, treatment, or policy."[2] Thus, HRQOL is a patient-perceived and patient-reported outcome, and has evolved as an indicator of health status in parallel with the Outcomes Movement and patient-focused care. It was used initially to measure health status based on the RAND Health Insurance Experiment[2] and is a multidimensional concept that covers the continuum of health from observable functional status (physical behaviors) to nonobservable quality-of-life factors (psychological and social manifestations).

## 1. Conceptual Underpinnings of HRQOL

Conceptual frameworks or models that link HRQOL, functional status, and clinical indicators are limited. Development and validation of HRQOL tools have used associations with symptoms, biological markers, and clinical indicators to confirm that tools measure the correct construct. Functional status appears to influence perceived HRQOL and is a subset of HRQOL. The most commonly referenced model for HRQOL, the Wilson and Cleary model, is proposed to relate objective indicators to subjective experience.[3] This model integrates both biological and psychological aspects of health outcomes. There are 5 different levels in the model belonging to objective indicators (physiological factors, symptom status, and functional health) and subjective experience (general health perceptions and overall quality of life). The model has been modified and tested for causal and bidirectional relationships between health, HRQOL, and functional status in various disease conditions such as HIV/AIDS and heart failure.[4,5,6,7]

## Functional Status and Its Measurement

Functional status (FS) is the extent to which individuals can perform normal or usual behaviors and activities, given their limitations due to health problems.[2] It is usually conceptualized as the ability to perform self-care, self-maintenance, and physical activities.[8] FS measures incorporate physical and cognitive aspects of functioning, and can be used to compare healthy individuals to those whose functioning has been altered by disease. The measurement of FS is common in conditions with differing degrees of physical and cognitive functional limitations, such as arthritis, cerebral palsy, and bipolar disorders.[8] In such conditions, FS is measured in combination with HRQOL as a means of confirming results of the impact of physical and cognitive limitations on HRQOL.[9]

Diseases or conditions that affect physical functioning, such as stroke, may affect FS measurement. Researchers commonly measure FS using metrics such as activities of daily living (ADL) or instrumental activities of daily living (IADL), the Barthel Index, or Dartmouth COOP Functional Health Assessment Charts. ADLs include activities performed as part of a person's daily routine, such as personal hygiene, walking, getting up from a chair, eating, drinking, and taking medication.[2] IADLs include driving, preparing meals, doing housework, shopping, managing finances, managing medication, or using the telephone. Numerical scales such as the Functional Independence Measure (FIM)[10] identify an individual's level of functioning.

## 2. Selected Health-Related Quality-of-Life Instruments

There are many published HRQOL instruments. To provide a glimpse of the scope of this field, we reviewed the literature using PubMed with the following keywords (independently and in combination): health status, HRQOL, instruments, health assessments, functional status, and measuring HRQOL. We identified articles published in the area from 1970 until 2008 that represent a range of disease conditions. (Table 1 includes a selection.) The literature review reveals that there are some commonly used generic tools (SF-36, the SF-series, and the EQ-5D) and various disease-specific instruments for prevalent and/or chronic conditions such as diabetes (Diabetes Quality of Life (DQOL), D-39), asthma (AQLQ), and cancer (European Organisation for Research and Treatment of Cancer (EORTC)). We categorized the literature based on development, validation, and application.

## Validation of Health-Related Quality-of-Life Tools

Measurement of multidimensional concepts such as HRQOL presents some challenges because these concepts are patient-perceived and subjective but need to be interpreted by the clinician or researcher. HRQOL tools are validated by testing their psychometric properties such as reliability; content, construct, and concurrent validity; and responsiveness (described in the previous chapter). Measuring changes in quality of life is paramount. Changes in HRQOL have traditionally been measured as the difference between measurement scores at two different times.

There have been several attempts in the literature to correlate this change with clinical indicators in order to identify the need for modification of therapy and to evaluate the effect of an intervention. A challenge in measuring HRQOL change is that any observable change may be statistically significant but not clinically significant. In addition, 2 patients may have a numerically identical measurement of change in HRQOL yet, due to the subjective nature of "quality," may not feel the same sense of impact of an improvement or dissatisfaction over a decline in HRQOL.

## Clinical Significance of Change

Clinical significance has been defined by Sackett and colleagues as the importance of a difference in clinical outcomes between the experimental and control groups, and equated to the magnitude of a study result.[11] Two concepts associated with change of HRQOL scores are responsiveness and minimally clinical important difference (MCID). Responsiveness, or the "the ability of an instrument to detect small but important clinical changes," is directly related to the magnitude of change in subject scores, which constitutes a clinically important change.[12] Although responsiveness has been used as a proxy measure of change, MCID is best measured using patient reports. Better understanding of the concepts of responsiveness and minimally important difference (MID) is useful in selecting appropriate HRQOL instruments for health and disease management evaluations. For people with chronic conditions, it is important to monitor the trajectory of HRQOL scores alongside the treatment regimens.

Part of defining an MCID is to assess the MID that is obtained when patients judge their health status relative to their memories (the conventional method) as well as relative to others with a similar condition.[13,14] For example, Juniper and colleagues measured MID in asthma using the asthma quality-of-life questionnaire.[15] Persons with asthma were asked to complete the questionnaire and 4 global rating of change questions on a 14-point response scale that asked if there had been any change in their activity limitations, symptoms, emotions, or overall quality of life since their last clinic visit. The researchers found that a change of 0.5 units indicated an MID as perceived by the patient; a difference of 1.0 indicated moderate change and any difference greater than 1.5 indicated a large change. The results of this study show how to translate a patient-perceived change into a clinically important change.[16]

## Measurement of Health-Related Quality of Life

HRQOL can be measured using the health index or health profile approach.[17] A profile approach provides scores for each domain used to build the profile, while the index approach computes one score to summarize the HRQOL value.

HRQOL can also be measured using a generic or disease-specific approach. A generic quality-of-life instrument is intended to measure overall health-related quality of life from a broad perspective, applicable across diseases and health conditions, populations, and health care interventions and summarizes the quality of an individuals' health across various domains. Examples include the SF-36 (Short Form 36) Health Status Questionnaire, the Sickness Impact Profile, the Quality of Well-Being Questionnaire, and the EuroQol instrument.[2] The disease-specific approach focuses on health as modified by a particular condition such as migraines or diabetes. Disease-specific quality-of-life instruments measure health-related quality of life and are designed to be applicable to a single disease or health condition. They summarize an individual's health in the various areas most important to that clinical condition.[2] Both generic and disease-specific instruments can provide an index measure or a profile of health status using several domains.

Generic and disease-specific instruments, by design, measure different aspects of HRQOL. Generic instruments are broad and many are suitable in large populations. They can be used to compare HRQOL between diseases, and to establish norms for healthy individuals and populations within and across countries. However, their breadth makes it difficult to be sensitive and specific to attributes of health affected by a certain condition. On the other hand, disease-specific instruments are both sensitive and specific for a certain condition. The instruments are useful in measuring impact on HRQOL of interventions to treat or manage conditions, and to compare within and between patients, treatments, or management approaches. These differences between generic and disease-specific instruments present certain challenges in measurement of health and disease management programs.

## Health Profile Approach

Typically, in the health profile approach, a generic instrument (such as the SF-36) includes domains that encompass many features of an individual's health physical, emotional, and social, and the impact of disease on daily roles, levels of pain and energy, and overall health. Disease-specific instruments tend to include some of the same domains but probe specific attributes of the disease. For example, the asthma quality-of-life questionnaire includes domains specific to asthma that probe key attributes of this chronic condition. Researchers can use various scales to obtain responses from patients in either generic or disease-specific instruments, such as a Likert or rating scale that is worded using limitation, extent, or agreement. The data collected could be scored and transformed differently; for example, the SF-36 uses a transformation based on the scale range of scores and standardizes each domain score on a scale of 100 for comparison purposes. The result of a health profile approach is a domain-specific score. Users can obtain health status profiles for the general population and for populations with certain health conditions.

## Health Index Approach

The health index approach for measuring HRQOL uses utility as the measure of preference. In understanding preference-based measurement of health, patient preferences are defined as values that persons with a clinical condition assign to their health.[2] Community preferences are values assigned to a clinical condition by representatives of the general population, where the representative cohort includes persons with clinical conditions in general proportion to the prevalence of those conditions in the overall populations.[2]

Utility is a measurement of the desirability of, or preference for, a particular health outcome or health state across various states or levels of health. This information is typically used to evaluate the value assigned to obtaining a suboptimal outcome relative to an optimal outcome, such as excellent health.[2] Usually, utility values are measured on a scale of 1.0 (perfect health) to 0.0 (dead), where the maximum and minimum levels are known as the anchors (or anchor states).[2] Thus, utilities are quantitative or numerical expressions; that is, they describe both that one outcome is preferred to another, and how much more the first is preferred to the second. Patient preference for different aspects of a condition or the condition itself is assessed using various methods such as standard gamble, time trade-off, or rating scales.[18]

Utility is used to measure quality-adjusted life years (QALYs) where the quality of life is taken into account in the remaining years of life gained from a health care intervention. The Q measures the value or quality associated with life per se or as modified by a condition. It is multiplied by a time factor (life years, LY) to obtain a QALY. In general, although QALY is convenient to use, measurement issues and difficulty in interpretation of individual domains of health have led to a wider use of the health profile approach, especially in disease and population health management.

## 3. Health and Disease Management

Health and disease management (HDM) programs typically manage care for persons with chronic conditions who require high-resource utilization, have a potential for lifestyle modification to improve outcomes, and are at high risk for poor outcomes. Common chronic conditions targeted by HDM programs include asthma, diabetes, hypertension, osteoporosis, and hyperlipidemia. HDM programs require an understanding of the progression of a disease and a targeting of interventions at critical points using evidence-based practices; their purpose is to improve outcomes and to delay or prevent morbidity and mortality.[19]

HDM programs use a systematic approach to attain coordinated care with the goals of decreasing the overall costs of a chronic disease and improving outcomes.

In order to be successful, an effective program requires a collaborative effort from patients, physicians, and other health care professionals, as well as well-organized program, information, and financial management. HDM programs can be conducted in various settings (for example, community clinics and pharmacies) by various providers (nurses, physicians, or pharmacists) through several modes (face-to-face, over the telephone, or by mail).

HDM programs activities may include assessment of medical or medication history, baseline health status, and other measurements, including HRQOL. Visits after an initial assessment are typically shorter and involve completion of selected assessments measuring various clinical parameters of interest and HRQOL. In addition to the time involved, having numerous assessments at each visit causes an administrative burden as well as respondent fatigue.

For high-risk patients with multiple chronic conditions, some HDM providers utilize a case management approach rather than treating specific diseases. This approach has implications on the measurement of effectiveness of HDM programs, as well as the decision to use generic versus disease-specific HRQOL instruments.

## Use of Health-Related Quality-of-Life Tools in Health and Disease Management

HRQOL can help measure the impact of an HDM intervention from the patient's perspective. HDM programs usually measure HRQOL and patient satisfaction, but functional status is less commonly measured because HDM typically involves treating persons with chronic conditions and functional status is a generic measure.

A variety of generic and disease-specific instruments have been used in HDM program evaluations for diseases such as diabetes,[20,21] hypertension,[22] dyslipidemia,[23] asthma,[24,25] COPD,[26] chronic heart failure,[27,28,29] obesity,[30,31] and depression.[32] The SF-36 and the family of SF tools are used most frequently to measure HRQOL because they are generic instruments and have been validated across many diseases, languages, and cultures. It also remains the standard against which newly developed instruments are often validated.[33] Scoring algorithms and population norms for SF-36 are also well established, making it easier to interpret results.[34]

## Issues with Health-Related Quality-of-Life Measurement Relevant to Health and Disease Management

The subjective nature of HRQOL lends itself to certain biases. Hence, validation of HRQOL has traditionally been conducted by correlating the outcomes with common clinical indicators. For example, one might examine the correlation of changes in blood pressure to HRQOL to validate its measurement for persons with hypertension. However, as more instruments in the area are validated and used, HRQOL is also measured as a standalone indicator. Whether HRQOL is evaluated alone or in conjunction with a clinical measure depends on the intent of the evaluation. For example, a clinical indicator is necessary when HRQOL is used to measure impact of a clinical or educational intervention. However, a clinical indicator may not be needed when an evaluator is comparing HRQOL change between programs.

When choosing an appropriate HRQOL measure for an HDM program, a number of issues must be addressed. First, researchers must decide whether to use an existing instrument or develop one customized for the program or intervention of interest. The precision of a customized instrument must be balanced against the cost of development and validation. Secondly, the study team must decide whether to use a generic or disease-specific instrument. Alternatively, because these 2 types of instruments complement each other's strengths and weaknesses, researchers might choose to use them in combination to measure the effectiveness of HDM programs.[35] However, combining instruments has its own limitations, such as respondent fatigue, that evaluators should consider before making a final design choice.

Other items that must be taken into account in HRQOL instrument selection are patient social and psychological factors that affect HRQOL, such as perceived social constraints, social support, social desirability, and personality traits. There is the potential for response shift due to internal changes in values within a patient group or between groups that impacts HRQOL.[36] Cultural translation and, in particular, validation of an instrument are critical when using an instrument outside of the language in which it was developed. Administration issues such as mode (in person, on paper, or electronically) and the use of a proxy (key in pediatric and behavioral health studies) also require careful consideration.

With the growing interest in international and cross-cultural comparisons of HRQOL, there is a need to standardize and translate validated instruments to different language or cultural versions. The vast majority of existing instruments are developed in European and Anglo-American countries. To facilitate the comparisons of HRQOL across different cultural or ethnic groups, many organizations and professional associations have issued translation guidelines.[37]

Cultural validation is an area of importance when translating HRQOL instruments. The perception of higher or lower quality of life can differ markedly across cultures. If a HRQOL instrument is translated but not culturally validated, findings will be biased because the instrument measures a specific cultural measure of quality of life that may not apply directly to the group to which the tool is now being administered. Therefore, it is imperative to develop country-specific normative values.

## Response Shift in HRQOL Measurement

Patients may perceive the meaning or structure of HRQOL differently over time due to the progression of a health condition. This phenomenon, known as response shift, can have a negative impact on the validity in the measurement of change in HRQOL. Response shift can occur as a result of 1) a change in the respondent's internal standards of measurement (scale recalibration), 2) a change in the respondent's values (the importance of component domains constituting the target construct), or 3) a redefinition of the target construct (reconceptualization).[37]

Recalibration occurs when individuals adjust their expectations to enable them to be satisfied with a different objective standard of circumstances. For example, after adjustment to the onset of a cancer, a cancer survivor may reclassify mental health measured by the item "calm and peaceful" as "most of the time," while prior to cancer the same level of mental health would only be rated as "a little of time." *Reprioritization* refers to reweighting the importance of different domains within HRQOL. For example, a cancer survivor may come to place greater value on spirituality and de-emphasize their value on other types of relationships. In reprioritization, subjects change their relative importance of domains of HRQOL. *Re-conceptualization*, however, implies that subjects may discard some domains and/or new ones may emerge.

Accounting for response shift in a longitudinal HRQOL study is important in ensuring that the same construct is compared on any 2 occasions, both to monitor adjustment and to assess how successful adjustment may be achieved. Evidence suggests that if potential response shift was not considered, the finding of significant age-related drops in HRQOL may be misleading.[38,39] Therefore, establishing whether the reported increase of decrease in HRQOL is a real effect, or a result of a change in recalibration, reprioritization, or re-conceptualization of the construct, is important in building confidence in the interpretation of findings.

## Social Desirability Issues

Social desirability (including personality traits) has been shown to influence the report of HRQOL via indirect, mediating, and moderating effects. When administering HRQOL measures, it is likely that a person may offer a socially desirable answer to "look good" and to report better HRQOL scores. A socially desirable answer is often linked to personal characteristics and many studies report that these characteristics were stronger determinants of HRQOL than sociodemographic and clinical factors, age,[40] illness appraisal,[41] social integration,[42] income,[42] comorbidity,[42] CD4+ counts and HIV disease stage,[41] seizure outcome after epilepsy surgery,[43] and seizure relief.[44] Hooker and colleagues found that neuroticism explained 39% of the variance in psychological HRQOL, but less than 30% for physical HRQOL.[45]

Kempen and colleagues found that neuroticism, mastery, and self-efficacy explained 31 to 38% of variance in mental health but less than 10% for physical functioning or pain.[46] Evidence suggests that personal characteristics such as coping style[47] and social support[48] were indirectly associated with HRQOL, while optimism mediated this effect.[49] Given the influence of psychological factors such as social desirability on HRQOL measures, it is useful to evaluate social desirability and personality traits to help interpret HRQOL scores.

## Proxy Issues in HRQOL Measurement

Discordance between the patient and proxy reports of HRQOL are well documented.[50,51,52,53] Lower levels of agreement were found predominantly in studies employing a small sample size (approximately 50 patient-proxy pairs or fewer). In larger studies comparing patients and their significant others, median correlations were between 0.60-0.70 for physical HRQOL domains and about 0.50 for psychosocial domains.

In pediatric HRQOL studies, the agreement between parents' or guardians' and children's ratings, are inconsistent.[54] Some studies show that parents report higher HRQOL scores than do their children across all domains.[55,56] However, others show that compared to children's self-ratings, parents tend to report better physical and social functioning, but more depression and bodily pain. In contrast to children's own ratings, parents may underestimate HRQOL for sick children,[57] but overestimate for healthy children.[58]

Analytically, patients' self-rated or proxy-rated HRQOL may be compared using t-tests or regression methods.[59,60,61,62] Some of these methods of comparison are limited because they cannot assure whether or not HRQOL measures between the dyads are comparable. It is possible that patients and proxies perceive the construct of HRQOL or meanings of specific items differently. Unless the instrument is validated for use in proxies, interpretation of proxy results should be made with caution. Mixed results were reported in studies comparing patients and their health care providers as proxies, but most of these studies employed a relatively small sample size.[53] Proxy raters tended to report more HRQOL problems than patients themselves, but the magnitude of observed differences was modest (median standardized differences of about 0.20).[53]

## 4. Summary

HRQOL has been measured in HDM programs to capture humanistic outcomes or PROs. Measurement of HRQOL is an important aspect of program evaluation in HDM because it incorporates patient perceptions of health and change due to intervention. However, several measurement issues in HRQOL, including subjectivity in measurement, have kept it secondary to clinical measurements and changes in HRQOL are reported alongside clinical changes to give them relevance. Because there are a number of HRQOL instruments available, care should be taken in selecting the optimal instrument for any specific disease management study. In general, a combination of generic and disease-specific instruments may be recommended in evaluating an HDM program.

Health-Related Quality of Life/Functional Status and Health and Disease Management

TABLE 1. Select HRQOL instruments from literature

| Reference | Study Type* | Disease | Methodology** | Patient-Reported Outcome Type*** | Instruments |
|---|---|---|---|---|---|
| 63 | R | Cancer | M | Dz specific | European Organisation for Research and Treatment of Cancer (EORTC) quality-of-life questionnaire core-30 (QLQ-C30) and the EORTC brain cancer module (EORTC BN-20). |
| 64 | P | Cancer | | Generic | RAND-36 Health Status Inventory |
| 65 | A | Head and neck cancer | M | HRQOL | EORTC (European organisation for Research and Treatment of Cancer/ Radiation Therapy Oncology Group) late radiation-induced morbidity scoring system C30 |
| 66 | V | Stroke | M | Utility | EuroQol Index (EQ-5D) and the Health Utility Index 2 and 3 (HUI2/3). |
| 67 | A | Stroke | M | HRQOL; Dz specific | Stroke-impact profile and 2 stroke-specific scales (stroke impact scale and stroke-specific quality-of-life scale) |
| 68 | A | Acute MI | | Dz specific | Seattle Angina Questionnaire |
| 69 | P | Heart failure | M | Dz specific | Minnesota Living With Heart Failure Questionnaire and the Dyspnea-Fatigue Index |
| 70 | A | Chronic heart failure | A | HRQOL; Dz specific | SF-36; disease-specific HRQOL with the Kansas City Cardiomyopathy Questionnaire, depression measured with self-reported patient health questionnaire |
| 71 | M | Diabetes | A | HRQOL; Generic | Ontario Health Survey |
| 72 | P/V | Acute otitis media | | HRQOL | RAND general health rating index; Functional Status Questionnaire (FSQ Generic and FSQ Specific);TNO-AZL Infant Quality of Life (TAIQOL) |
| 73 | A/M | Celiac disease | A | Dz specific | Gastrointestinal quality-of-life index (GIQLI) and the EuroQol Index (EQ-5D). |
| 74 | A | COPD | M | HRQOL; Dz specific | The Chronic Respiratory Disease Questionnaire (CRQ), the Medical Outcomes Study Short Form 36-item survey (SF-36, version 2.0) |
| 75 | P | COPD | M | HRQOL | St. George's respiratory questionnaire (SGRQ) and the new 8-item visual simplified respiratory questionnaire (VSRQ) |
| 76 | REV | Rheumatology | M | HRQOL | QALY |

Part 3: Patient-Reported Outcomes

TABLE 1. Select HRQOL instruments from literature

| Reference | Study Type* | Disease | Methodology** | Patient-Reported Outcome Type** | Instruments |
|---|---|---|---|---|---|
| 77 | P | Osteoporosis | | Generic | EQ-5D questionnaire |
| 78 | P | Kidney | M | Dz specific | Kidney Disease Quality-of-Life Short-Form questionnaire (primary outcome) and the Health Utilities Index Mark 2 (secondary outcome) |
| 79 | A | Dialysis | M | Generic | HRQOL |
| 80 | P | BMI | A | Generic | EQ-5D/EQ-VAS, Health Utilities Index (HUI2 & HUI3); SF-6D. |
| 81 | A/V | Migraines | A | Dz specific & Generic; utility | Migraine-specific disability questionnaire, and the Health Utilities Index Mark 3 (HUI3). |
| 82 | P | Irritable Bowel Syndrome | M | HRQOL; | SF-36; Functional Bowel Disease Severity Index |

*A=Assessment; V=Validation; D=Development; R=Reliability; REV=Review **M=Measurement P=Application

# References

1. Preamble to the Constitution of the World Health Organization as adopted by the International Health Conference, New York, 19-22 June, 1946; signed on 22 July 1946 by the representatives of 61 States (Official Records of the World Health Organization, no. 2, p. 100) and entered into force on 7 April 1948. Available at: http://www.who.int/about/definition/en/print.html. Accessed August 26, 2009.
2. Brook RH, Ware JE, Rogers WH, et al. The effect of coinsurance on the health of adults. Results from the RAND Health Insurance Experiment. Santa Monica, CA: RAND Corporation, 1984. Report R-3055-HHS. ISBN 0-8330-0614-2.
3. Wilson IB, Cleary PD. Linking clinical variables with health-related quality of life: a conceptual model of patient outcomes. *JAMA*. 1995;273:59-65.
4. Mathisen L, Andersen MH, Veenstra M, Wahl AK, Hanestad BR and Fosse E. Quality of life can both influence and be an outcome of general health perceptions after heart surgery. *Health Qual Life Outcomes*. 2007;5:27.
5. Krethong P, Jirapaet V, Jitpanya C, Sloan R. A causal model of health-related quality of life in Thai patients with heart-failure. *J Nurs Scholarsh*. 2008;40(3):254-260.
6. Ulvik B, Nygård O, Hanestad BR, Wentzel-Larsen T, Wahl AK. Associations between disease severity, coping and dimensions of health-related quality of life in patients admitted for elective coronary angiography: a cross sectional study. *Health Qual Life Outcomes*. 2008;6:38.
7. Osoba D. Translating the science of patient-reported outcomes assessment into clinical practice. *J Natl Cancer Inst Monogr*. 2007;(37):5-11.
8. National Committee on Vital and Health Statistics: Classifying and Reporting Functional Status; 2000. Available at: http://www.ncvhs.hhs.gov/010617rp.pdf. Accessed July 10, 2009.
9. Romberg A, Virtanen A, Ruutiainen J. Long-term exercise improves functional impairment but not quality of life in multiple sclerosis. *J Neurol*. 2005;252(7):839-845.
10. Houlden H, Edwards M, McNeil J, Greenwood R. Use of the Barthel Index and Functional Independence Measure during early inpatient rehabilitation after single incident brain injury. *Clin Rehabil*. 2006;20(2):153-159.
11. Sackett DL, Haynes RB, Tugwell P. *Clinical Epidemiology: A Basic Science for Clinical Medicine*. Boston, MA: Little, Brown & Co.; 1985:181-182.
12. Deyo RA, Diehr P, Patrick DL. Reproducibility and responsiveness of health status measures. *Control Clin Trials*. 1991;12:142S-158S.
13. Redelmeier DA, Guyatt GH, Goldstein RS. Assessing the minimal important difference in symptoms: A comparison of two techniques. *J Clin Epidemiol*. 1996;49(11):1215-1219.
14. Wright J. The minimal important difference: who's to say what is important?. *J Clin Epidemiol*. 1992;49(11):1221-1222.
15. Juniper EF, Guyatt GH, Willan A, Griffith LE. Determining a minimal important change in a disease-specific quality of life questionnaire. *J Clin Epidemiol*. 1994;47(1):81-87.
16. Copay AG, Subach BR, Glassman SD, Polly DW Jr, Schuler TC. Understanding the minimum clinically important difference: a review of concepts and methods. *Spine J*. 2007;7(5): 541-546.
17. Walker SR and Rosser R, eds. *Quality-of-Life Assessment: Key Issues in the 1900s*. Norwell, MA: Kluwer Publishers; 1993: 209-220.
18. Torrance GW. Utility approach to measuring health-related quality of life. *J Chronic Dis*. 1987;40(6):593-600.
19. Gurnee MC, DaSilva RV. Constructing disease management programs. *Managed Care*. June 1997. Available at: http://www.managedcaremag.com/archives/9706/9706.disease_man.shtml. Accessed June 10, 2001.
20. Honish A, Westerfield W, Ashby A, Momin S, Phillippi R. Health-related quality of life and treatment compliance with diabetes care. *Dis Manag*. 2006;9(4):195-200.
21. Cranor CW, Bunting BA, Christensen DB. The Asheville Project: long-term clinical and economic outcomes of a community pharmacy diabetes care program. *J Am Pharm Assoc (Wash)*. 2003;43(2):173-184.

## Part 3: Patient-Reported Outcomes

22. Okamoto MP, Nakahiro RK. Pharmacoeconomic evaluation of a pharmacist-managed hypertension clinic. *Pharmacotherapy*. 2001;21(11):1337-1344.
23. Bunting BA, Smith BH, Sutherland SE. The Asheville Project: clinical and economic outcomes of a community-based long-term medication therapy management program for hypertension and dyslipidemia. *J Am Pharm Assoc*. 2008;48(1):23-31.
24. Bunting BA, Cranor CW. The Asheville Project: long-term clinical, humanistic, and economic outcomes of a community-based medication therapy management program for asthma. *J Am Pharm Assoc*. 2006;46(2):133-147.
25. Shelledy DC, Legrand TS, Gardner DD, Peters JI. A randomized, controlled study to evaluate the role of an in-home asthma disease management program provided by respiratory therapists in improving outcomes and reducing the cost of care. *J Asthma*. 2009;46(2):194-201.
26. Campos MA, Alazemi S, Zhang G, Wanner A, Sandhaus RA. Effects of a disease management program in individuals with alpha-1 antitrypsin deficiency. *COPD*. 2009;6(1):31-40.
27. Martin M, Blaisdell-Gross B, Fortin EW, et al. Health-related quality of life of heart failure and coronary artery disease patients improved during participation in disease management programs: a longitudinal observational study. *Dis Manag*. 2007;10(3):164-178.
28. Choo J, Burke LE, Pyo Hong K. Improved quality of life with cardiac rehabilitation for post-myocardial infarction patients in Korea. *Eur J Cardiovasc Nurs*. 2007;6(3):166-171.
29. Elliott D, Lazarus R, Leeder SR. Health outcomes of patients undergoing cardiac surgery: repeated measures using Short Form-36 and 15 Dimensions of Quality of Life questionnaire. *Heart Lung*. 2006;35(4):245-251.
30. Modi AC, Loux TJ, Bell SK, Harmon CM, Inge TH, Zeller MH. Weight-specific health-related quality of life in adolescents with extreme obesity. *Obesity* (Silver Spring). 2008;16(10):2266-2271.
31. Yackobovitch-Gavan M, Nagelberg N, Demol S, Phillip M, Shalitin S. Influence of weight-loss diets with different macronutrient compositions on health-related quality of life in obese youth. *Appetite*. 2008;51(3):697-703.
32. Sherbourne CD, Weiss R, Duan N, Bird CE, Wells KB. Do the effects of quality improvement for depression care differ for men and women? Results of a group-level randomized controlled trial. *Med Care*. 2004;42(12):1186-1193.
33. Ahlgren SS, Shultz JA, Massey LK, Hicks BC, Wysham C. Development of a preliminary diabetes dietary satisfaction and outcomes measure for patients with type 2 diabetes. *Qual Life Res*. 2004;13(4):819-832.
34. Short Form-36. Available at: http://www.sf-36.org. Accessed July 10, 2009.
35. Hart HE, Redekop WK, Bilo HJ, Meyboom-de Jong B, Berg M. Health related quality of life in patients with type I diabetes mellitus: generic & disease-specific measurement. *Indian J Med Res*. 2007;125(3):203-216.
36. Schwartz CE, Andresen EM, Nosek MA, Krahn GL; RRTC Expert Panel on Health Status Measurement. Response shift theory: important implications for measuring quality of life in people with disability. *Arch Phys Med Rehabil*. 2007;88(4):529-536.
37. Acquadro C, Conway K, Hareendran A, Aaronson N; European Regulatory Issues and Quality of Life Assessment (ERIQA) Group. Literature review of methods to translate health-related quality of life questionnaires for use in multinational clinical trials. *Value Health*. 2008;11(3):509-521.
38. Brossart DF, Clay DL, Willson VL. Methodological and statistical considerations for threats to internal validity in pediatric outcome data: response shift in self-report outcomes. *J Pediatr Psychol*. 2002;27(1):97-107.

39. Drukker M, Kaplan C, Schneiders J, Feron FJ, van Os J. The wider social environment and changes in self-reported quality of life in the transition from late childhood to early adolescence: a cohort study. *BMC Public Health.* 2006;6:133.
40. Cederfjall C, Langius-Eklof A, Lidman K, Wredling R. Gender differences in perceived health-related quality of life among patients with HIV infection. *AIDS Patient Care and STDs.* 2001;15(1):31-39.
41. Nesbitt BJ, Heidrich SM. Sense of coherence and illness appraisal in older women's quality of life. *Res Nurse Health.* 2000;23(1):25-34.
42. Allison PJ, Guichard C, Gilain L. A prospective investigation of dispositional optimism as a predictor of health-related quality of life in head and neck cancer patients. *Qual Life Res.* 2000;9(8):951-960.
43. Canizares S, Torres X, Boget T, Rumia J, Elices E, Arroyo S. Does neuroticism influence cognitive self-assessment after epilepsy surgery? *Epilepsia* 2000;41(10):1303-1309.
44. Rose KJ, Derry PA, McLachlan RS. Neuroticism in temporal lobe epilepsy: assessment and implications for pre- and postoperative psychosocial adjustment and health-related quality of life. *Epilepsia.* 1996;37(5):484-491.
45. Hooker K, Monahan D, Shifren K, Hutchinson C. Mental and physical health of spouse caregivers: the role of personality. *Psychol Aging.* 1992;7(3):367-375.
46. Kempen GI, Jelicic M, Ormel J. Personality, chronic medical morbidity, and health-related quality of life among older persons. *Health Psychology.* 1997;16(6):539-546.
47. Burgess AP, Carretero M, Elkington A, Pasqual-Marsettin E, Lobaccaro C, Catalan J. The role of personality, coping style and social support in health-related quality of life in HIV infection. *Qual Life Res.* 2000;9(4):423-437.
48. Lara ME, Leader J, Klein DN. The association between social support and course of depression: is it confounded with personality? *J Abnormal Psychol.* 1997;106(3):478-482.
49. Amir M, Roziner I, Knoll A, Neufeld MY. Self-efficacy and social support as mediators in the relation between disease severity and quality of life in patients with epilepsy. *Epilepsia.* 1999;40(2):216-224.
50. Grootendorst PV, Feeny DH, Furlong W. Does it matter whom and how you ask? inter- and intra-rater agreement in the Ontario Health Survey. *J Clin Epidemiol.* 1997;50(2):127-135.
51. Pierre U, Wood-Dauphinee S, Korner-Bitensky N, Gayton D, Hanley J. Proxy use of the Canadian SF-36 in rating health status of the disabled elderly. *J Clin Epidemiol.* 1998;51(11):983-990.
52. Sneeuw KC, Sprangers MA, Aaronson NK. The role of health care providers and significant others in evaluating the quality of life of patients with chronic disease. *J Clin Epidemiol.* 2002;55(11):1130-1143.
53. Sprangers MA and Aaronson NK. The role of health care providers and significant others in evaluating the quality of life of patients with chronic disease: a review. *J Clin Epidemiol.* 1992;45(7):743-760.
54. De Civita M, Regier D, Alamgir AH, Anis AH, Fitzgerald MJ, Marra CA. Evaluating health-related quality-of-life studies in paediatric populations: some conceptual, methodological and developmental considerations and recent applications. *PharmacoEconomics.* 2005;23(7): 659-685.
55. Sturms LM, van der Sluis CK, Groothoff JW, ten Duis HJ, Eisma WH. Young traffic victims' long-term health-related quality of life: child self-reports and parental reports. *Arch Phys Med Rehabil.* 2003;84(3):431-436.
56. Theunissen NC, Vogels TG, Koopman HM, et al. The proxy problem: child report versus parent report in health-related quality of life research. *Qual Life Res.* 1998;7(5):387-397.
57. Ennett ST, DeVellis BM, Earp JA, Kredich D, Warren RW, Wilhelm CL. Disease experience and psychosocial adjustment in children with juvenile rheumatoid arthritis: children's versus mothers' reports. *J Pediatr Psychol.* 1991;16(5):557-568.

**Part 3: Patient-Reported Outcomes**

58. Russell KM, Hudson M, Long A, Phipps S. Assessment of health-related quality of life in children with cancer: consistency and agreement between parent and child reports. *Cancer.* 2006;106(10):2267-2274.
59. Britto MT, Kotagal UR, Chenier T, Tsevat J, Atherton HD, Wilmott RW. Differences between adolescents' and parents' reports of health-related quality of life in cystic fibrosis. *Pediatr Pulmonol.* 2004;37(2):165-171.
60. Chang PC, Yeh CH. Agreement between child self-report and parent proxy-report to evaluate quality of life in children with cancer. *Psychooncology.* 2005;14(2):125-134.
61. Klassen AF, Miller A, Fine S. Agreement between parent and child report of quality of life in children with attention-deficit/hyperactivity disorder. *Child Care Health Dev.* 2006;32(4): 397-406.
62. Robitail S, Simeoni MC, Ravens-Sieberer U, Bruil J, Auquier P; the KIDSCREEN Group. Children proxies' quality-of-life agreement depended on the country using the European KIDSCREEN-52 questionnaire. *J Clin Epidemiol.* 2007;60(5):469-478.
63. Taphoorn MJ, Stupp R, Coens C, et al. Health-related quality of life in patients with glioblastoma: a randomised controlled trial. *Lancet Oncol.* 2005;6(12):937-944.
64. Blanchard CM, Courneya KS, Stein K; American Cancer Society's SCS-II. Cancer survivors' adherence to lifestyle behavior recommendations and associations with health-related quality of life: results from the American Cancer Society's SCS-II. *J Clin Oncol.* 2008;26(13):2198-2204.
65. Langendijk JA, Doornaert P. Impact of late treatment-related toxicity on quality of life among patients with head and neck cancer treated with radiotherapy. *J Clin Oncol.* 2008;26(22): 3770-3776.
66. Haacke C, Althaus A, Spottke A, Siebert U, Back T, Dodel R. Long-term outcome after stroke: evaluating health-related quality of life using utility measurements. *Stroke.* 2006;37(1): 193-198.
67. Salter KL, Moses MB, Foley NC, Teasell RW. Health-related quality of life after stroke: what are we measuring? *Int J Rehabil Res.* 2008;31(2):111-117.
68. Ho PM, Eng MH, Rumsfeld JS, et al. The influence of age on health status outcomes after acute myocardial infarction. *Am Heart J.* 2008;155(5):855-861.
69. Heo S, Doering LV, Widener J, Moser DK. Predictors and effect of physical symptom status on health-related quality of life in patients with heart failure. *Am J Crit Care.* 2008;17(2):124-132.
70. Faller H, Stork S, Schowalter M, et al. Is health-related quality of life an independent predictor of survival in patients with chronic heart failure? *J Psychosom Res.* 2007;63(5):533-538.
71. Manuel DG, Schultz SE. Health-related quality of life and health-adjusted life expectancy of people with diabetes in Ontario, Canada, 1996-1997. *Diabetes Care.* 2004;27(2):407-414.
72. Brouwer CN, Schilder AG, van Stel HF, et al. Reliability and validity of functional health status and health-related quality of life questionnaires in children with recurrent acute otitis media. *Qual Life Res.* 2007;16(8):1357-1373.
73. Casellas F, Rodrigo L, Vivancos JL, et al. Factors that impact health-related quality of life in adults with celiac disease: a multicenter study. *World J Gastroenterol.* 2008;14(1):46-52.
74. Wyrwich KW, Metz SM, Kroenke K, Tierney WM, Babu AN, Wolinsky FD. Measuring patient and clinician perspectives to evaluate change in health-related quality of life among patients with chronic obstructive pulmonary disease. *J Gen Intern Med.* 2007;22(2):161-170.
75. Tonnel AB, Perez T, Grosbois JM, Verkindre C, Bravo ML, Brun M; TIPHON study group. Effect of tiotropium on healt-related quality of life as a primary efficacy endpoint in COPD. *Int J Chron Obstruct Pulmon Dis.* 2008;3(2):301-310.

76. Bakker CH, Rutten-van Mölken M, van Doorslaer E, Bennett K, van der Linden S. Health related utility measurement in rheumatology: an introduction. *Patient Educ Couns*. 1993;20(2-3):145-152.
77. Oskar S, Borgstrom F, Zethraeus N, et al. Long-term cost and effect on quality of life of osteoporosis-related fractures in Sweden. *Acta Orthop*. 2008;79(2):269-280.
78. Wang W, Tonelli M, Hemmelgarn B, et al; Alberta Kidney Disease Network. The effect of increasing dialysis dose in overweight hemodialysis patients on quality of life: a 6-week randomized crossover trial. *Am J Kidney Dis*. 2008;51(5):796-803.
79. Moist LM, Bragg-Gresham JL, Pisoni RL, et al. Travel time to dialysis as a predictor of health-related quality of life, adherence, and mortality: the Dialysis Outcomes and Practice Patterns Study (DOPPS). *Am J Kidney Dis*. 2008;51(4):641-650.
80. Wee HL, Cheung YB, Loke WC, et al. The association of body mass index with health-related quality of life: an exploratory study in a multiethnic Asian population. *Value Health*. 2008;11(suppl 1):S105-S114.
81. Brown JS, Neumann PJ, Papadopoulos G, Ruoff G, Diamond M, Menzin J. Migraine frequency and health utilities: findings from a multisite survey. *Value Health*. 2008;11(2):315-321.
82. Rey E, Garcia-Alonso MO, Moreno-Ortega M, Alvarez-Sanchez A, Diaz-Rubio M. Determinants of quality of life in irritable bowel syndrome. *J Clin Gastroenterol*. 2008;42:1003-1009.

CHAPTER 16

# Work Outcomes in Health and Disease Management

Jayashri Sankaranarayanan, MPharm, PhD; Sue Jennings, MAEd, MPH, PhD; and Teresa Hartman, MLS

The impact of disease and medical treatments on the ability to work and be productive at work are important to many stakeholders, including employers, pharmaceutical developers and manufacturers, health and disease management firms, and society at large. In particular, employers are keenly interested in work outcomes of sick and injured employees, and have a stake in understanding the economic burden of medical conditions and the value of health improvement initiatives.[1]

## 1. The Importance of Work Outcomes

About US$260 billion is lost in workplace productivity by patients every year in the United States because of health-related problems.[2] Studies may differ in the precise definition of a work outcome, but estimates of the annual cost of health-related productivity loss are large and attributable to 2 factors: absenteeism (time lost from work because of illness-related absences, short- and long-term disability, or reduced productivity) and presenteeism (decreased on-the-job productivity).[3] Studies suggest the cost of lost productivity may be several times greater than direct medical costs and that productivity losses related to presenteeism may account for a larger proportion of those losses.[4,5] A meta-analysis estimated the overall cost of presenteeism at one-fifth to three-fifths of the total amount lost to the 10 most costly medical conditions.[5] Studies have estimated productivity losses of US$3 billion from anxiety disorders,[6] US$58 billion in indirect costs from diabetes,[7] US$51.5 billion from depression, and US$12 billion from migraine.[8]

For several reasons, productivity is a focus of the work outcomes literature in the US. First, employers in their role as payers have moved to the center of many health care benefit decisions, focusing on workforce productivity.[9] Second, employees recognize that their career and salary trajectories are affected by their health status. Employees understand how treatment decisions affect not only their survival and quality of life, but also their on-the-job productivity, job status, and position and compensation. Third, as the effectiveness of available health interventions improves, workers are less likely to leave the labor market because of illnesses. Instead, an increasing number of workers will encounter difficulty in managing their chronic illnesses while employed. Consequently, for many individuals with chronic illnesses, eligibility for health insurance can be an important motivation for employment.

Over the last 3 decades, employers have carried out programs to improve employees' current health status, prevent or delay the onset of costly chronic conditions, and better manage existing chronic conditions. As a result, there is notable interest in developing suitable methods for assessing the complete impact of these programs on work outcomes.[10,11] This chapter provides an assessment of work outcomes terminology, measures, data sources, and methods of measurement. It also includes a summary of the measurement challenges involved with linking work absence to disease, and assigning a monetary value to changes in productivity. Lastly, it provides guidance on selecting work outcome measures and the use of these measures to assess the impact of worksite health programs, including disease management and population wellness management.

## 2. Work Outcomes

*Work outcomes* are defined as the degree to which a person's health status or health-related medical interventions influence the quantity and/or quality of a person's participation in the labor market.[1] This definition, as well as the use of this term in this chapter, is focused on paid work outside the home. When defining work outcomes, 3 major concepts are considered:

- work role, including employment status and functional limitations;

- work disability, or the inability to function in a social role (for example, teaching or parenting); and

- work productivity, including absenteeism, time loss, and presenteeism

### Work Role Measures

Work role-related outcomes measure either an ability to perform specific demands of work (for example, climbing stairs or attending meetings), using job classifications (for example, employment status), or the impact of health problems on work using global indicators.[1]

### Employment Status

Employment status is often measured using questionnaires to assess a person's participation in the labor force during a given period or changes in workforce participation. In studying populations with recent interruptions in work after a health episode (for example, heart attack), it is important to distinguish whether or not an individual has returned to his/her usual type or level of work activity. In such cases, employment status is collected by asking the primary tasks a respondent was engaged in during a specific period, postepisode, postepisode job loss, or post-treatment return to work. Thus, pre-event and postevent employment status questions can assess changes in full-time or part-time work, changes in occupation, and job adjustments.[1]

The advantages of employment status as a work outcome measure are that it is objective and easy to identify. Employment categories are economically meaningful to the individual, the employer, and society. Researchers can use these data to benchmark and compare working populations with regards to productivity loss and associated costs.[1]

Several limitations make employment status a one-dimensional measure for defining work outcomes. One limitation is in the various methods for classifying and describing jobs and occupations by specific needs or demands. The challenge in using comparative data across job categories is that occupations with the same name can differ by organizational setting and can consist of different activities and rewards. Second, employment status may misrepresent the success of the outcome by masking partial disabilities and the quality of work experiences from the worker's perspective. These masked work disabilities lead to decreased productivity or job satisfaction.

Third, loss of employment or certain occupational transitions may be interpreted as unsuccessful outcomes, although they may not be related to the worker's health. For example, individuals may experience a change in occupation due to a long-distance move and not because of an underlying illness. Thus, the validity of employment status measures is a concern when there is no comparison group, and when reasons assigned by respondents are unclear. Finally, employment status categories cannot be applied to individuals who were unemployed before or after an illness event.[1]

## Functional Limitations

Questionnaires on functional limitations measure the degree to which health conditions affect an individual's ability to work. Some health status instruments that assess functional limitations include items on work outcomes (see Appendix 1 for details). Examples of global work indicators of functional limitations are the health profile measures of the Medical Outcome Study 36-Item Short Form (SF-36) role questions,[12-14] the preference-based measures of EuroQol,[12,15] the Quality of Well-Being Scale (QWB),[12,16] and the Sickness Impact Profile (SIP).[12,17]

The SF-36 is a multipurpose, short-form health survey with 36 questions[12-14] on activity limitations (commonly referred to as physical role limitation) and the emotional health scale (commonly referred to as the emotional role limitation scale).[12,13] The EuroQol Instrument, referred to as the EQ-5D, is a standardized, nondisease-specific, global health-related, quality-of-life measure developed for describing and valuing health-related quality of life. It provides self-reported data on limitations in routine activities using a 3-level response scale to grade ability to perform work.[15] The items on the QWB are from the activity limitation questions of the National Health Interview Survey (NHIS) and other related surveys such as the Current Population Survey conducted by the US Census Bureau.[16] The NHIS is a national survey that records the health of civilian noninstitutionalized populations in the US and is one of the major data collection programs of the National Center for Health Statistics (NCHS), part of the Centers for Disease Control and Prevention

(CDC).[18] The NHIS asks respondents to name the condition(s) that caused any activity limitations, creating estimates of the proportion of the US population with severe work limitations (that is, inability to work) or partial limitations (limits in the amount or kind of work performed).[12,18] The SIP contains a separate series of paid-work questions.[17]

Advantages of these functional measures are that they are brief, practical, easy to administer, and usually available in several formats (for example, phone and mail). They provide summary information that can identify proportions of populations with limitations in performing work, which is helpful in designing health-improvement programs. The role scales contained in all 4 measures (EuroQol, QWB, SF-36, and SIP) generally have a high degree of validity as measures of change in employment status.[12-17]

The disadvantages of the functional limitation measures (except for the QWB) as work outcome measures are that they focus on the human burden of health concerns, not economic implications. Further, these measures do not always specify the meaning of work or work activities and do not differentiate among social roles. Except for the SIP, the scales pose global questions (for example, "Were [you] limited in type of work or other activities?"). They do not distinguish between paid and unpaid work and the respondent has to identify the exact nature of his or her work role.

This lack of specificity introduces measurement error. Role-level questions do not ask the manner in or degree to which health problems have affected work performance or work activities. In addition, some scales do not differentiate between levels of work activity (for example, severe or partial limitations), leaving few employed respondents to report unable to work,[12] skewing responses to higher functioning levels. The role-functioning questions in the SF-36 include work along with other activities, clouding responses even more. In addition, paid work is distinguished from other work activities in the SF-36 questions, introducing noise in the response. Thus, it may be preferable to use functional status measures and work role measures in a complementary way when studying the impact of health care interventions on work outcomes.

## Work Disability

Work disability refers to a person's limitations in a social context—or the gap between a person's capabilities and the demands of their roles in their physical and social environments. Functional measures (for example, the QWB, SF-36, and SIP) also assess disability, but this should not be confused with work disability. Functional limitations are a person's inability to perform tasks in different settings (for example, climbing stairs or reading), while disability is a person's inability to perform in social roles. For example, individuals cognitively impaired by stroke can manage a house but may be disabled in their role as professor. A disability is adjusted, reduced, or removed by initiating health interventions, changing role demands, improving supports, providing job retraining services, and creating job accommodations.

Accessing the information on disability and workers compensation from administrative records of employers may be problematic for conducting national or regional comparisons because access to such data may differ from state to state. In addition, the accuracy of the archival data may be questionable because these data assume that each individual's on-the-job productivity is determined by itself, when in reality, productivity is interdependent among employees. For example, some teammates contribute more in the short run to make up for the illness-related productivity loss of a coworker. Thus, interdependence among employees can affect the objective measurement of productivity. Another disadvantage is when workers are aware that their productivity is being monitored, and change their behavior accordingly.[9]

## Work Productivity

Work productivity is the third work outcome of interest. Productivity losses can occur in several ways, including when an individual stops working entirely, is absent from work due to illness, is prevented from working (for example, by workplace safety rules), performs less than optimally when working while ill or is anxious or worried about a dependent's health (presenteeism), or reduces the time or effort spent on work activities (for example, because of back pain, arthritis, or a migraine).

Work productivity measurements differ for various reasons.[1] For the individual employee, work productivity usually refers to the goods and services produced through paid work activity or the physical output of the employee. For the employer, work productivity is a ratio of physical outputs to input resources (for example, labor hours, materials, and management time). For the health care industry, comparing measures across employers and industries becomes important.[1]

Selecting the appropriate perspective is the first step in selecting a suitable approach to data collection. The following discussion focuses on 2 areas of productivity—absenteeism/time loss from work, and presenteeism. Several instruments designed to measure absenteeism and presenteeism exist, and a number of articles describe and assess these instruments.[1,19-21] Appendix 2 provides information on some of the more well-known and frequently used instruments that measure absenteeism and presenteeism.

### Health-Related Absenteeism or Time Loss from Work

Health-related absenteeism is the time missed from work because of a health condition or its treatment. Conceptually, it is straightforward to confirm self-reported measures of absenteeism against factual data of workplace presence or absence. There are 2 primary sources of absenteeism data: self-reported data, such as that solicited on national surveys (for example, the NHIS),[18] and employer data on absenteeism, short- and long-term disability, and workers compensation. The NHIS asks respondents about the number of whole and partial days missed from work, the number of days respondents were late for work or left work early, and the number of whole or partial days spent in bed due to a health condition.

In retrospective studies, respondents are asked to recall frequency of work missed during long time periods. In clinical research studies, respondents are asked to report the quantity of time missed from work. Several of the instruments in Appendix 1 also request respondents to report whole or partial days missed from work. The recall time frame ranges from days to months, depending on health problem or treatment period. For example, the recall period may be days for migraine episodes or months for chronic stable angina.

A primary disadvantage of self-reported responses is recall bias, which can arise when respondents either omit instances of time missed within the reference period or include some time missed that occurred before or after the reference period.[1] In addition to pretesting measures, using time-loss diaries and shorter recall periods can reduce bias. However, diaries are expensive to analyze and respondents frequently need reminders to complete them on time.[1] Short recall periods (for example, 1- or 2-week intervals) have been reliable and valid as a reasonable alternative for lost time data.[1,19-22] However, short recall periods can skew the data towards no time loss because little or no work time is missed or in the opposite direction because work time was missed at the time of the survey, but not before.

Employer administrative records that distinguish between sickness, vacation, absenteeism, short- and long-term disability and workers compensation may also be used. However, not all employer data differentiate between absence due to illness or treatment, and absence associated with care-giving or vacation. Employer-based administrative absenteeism data also rarely identify a specific medical condition.

## Presenteeism

Several definitions of presenteeism exist in the scientific, business, and popular literature. In these definitions, the concept is defined both negatively (ie, being unproductive while at work) and positively (being fully present and productive while at work). In this chapter we define *presenteeism* as "decreased on-the-job productivity associated with health concerns/problems."[3] This definition focuses on work outside the home and on the association between health-related issues and productivity decline.[23]

While there is no consensus on assessing presenteeism using self-reported questionnaires, productivity survey instruments assess presenteeism in 1 of 3 ways: (1) self-assessed overall impairment, (2) comparative productivity, performance, and efficiency (with those of others and with one's norm), and (3) respondent estimates of unproductive time while at work.[19] A review of 17 presenteeism instruments found that several questionnaires on presenteeism loss address the relationship of weakened ability to function while at work with general health reasons.[19] Most survey instruments specifically measure productivity loss within the domain of paid work. The Care Continuum Alliance keeps a periodically updated list of presenteeism instruments with added information about each.[24]

Fourteen selected instruments available through public or proprietary access

### Part 3: Patient-Reported Outcomes

are listed in Appendix 2. These instruments have varying characteristics that may impact the data collected. For example, recall periods of the instruments vary from 1 week to 52 weeks, and the instruments vary by length from 4 to 44 questions. Of the 14 instruments in Appendix 2, 10 are generic instruments while 4 are disease-specific instruments. There are 9 productivity instruments that are proprietary and can be used across various general medical conditions: the 6-item American Productivity Audit and Work and Health Interview;[25,26] 25-item Endicott Work Productivity Scale (19-21); 30-item Health and Labor Questionnaire;[19-21,27] 44-item Health and Productivity Questionnaire[19,28] or 24-item Health and Work Questionnaire;[19-,29,30] 9-item Health-Related Productivity Questionnaire Diary;[19,31] Stanford Presenteeism Scale;[20,32-34] 25-item Work Limitations Questionnaire (WLQ);[19-,35,36] and the 4-item Work Productivity Short Inventory.[19,37,38]

Some instruments focus on the impact of specific health conditions and give subjective assessments of the effectiveness in performing work activities and work-related productivity loss in studies of migraine headaches.[39] Two productivity instruments that are proprietary for specific diseases are the 28-item Migraine Work and Productivity Loss Questionnaire;[19-21,39] and the 17-item Angina-Related Limitations at Work Questionnaire.[19,20,40] One productivity instrument in the public domain is the 6-item Work Productivity and Activity Impairment Questionnaire (WPAI)[19-21,41,42] that is also available for specific health problems like allergic rhinitis, gastroesophageal reflux disease and chronic hand dermatitis.[19,21,43]

Two productivity instruments that are in the public domain for specific diseases are the 9-item Work Productivity and Activity Impairment Questionnaire–Allergy Specific;[19,21,43] and the Migraine Disability Assessment Questionnaire.[19,21,44] These surveys request respondents to rate their on-the-job effectiveness on days they were symptomatic (for example, during a migraine-headache episode). Ratings scales range from 0 percent (not at all effective) to 100 percent (completely effective). Often, this information is combined with time-loss data (for example, sickness absence data). Three of these 14 instruments (the Health and Work Questionnaire, Stanford Presenteeism Scale and WLQ) do not measure absenteeism.

Four commonly used instruments include the Health and Labor Questionnaire, the Work Productivity and Activity Impairment Questionnaire, the Work Limitations Questionnaire, and the Stanford Presenteeism Scale. The Health and Labor Questionnaire[19-21,27] provides a comprehensive method for evaluating loss in health-related productivity and includes 4 modules: work absences, reduced on-the-job performance, the degree of trouble in performing paid work, and productivity in unpaid work. The Work Productivity and Activity Impairment Questionnaire includes a general health version (WPAI:GH) and a specific health problem version (WPAI:SHP). These instruments, created simultaneously using the same template, are patient-reported quantitative assessments of the absenteeism, presenteeism, and daily activity impairment attributable to general health and specific health problems, respectively.[19-21,41-43]

The WLQ is a validated 25-item, self-administered, self-reported instrument that measures on-the-job work disability and productivity loss.[19-21,35,36] Four scales reflect the multidimensional character of work roles: a 5-item time scale on time and scheduling demands; a 6-item physical scale covers job tasks that involve bodily strength, movement, endurance, coordination and flexibility; a 9-item mental-interpersonal scale on cognitive and social tasks; and a 5-item output scale on decreased work productivity. Scale scores ranging from 0 (limited none of the time) to 100 (limited all of the time) represent the percentage of time in the past 2 weeks respondents experienced job performance limitations. Using an empirically derived algorithm, the work limitation data from the WLQ can be converted into productivity loss score. The Stanford Presenteeism Scale introduces another important distinction by assessing presenteeism as being present on the job in both knowledge- and production-based jobs.[20,32-34] The WPAI and WLQ offer significant advantages over other instruments because of their reported psychometric properties and their use in various populations (clinical and employee).[21]

## Summary of Measurement Challenges with Work Outcomes

Data from self-reported instruments can be collected broadly from many different subpopulations and for various disease states in epidemiological and clinical trials. Besides the usual recall issues associated with self-reporting, the ability to make causal inferences about the role of health status as a determinant of these workplace outcomes may be questionable.[9] Furthermore, questions that can be seen as sensitive or threatening, such as those about personal productivity or impact of an illness on work productivity, may affect the accuracy of responses and productivity estimates. In addition, the timing of questions, the time frame, the type of position, firm or industry can affect the response and productivity estimate accuracies.

Conceptually, it is easier to validate self-reported absenteeism measures against factual data of workplace presence or absence. A worker may experience problems carrying out certain role tasks for a short period. Archival records (administrative databases) can be used to quantify employee performance. Also, there are few objective measures of presenteeism that are applicable for many different types of workers. Although call center and manufacturing jobs do have a distinct, measureable output, the output of the white collar labor force is very difficult to quantify. Measurement concerns arise with each case (whether self-reported or archival data). The validity of productivity instruments has been difficult to prove because of the differences in how the data are collected, the complexity of the data collected, the variety of work settings assessed, and the absence of a gold standard against which to evaluate the instrument's findings of employee performance. In summary, while they are easy to use, validation of the presenteeism measures is limited to a handful of published validation studies.[19,45]

## Methods to Estimate Costs of Productivity Losses

Despite these challenges in using presenteeism instruments, there is much interest in assigning a monetary value to lost productivity.[19,45] Mattke and colleagues[19] summarize the 3 primary methods used to estimate the cost of lost productivity (although none appears to be validated):

1. *Salary Conversion Methods*, also known as the human capital approach, use self-reported information on missed work, unproductive hours, and salary to estimate the cost for lost productivity. It expresses the loss as the product of missed workdays, or self-reported unproductive hours or self-reported percentage decline of performance, multiplied by salaries.[19,36,46,47] Actual salaries of the respondents,[19,26,36,46,47] mean salaries for the corporation[48] or national median wages[5] have been used for the conversion. This is the most commonly used method.

   While this method is computationally easy, and intuitive, it may both underestimate and overestimate the cost. In some work situations, the interdependence of workers may be so high that the absence of a key employee may limit the productivity of other workers, thus underestimating the cost of the lost time. In contrast, this method may overestimate the cost by not considering that employees may make up for unproductive time though uncompensated overtime.

2. *Introspective Methods* use survey response to structure thought experiments. This allows employers to estimate the extent of their lost productivity rather than a specific dollar amount. However, these methods are more difficult to perform and less intuitive to explain.

3. *Firm-Level Methods* ask managers to estimate the impact of survey findings on their company-level productivity and the costs of any repairs they undertake as a result.[19]

A lack of a proven and validated method to obtain monetary estimates of the cost of lost productivity is a drawback of measuring presenteeism. Applying a salary conversion method seems easier even if it provides a lower-bound estimate of the cost of lost job productivity. However, before salary conversion becomes the basis for policy and managerial decisions, a thorough evaluation of this method and its alternatives is needed. Benchmarking the different methods will determine if and to what degree cost estimates of productivity losses differ based on these methods. Operational standards for using different methods should consider the difficulty of job productivity measurements in white collar occupations and reflect the interest of various stakeholders.[19]

## 3. Guidance on Selecting Work Outcome Measures

Evaluations of disease management and population health programs implemented at the worksite benefit from various outcome measures, including modifiable risk factors, health status, clinical outcomes, indicators of behavior change, utilization process measures, medical costs, and work outcomes in the short-, medium-, and long-term.[24] Work outcome measures such as absenteeism and presenteeism are especially important given that they may change soon after the program's introduction and more rapidly than health care service use or costs.[24] In 2008, the Care Continuum Alliance recommended that productivity measures be included in evaluations of worksite wellness and disease management programs.[24] Given the lack of consensus on a gold standard for productivity instruments and the variability of environments in which the programs are carried out, choosing a suitable work outcome measure when planning studies requires knowledge of available instruments, characteristics of the worksite and employee population, and goals and limitations of the study.

When selecting an instrument, researchers should consider important questions, including:

- What evidence is there in the literature of the instrument's reliability and validity?
- Is the instrument suitable for the target population, including the type of workforce and work setting, languages in use, and reading level?
- Does the instrument capture the work-related outcomes the intervention is hypothesized to impact?
- What is the time frame when these hypothesized effects occur, and how long do they last; that is, are they impacting short- or long-term outcomes?
- What recall period is used in the instrument and will these periods capture the impact of an intervention, be representative of the reporting period, and reduce recall bias in findings?
- What are the logistics of giving the instrument or gathering the data, including the cost of licensing and administration, the length of the survey, and the ability to integrate these measures into existing evaluation strategies?
- How important is it to be able to assign financial costs to these effects and does the measurement tool collect suitable information to do this?
- Are guidelines or comparison data available for interpreting scores of work outcomes?

For example, if one were planning to evaluate a worksite health promotion program at a large site, the measurement tool must be designed to assess productivity for all the types of employees at the site, be available in all languages, and be written at a reading level that would be accessible to all participants. The cost of administration and licensing must also be within the budget of the evaluation.

## 4. Disease Management and Worksite Health Programs in Promoting Productivity

### Benefits to Stakeholders

Stakeholders want to realize benefits of promoting productivity from disease management and worksite health programs. Knowledge of the extent of productivity losses have made employers believe that better management of recovery from surgery, return to work after injury, or productivity loss because of acute or chronic conditions might help decrease their costs and improve employee health. Employers believe the health-related benefits their organizations provide (such as group health insurance, wellness programs, and disability insurance) are an investment in their employees. With the need to make the business case for quality improvement, payer policy makers see the opportunity to align the social welfare objective of improving care for chronic conditions. Therefore, payers launch health and disease management programs with the help of the expertise of wellness program-implementing organizations. However, payers also need to study the value of these initiatives for their impact on work outcomes.

### Potential Impact of Disease Management on Productivity

Several studies have documented the relationship between measures of health and measures of productivity.[5,25,49,50] The measures of health assessed include both health risks such as poor diet, alcohol or tobacco use, obesity, physical inactivity and stress, and disease states such as diabetes, migraine, arthritis, cancer, depression, and asthma. Findings suggest 2 important questions for those engaged in population health management activities: Can programs impact productivity measures by reducing risks and promoting better disease management? If they do, are evaluations of these programs that focus only on medical care utilization and associated costs underestimating the value of the programs to the purchasers, payers, and participants?

While most studies have focused on the association between health and productivity, few have used productivity measures to evaluate health management programs. There is increasing interest in including presenteeism in evaluations, especially of wellness and total population management programs, by program providers, purchasers, and payers. These measures offer the opportunity to be more comprehensive in assessing the impact of the program and provide a basis for assessing shorter-term outcomes rather than wait for the longer-term impact of risk decline on health service use and medical costs.

## Examples of Disease Management Affecting Presenteeism or Absenteeism

Given the relationship between health status and productivity, programs that focus on chronic disease management, health promotion, or risk reduction that intervene across the care continuum have the potential to impact productivity. Disease management programs are designed to encourage individuals with chronic conditions to improve self-management and adherence to medical regimens. It can be hypothesized that success in helping employees to better manage their condition may be associated with improved productivity. For example, an asthma disease management program that helps to improve an employee's asthma-related symptoms may reduce emergency room visits and hospitalizations, reducing absenteeism associated with the condition.

The Asheville Project, a pharmacist-run disease management program in North Carolina,[51-53] has documented an increase in productivity and a decrease in disease-related absenteeism for diabetes and other chronic conditions. Musich, et al.[48] examined outcomes for disease management programs in various settings (such as workplace, health plan, and community) for arthritis, asthma, cancer, depression, diabetes, cardiovascular disorders, and migraines, and found that for each condition there were positive health outcomes, declines in utilization/medical costs, and improved productivity. Several studies have found a positive association between risk reduction interventions and reduced absenteeism/disability days,[54-57] and others have found a correlation between the uses of drugs designed to reduce the impact of allergies and improvements in work impairment.[58] A 2009 Cochrane review identified 6 randomized controlled trials that tested the relationship between workplace interventions and work disability for musculoskeletal and mental health disorders.[59] They found moderate-quality evidence for a reduction in sickness-related absence because of workplace interventions for musculoskeletal disorders. But, the authors were unable to draw conclusions for mental health or other disorders.

Positive outcomes associated with productivity are substantially limited compared with positive outcomes associated with health care use, cost, and clinical indicators. This may be a function of the infrequency with which disease management programs include productivity measures among the metrics to evaluate their programs rather than a failure of the programs to improve productivity. As mentioned above, there have been several studies that link health risks to measures of productivity.[50,60,61] There have been fewer studies, however, that examine the relationship between changes in risk factors and changes in productivity, especially presenteeism.

Pelletier and colleagues[62] assessed the association of changes in risk status with changes in absenteeism and presenteeism in a nonexperimental, pre-post study of employed individuals taking a health risk appraisal. The authors found that reducing risk was associated with declines in absenteeism and presenteeism. They did not find, however, an association between increases in risk and reduced productivity. In another study, researchers used a prospective, controlled design to assess the impact of a workplace health promotion program on presenteeism, one of the few available studies to have specifically addressed this relationship.[63] It found significant declines in measured health risks and in absenteeism days and an increase in work performance (presenteeism) in the intervention group relative to the comparison group.

Because of the several limitations of the various studies, caution is recommended in interpreting the results of the studies given a low-response rate and problems in matching participant and comparison group members.[63] Also, a Cochrane review study including randomized control trials of workplace interventions was limited to musculoskeletal and mental health.[59] However, when the review considered all the types of work disability together, only lower-quality evidence indicated that workplace interventions are more effective than usual care in reducing sickness-related absence.

Integrating pharmacy and medical claims could also help understand health-related productivity losses. Using the Health and Work Performance Questionnaire combined with medical and pharmacy claims, one study demonstrated a link between health and productivity losses among 10 employers with 51,648 employee respondents (64). Health-related productivity costs were significantly higher than medical and pharmacy costs alone (on average 2.3 to 1). Important correlates of productivity loss were chronic conditions such as depression/anxiety, obesity, arthritis, and back/neck pain, and comorbidities.

## 5. Summary

Valid and reliable measures of work outcomes related to work roles (employment status and functional limitations), work disability, and productivity (absenteeism and presenteeism) are available. However, estimating costs of lost productivity needs further study; the estimates, though, should reflect the perspective (corporate or social welfare) of various stakeholders. The available work outcome measures have the potential to complement existing strategies for evaluating health management programs. This potential will have a greater opportunity to be realized if stakeholders (employers, payer policy makers, employees, and organizations implementing wellness programs) adapt their initiatives to understand comprehensively the relationship of changes in risk status or health and disease management with productivity, and the associated cost-effectiveness. This will inform and enable stakeholder decisions in developing, delivering, and evaluating health and disease management interventions that promote health and productivity.

**APPENDIX 1.** Functional limitation instruments that assess work outcomes

| Instrument | Work Outcome Items | Administration and Response Scales | Measures |
|---|---|---|---|
| The Medical Outcome Study 36-Item Short Form (SF-36)[12-14] | • Role activity limitation items of national surveys (ie, inability to accomplish as much as usual, and difficulty performing roles described as requiring extra effort), <br>• role-physical health scale, <br>• emotional health scale adds a criterion; being unable to work as carefully as usual | • Self-report of role limitation in the past week <br>• Uses 5-point Likert response scale ranging from all, most, some, a little and none of the time | • Paid work is not addressed separately from other work activities <br>• Yields an 8-scale profile of functional health and well-being scores, psychometrically based physical and mental health summary measures <br>• Version 2 has better phrased role-functioning items |
| EuroQol (now referred to as the EQ-5D)[12,15] | • A single set of items across 5 dimensions; mobility, self-care, usual activities, pain/discomfort, and anxiety/depression simultaneously grades multiple-role levels (ie, ability in performing employment, housework, schoolwork, family life, and leisure) | • Self-report <br>• Uses a 3-level response scale: have no problems, some problems, unable to perform | • Global health-related quality of life |
| Quality of Well Being Scale (QWB)[12,16] | • Items on limitations in activity performance for the past 4 days based on the National Health Interview Survey (NHIS) | • Interview in a semi-structured format <br>• Uses yes/no response scale | • Overall score of activity limitations; scale items weighted to reflect health-state preferences; estimates US populations with severe, or partial limitations in work performed |
| Sickness Impact Profile (SIP)[12,17] | • Activity limitation items of national surveys; series of paid-work questions: 8 items including 2 items on the work done (working shorter hours, and doing part of job at home, 2 items address the kind of work (ie, doing light work and working with some changes), 1 item on accomplishments, 1 item on care in doing work, irritability toward others and interrupted work <br>• Role limitation criteria in the SIP overlaps with items in the SF-36 | • Self-report <br>• Scored by number and type of items checked by respondents with their health | • Contains separate paid work questions <br>• Reports a scale score to assess any disability <br>• Overall, category, and dimension scores can be calculated |

## Part 3: Patient-Reported Outcomes

APPENDIX 2. Selected productivity instruments that assess presenteeism and absenteeism*

| Instrument | Recall Period, Week(s) | Presenteeism Questions |
|---|---|---|
| **Proprietary access for general conditions** | | |
| 1. American Productivity Audit and Work and Health Interview[25,26] | 2 | 6 |
| 2. Endicott Work Productivity Scale[19-21] | 1 | 25 |
| 3. Health and Labor Questionnaire[19-21,27] | 2 | 30 |
| 4. Health and Productivity Questionnaire[19,28] or Health and Work Performance Questionnaire | 1 (clinical), 4 (employer) | 44 |
| 5. Health and Work Questionnaire[19-21,29,30] | 1 | 24** |
| 6. Health-Related Productivity Questionnaire Diary[19,31] | 1 | 9 |
| 7. Stanford Presenteeism Scale[20,32-34] | 4 | 6** |
| 8. Work Limitations Questionnaire[19-21,35,36]*** | 2 | 25** |
| 9. Work Productivity Short Inventory[19,37,38]**** | 2/12/52 | 4 |
| **Proprietary access for specific diseases** | | |
| 1. Migraine Work and Productivity Loss Questionnaire[19-21,39] | Most recent episode | 28 |
| 2. Angina-Related Limitations at Work Questionnaire[19,20,40] | 4 | 17 |
| **Public access for general and specific diseases** | | |
| 1. Work Productivity and Activity Impairment Questionnaire[19,21,41,42] | 1 | 6 |
| 2. Work Productivity and Activity Impairment Questionnaire–Allergy Specific[19,21,43] | 1 | 9 |
| 3. Migraine Disability Assessment Questionnaire[19,21,44] | 12 | 7 |

*Adapted from references.[19-21] ** Do not assess absenteeism ***for General Chronic
****>12 conditions from allergies, respiratory infections, arthritis, asthma, anxiety disorder, depression and bipolar disorder, stress, diabetes mellitus, hypertension, migraines, coronary heart disease or high cholesterol, and 4 caregiving conditions.

# References

1. Lerner DJ, Bungay KM. Measuring work outcomes. In: Grauer DW, Lee J, Odom TD, et al, eds. *Pharmacoeconomics and Outcomes: Applications for Patient Care*. 2nd ed. Kansas City, MO: American College of Clinical Pharmacy; 2003.
2. Davis K, Collins SR, Doty MM, et al. Health and productivity among U.S. workers. *Issue Brief* (Common Fund) 2005;(856):1-10.
3. Schultz AB, Edington DW. Employee health and presenteeism: a systematic review. *J Occup Rehabil*. 2007;17:547-579.
4. Loeppke R, Hymel PA, Lofland JH, et al. Health-related workplace productivity measurement: general and migraine-specific recommendations from the ACOEM Expert Panel. *J Occup Environ Med*. 2003;45:349-359.
5. Goetzel RZ, Long SR, Ozminkowski RJ, et al. Health, absence, disability, and presenteeism cost estimates of certain physical and mental health conditions affecting U.S. employers. *J Occup Environ Med*. 2004;46:398-412.
6. Mychaskiw MA, Sankaranarayanan J. A national estimate of indirect costs associated with anxiety disorders. *Value Health*. 2003;6:350.
7. American Diabetes Association. Economic costs of diabetes in the U.S. in 2007. *Diabetes Care*. 2008;31:596-615.
8. Hawkins K, Wang S, Rupnow MF. Indirect cost burden of migraine in the United States. *J Occup Environ Med*. 2007;49:368-374.
9. Greenberg PE, Birnbaum HG, Kessler RC, et al. Impact of illness and its treatment on workplace costs: regulatory and measurement issues. *J Occup Environ Med*. 2001;43:56-63.
10. Goetzel RZ, Ozminkowski RJ. The health and cost benefits of work site health-promotion programs. *Annu Rev Public Health*. 2008;29:303-323.
11. Mattke S, Serxner SA, Zakowski SL, et al. Impact of 2 employer-sponsored population health management programs on medical care cost and utilization. *Am J Manag Care*. 2009;15: 113-120.
12. Coons SJ, Rao S, Keininger DL, et al. A comparative review of generic quality-of-life instruments. *Pharmacoeconomics*. 2000;17:13-35.
13. Ware JE. SF-36 Health Survey Update. http://www.sf-36.org/tools/sf36.shtml#VERS2. Accessed March 31, 2010.
14. Ware JE, Kosinski M, Keller SD, eds. SF-36 *Physical and Mental Health Summary Scales: A User's Manual*. Boston, MA: The Health Institute; 1994.
15. Euroquol Group. EQ-5D: A standardised instrument for use a measure of health outcome. Available at: http://www.euroqol.org/. Accessed January 5, 2010.
16. Kaplan RM, Ganiats TG, Sieber WJ, et al. The Quality of Well-Being Scale: critical similarities and differences with SF-36. *Int J Qual Health Care*. 1998;10:509-520.
17. Bergner M, Bobbitt RA, Carter WB, et al. The Sickness Impact Profile: development and final revision of a health status measure. *Med Care*. 1981;19:787-805.
18. National Center for Health Statistics. About the National Health Interview Survey. http://www.cdc.gov/nchs/nhis/about_nhis.htm. Accessed February 23, 2010.
19. Mattke S, Balakrishnan A, Bergamo G, et al. A review of methods to measure health-related productivity loss. *Am J Manag Care*. 2007;13:211-217.
20. Lofland JH, Pizzi L, Frick KD. A review of health-related workplace productivity loss instruments. *Pharmacoeconomics*. 2004;22:165-184.
21. Prasad M, Wahlqvist P, Shikiar R, et al. A review of self-report instruments measuring health-related work productivity: a patient-reported outcomes perspective. *Pharmacoeconomics*. 2004;22:225-244.
22. Revicki DA, Irwin D, Reblando J, et al. The accuracy of self-reported disability days. *Med Care*. 1994;32:401-404.
23. DMAA: The Care Continuum Alliance. http://www.carecontinuumalliance.org/. Accessed April 24, 2013.
24. DMAA: The Care Continuum Alliance. *Outcomes Guideline Report*. 2008;3:76.

**Part 3: Patient-Reported Outcomes**

25. Stewart WF, Ricci JA, Chee E, et al. Lost productive work time costs from health conditions in the United States: results from the American Productivity Audit. *J Occup Environ Med*. 2003;45:1234-1246.
26. Stewart WF, Ricci JA, Chee E, et al. Cost of lost productive work time among US workers with depression. *JAMA*. 2003;289:3135-3144.
27. Hakkart-van Roijen L, Essink-Bot ML. Manual: the health and labour questionnaire. http://www.imta.nl/publications/0052.pdf. Accessed March 31, 2010.
28. Wang PS, Beck A, Berglund P, et al. Chronic medical conditions and work performance in the health and work performance questionnaire calibration surveys. *J Occup Environ Med*. 2003;45:1303-1311.
29. Shikiar R, Halpern MT, Rentz AM, et al. Development of the Health and Work Questionnaire (HWQ): an instrument for assessing workplace productivity in relation to worker health. *Work*. 2004;22:219-229.
30. GlaxoSmithKline Group of Companies. Health and Work Questionnaire. http://tc.bmjjournals.com/cgi/data/10/3/233/DC1/1. Accessed March 31, 2010.
31. Kumar RN, Hass SL, Li JZ, et al. Validation of the Health-Related Productivity Questionnaire Diary (HRPQ-D) on a sample of patients with infectious mononucleosis: results from a phase 1 multicenter clinical trial. *J Occup Environ Med*. 2003;45:899-907.
32. Turpin RS, Ozminkowski RJ, Sharda CE, et al. Reliability and validity of the Stanford Presenteeism Scale. *J Occup Environ Med*. 2004;46:1123-1133.
33. Collins JJ, Baase CM, Sharda CE, et al. The assessment of chronic health conditions on work performance, absence, and total economic impact for employers. *J Occup Environ Med*. 2005;47:547-557.
34. Koopman C, Pelletier KR, Murray JF, et al. Stanford presenteeism scale: health status and employee productivity. *J Occup Environ Med*. 2002;44:14-20.
35. Ozminkowski RJ, Goetzel RZ, Chang S, Long S. The application of two health and productivity instruments at a large employer. *J Occup Environ Med*. 2004;46(7):635-648.
36. Lerner D, Amick BC III, Rogers WH, et al. The Work Limitations Questionnaire. *Med Care*. 2001;39:72-85.
37. Ozminkowski RJ, Goetzel RZ, Long SR. A validity analysis of the Work Productivity Short Inventory (WPSI) instrument measuring employee health and productivity. *J Occup Environ Med*. 2003;45:1183-1195.
38. Goetzel RZ, Ozminkowski RJ, Long SR. Development and reliability analysis of the Work Productivity Short Inventory (WPSI) instrument measuring employee health and productivity. *J Occup Environ Med*. 2003;45:743-762.
39. Lerner DJ, Amick BC III, Malspeis S, et al. The migraine work and productivity loss questionnaire: concepts and design. *Qual Life Res*. 1999;8:699-710.
40. Lerner DJ, Amick BC III, Malspeis S, et al. The Angina-related Limitations at Work Questionnaire. *Qual Life Res*. 1998;7:23-32.
41. Reilly MC, Zbrozek AS, Dukes EM. The validity and reproducibility of a work productivity and activity impairment instrument. *Pharmacoeconomics*. 1993;4:353-365.
42. Reilly MC. Work Productivity Studies - Work Productivity and Activity Impairment Questionnaire (WPAI). Available at: http://www.reillyassociates.net/Index.html. Accessed March 31, 2010.
43. Reilly MC, Tanner A, Meltzer EO. Work, classroom and activity impairment instruments: validation studies in allergic rhinitis. *Clin Drug Investig*. 1996;11:278-288.
44. Lipton RB, Stewart WF. Migraine Disability Assessment Test. http://www.uhs.berkeley.edu/home/healthtopics/pdf/assessment.pdf. Accessed March 31, 2010.
45. Mattke S, Balakrishnan A, Bergamo G, et al. A review of methods to measure Health-related Productivity Loss-Online Appendix. Am J Manag Care. 2007;13:a217-a218. Available at: http://www.ajmc.com/media/pdf/AJMC_07aprMattkeAppendix.pdf. Accessed January 5, 2010.
46. Allen HM Jr, Bunn WB III. Validating self-reported measures of productivity at work: a case for their credibility in a heavy manufacturing setting. *J Occup Environ Med*. 2003;45:926-940.

47. Allen HM Jr, Bunn WB III. Using self-report and adverse event measures to track health's impact on productivity in known groups. *J Occup Environ Med.* 2003;45:973-983.
48. Hemp P. Presenteeism: at work—but out of it. *Harv Bus Rev.* 2004;82:49,58,155.
49. Musich SA, Schultz AB, Edington DW. Overview of disease management approaches: implications for corporate-sponsored programs. *Dis Manage Health Outcomes.* 2004;12:299-326.
50. Musich S, Hook D, Baaner S, et al. The association of two productivity measures with health risks and medical conditions in an Australian employee population. *Am J Health Promot.* 2006;20:353-363.
51. Bunting BA, Cranor CW. The Asheville Project: long-term clinical, humanistic, and economic outcomes of a community-based medication therapy management program for asthma. *J Am Pharm Assoc.* 2006;46:133-147.
52. Bunting BA, Smith BH, Sutherland SE. The Asheville Project: clinical and economic outcomes of a community-based long-term medication therapy management program for hypertension and dyslipidemia. *J Am Pharm Assoc.* 2008;48:23-31.
53. Cranor CW, Bunting BA, Christensen DB. The Asheville Project: long-term clinical and economic outcomes of a community pharmacy diabetes care program. *J Am Pharm Assoc* (Wash). 2003;43:173-184.
54. Lynch WD, Golaszewski TJ, Clearie AF, et al. Impact of a facility-based corporate fitness program on the number of absences from work due to illness. *J Occup Med.* 1990;32:9-12.
55. Schultz AB, Lu C, Barnett TE, et al. Influence of participation in a worksite health-promotion program on disability days. *J Occup Environ Med.* 2002;44:776-780.
56. Serxner S, Gold D, Anderson D, et al. The impact of a worksite health promotion program on short-term disability usage. *J Occup Environ Med.* 2001;43:25-29.
57. Bertera RL. The effects of workplace health promotion on absenteeism and employment costs in a large industrial population. *Am J Public Health.* 1990;80:1101-1105.
58. Meltzer EO, Casale TB, Nathan RA, et al. Once-daily fexofenadine HCl improves quality of life and reduces work and activity impairment in patients with seasonal allergic rhinitis. *Ann Allergy Asthma Immunol.* 1999;83:311-317.
59. van Oostrom SH, Driessen MT, de Vet HC, et al. Workplace interventions for preventing work disability. *Cochrane Database Syst Rev.* 2009;(2):CD006955.
60. Goetzel RZ, Anderson DR, Whitmer RW, et al. The relationship between modifiable health risks and health care expenditures. an analysis of the multi-employer HERO health risk and cost database. *J Occup Environ Med.* 1998;40:843-854.
61. Burton WN, Conti DJ, Chen CY, et al. The role of health risk factors and disease on worker productivity. *J Occup Environ Med.* 1999;41(10):863-877.
62. Pelletier B, Boles M, Lynch W. Change in health risks and work productivity over time. *J Occup Environ Med.* 2004;46:746-754.
63. Mills PR, Kessler RC, Cooper J, et al. Impact of a health promotion program on employee health risks and work productivity. *Am J Health Promot.* 2007;22:45-53.
64. Loeppke R, Taitel M, Haufle V, et al. Health and productivity as a business strategy: a multi-employer study. *J Occup Environ Med.* 2009;51(4):411-428.

CHAPTER 17

# Patient Satisfaction and Health and Disease Management

Anandi V. Law, BPharm, PhD, FAACP, FAPhA;
and Mark Bounthavong, PharmD

This chapter on patient satisfaction begins with an historical perspective and then presents a conceptual framework of patient satisfaction and its measurement in health care settings. It also describes the relationship of patient satisfaction with other health care indicators such as clinical and economic outcomes before concluding with a description of the role of patient satisfaction in health and disease management.

## 1. Historical Perspective

Patient satisfaction began to gain attention in the medical and health care arena in the 1980s, around the beginning of the Outcomes Movement, which brought terms such as *accountability* and *quality* into the health care sector.[1-6] At that time, health care costs were escalating and the United States government had moved from investing financially and encouraging growth of health care facilities (between WWII and the 1960s) toward attempting to contain costs (beginning in the 1970s).[1] Managed care organizations (MCOs) and health maintenance organizations (HMOs) sprouted in the early 1980s and their dual mission of improving quality care while containing costs drove attempts to measure the cost-quality balance. These organizations realized in the 1980s and 1990s that to stay competitive and profitable, they had to develop methods to attract both individuals and large groups such as employers who were shopping for a health care provider.[5,6]

According to Pascoe, patient satisfaction is "a healthcare recipient's reaction to salient aspects of the context, process, and results of their service experience."[7] Moreover, this *reaction* stems from the patient's expectations and perception of quality, which remains a difficult concept to quantify, measure, and standardize. Unlike a consumer product, a health care service experience is intangible, perishable (it is based on recall of the service experience), and heterogeneous (in that it varies from one provider to another and the experience is viewed differently by different patients).

In other words, quality in health care depends on many subjective variables that are difficult to measure and generalize. One factor influencing health care quality is the patient's perception of quality, which can vary from one individual to another. But there is one certainty in that patients are the end user of health care and their perspectives must be included in any determination of quality. As a result, patient satisfaction is a patient-reported outcome (PRO) that is being used by many stakeholders to capture the patient's perception of health care quality.

## 2. Patient Satisfaction and Quality of Health Care

Traditional models of health care have dominated how researchers have measured patient satisfaction. These models centered on the idea that the provider was the authority and gave orders for the patient to follow.[8,9] The patient filled the passive and compliant sick role and adhered to the provider's instructions. Patient perception was largely ignored or not reported, and quality was based on how the patient responded to the physician's recommended treatment. This traditional model eventually became a liability for MCOs and HMOs once patients found themselves in a position to choose other health care delivery systems.

Patient-centered care has changed the way that health care administrators and providers view and treat patients. MCOs and HMOs can compete for a patient's business by providing statistics on their performance, but more importantly, they advertise their patient satisfaction report cards to attract potential customers.[10,11] Ware and colleagues demonstrated that patients use satisfaction scores as part of their decision-making process to select health care plans.[12] As a consequence, patients may decide to choose a plan with a high patient satisfaction score if all technical competencies are similar.[12,13] Therefore, facilities with higher scores can potentially influence the decision a patient makes when selecting a health care plan. Ware and colleagues also reported that medical facilities with high patient satisfaction were associated with higher profitability.[12] It is not surprising that health care plans continually monitor patient satisfaction to keep their patients happy, attract new patients, and maintain their business.

These same patient satisfaction reports are used not only by patients but also by employers who provide health care to their employees.[14] Although economic incentives and discounts play a large role in an employer's decision to select a health care plan for their employees, patient satisfaction reports provide meaningful data that might influence the employer's final decision. It would be unintuitive for an employer to reject a health care plan that provided good coverage and high patient satisfaction scores.

Conversely, it would also be unwise for an employer to select a health care plan that had poor coverage and low patient satisfaction scores. The health care plan with a higher patient satisfaction score could potentially sway the decision of the employer, affecting the health care plan's financial outlook. Conversely, if the health care plan has low patient satisfaction scores, competition with other plans would make the one with a lower patient satisfaction score unattractive, resulting in a loss of a potential customer. This relationship between patient satisfaction, employer decision making, and economic consequences is reflected in the study by Spanca and colleagues where consumers selected health care plans with high patient satisfaction scores even though these plans provided less coverage and cost more than plans with lower patient satisfaction scores that provided more coverage and cost less.[13] The results of this study suggest that patient satisfaction scores might supersede the benefits of increased coverage and lower costs, 2 variables that have historically been primary factors in the conventional customer's decision-making process.[13]

Further examples of the impact of patient satisfaction on economic outcomes can be demonstrated with providers who are rated highly by their patients. Providers with high patient satisfaction scores can potentially negotiate better contracts for themselves with MCOs, and advertise to patients that they are providing higher quality services than their competitors. On the other hand, dissatisfied patients could rate their providers negatively or look elsewhere to receive their health care, empowering them with the ability to choose the best plan. In some cases, enrollees of health plans are bound by the selections their employers make; however, they still have the freedom to choose a different provider within the health plan if they are dissatisfied with their experience. Providers with poor patient satisfaction ratings could find themselves at a disadvantage compared to providers with higher ratings.

The Joint Commission (previously the Joint Commission for Accreditation of Health System Organizations (JCAHO)), MCOs, and HMOs use patient satisfaction as a measurement of health care quality.[11,15,16] The Agency for Healthcare Research and Quality (AHRQ) has made available the Consumer Assessment of Healthcare Providers and Systems (CAHPS) program, which provides surveys that measure the patient's experience with health care.[15] Originally initiated under the Consumer Assessment of Health Plans Study (known as CAHPS I) in the 1990s, the program was updated as CAHPS II (2002-2007) and then again to CAHPS III. Under this version, the focus of the CAHPS program is to provide support to administer, conduct, and report the results of the surveys.[15] A unique tool in the CAHPS program is the Health Plans Survey that captures the patient's assessment of their own health care plan. The National Committee for Quality Assurance (NCQA) currently uses the CAHPS Health Plan Survey in their health care plan reports that are ultimately used for accreditation purposes.

The advent of satisfaction measures in health care has followed several shifts in paradigm: competitive marketplace in health care resulting in a drive for profitability and accountability; patient-centered care where the patient is an involved customer and decision maker rather than an uninformed and willing patient; and the role of accreditation and outcomes in health care. In addition, employers have a stake in their employees' health care and use patient satisfaction scores as an indicator of health care quality to select the best health care plan.

## 3. Framework for Patient Satisfaction

Quality in health care is a multidimensional component that is loosely based on clinical outcomes (for example, improvement in blood pressure, reduction in cholesterol, and prevention of a heart attack). However, other factors that include economic and humanistic outcomes also contribute to quality in health care. Donabedian first described health care quality as having 3 essential components: structure, process, and outcomes.[17] Structure refers to the infrastructure of any health care facility which includes buildings, personnel, environment, and tools. Process involves the operations and procedures in health delivery, such as standard operating procedures, guidelines, competency reports, and memoranda. Outcomes include the clinical, economic, and humanistic (ECHO) measurements (or patient-reported outcomes) that comprise the measurements of health care quality.[18] These 3 elements are essential in measuring the overall quality of health care; to neglect any of these components would provide an incomplete assessment.

Patient satisfaction has evolved from the basic concept of customer satisfaction to a measurable outcome with clinical and economic consequences. With patient satisfaction, we not only treat patients but also attempt to address certain satisfaction levels that the patients have established for themselves through expectations of medical care and services to which they are entitled. The disconfirmation of expectations model in customer satisfaction proposes that the difference between perceived performance ($P$) and expectation ($E$) results in dissatisfaction if $P < E$ and satisfaction, if $P \geq E$.[19] Satisfaction in medical care has been described as a multidimensional component that includes: explanation, consideration, technical competence, accessibility, financial aspects, product availability, and general satisfaction.[20,21] The traditional idea that patients are treated like customers is incomplete and requires further evaluation and measurement that includes expected outcomes and role identification of the patient as more than just a customer.

Customers are involved with business transactions in which an exchange of funds results in increased revenue for the business and a commodity for the buyer. Patient satisfaction could be similarly conceptualized in that it deals with the care and service provided in relation to health care. In the past, the business model of customer service was applied where patients were treated as customers and health care was purchased. However, the field has moved away from that model and has instead adopted a patient-centered model. Johnson and colleagues defined patient-centered care as "a construct that advocates simplifying the care at the bedside in the acute care setting by focusing on the expected outcomes for the patient rather than the multiplicity of tasks of each department."[22]

A patient-focused approach should produce an efficient and effective system to provide quality health care to patients rather than burden them with unnecessary nonclinical essentials such as making appointments, travel, and costs. Moreover, patient satisfaction should measure the patient's experience, which includes both the clinical and nonclinical aspects of health care. For example, patient satisfaction with pharmacy services has shifted from measuring the business components, such as costs, wait times, and convenience, to more cognitive features of a patient's experience, such as patient understanding, patient empowerment, and pharmacist competency or knowledge.[23-25]

## 4. Measurement of Patient Satisfaction in Health Care

Health care assessments based solely on the technical aspects of care do not capture the patient perspective, creating a gap in the measurement of patient satisfaction. According to Ware and colleagues, patient satisfaction can encompass the characteristics of the providers, their services, and expectations of care.[21]

In developing patient satisfaction instruments, it is important to realize that instruments used to measure patient satisfaction are not universal and specific elements are only applicable to the research question(s) being studied.[21] Therefore, the context of the research should drive the type of patient satisfaction instrument used and, if necessary, direct researchers to develop novel instruments to fit the design and purpose of the research question(s). For example, when measuring patient satisfaction with different providers, an instrument will have to include questions that are unique to each encounter. The following section will describe the development of instruments that measure patient satisfaction in different contexts.

## Measurement of Patient Satisfaction with Services

### Clinician Services

Ware and colleagues identified 4 primary dimensions of patient satisfaction with physician services: physician conduct, availability of services, continuity and convenience of care, and access mechanisms.[26] Physician conduct was correlated with items that pertained to caring (labeled as humanness) and cure (labeled as quality and competence). Quality and competence included items that focused on providing important information, thoroughness in information gathering, preventative measures, and prudence (avoiding patient risk); humanness included items that focused on reassurance, consideration, and courtesy.

Availability of care focused on areas of medical resources in the forms of hospitals, specialists, family doctors, and office facilities that are readily available. Continuity and convenience of care were associated with coordination of services and the presence of a regular family doctor. Access mechanisms were strongly associated with the financial aspects of medical care (for example, cost, insurance, and payment mechanisms) and availability of emergency care. These dimensions of patient attitudes represent the current approach to measuring patient satisfaction with physician services in the literature, further supporting the idea that patient satisfaction is a multidimensional concept and cannot be simplified or based solely on clinical outcomes.

Research in patient satisfaction with providers has also included nurses.[27] Grogan and colleagues developed an instrument, the Patient Satisfaction Questionnaire (PSQ), to measure patient satisfaction with general practitioners' services that relied on previous research, and added an additional dimension to include an assessment of nurses.[27] The instrument includes 5 subscales (doctors, access, nurses, appointment, and facilities) and provides an instrument that captures the patient's perception of health care quality.[28] Research in patient satisfaction with medical services revealed a complex relationship between providers, nurses, and patients' expectation of the service they expect and receive.

## Pharmacy Services

Patient satisfaction measurements in the field of pharmacy were initially based on business components and physical facilities.[29] As pharmacy shifted to a more cognitive patient-focused profession, patient satisfaction measurements evolved to include pharmacist services. Several instruments measuring patient satisfaction with pharmacist services have been developed and validated.[28-30] MacKeigan and Larson[24] developed a patient satisfaction questionnaire using a framework similar to the one previously proposed by Ware.[21] The instrument is a 44-item Likert scale tool that measures 9 dimensions of patient satisfaction: access to care, availability, continuity with the pharmacy, interpersonal manner, technical competence, finances, efficacy of medication, general satisfaction, and satisfaction with medical care.[24] A shorter version of this instrument focuses on specific elements of pharmaceutical care.[25]

Researchers have identified 2 primary dimensions of this survey from factor analysis: friendly explanation (including items related to friendliness of care, the setting of care, and medication counseling) and managing therapy (items dealing with the concept of pharmaceutical care-managing drug therapy and solving therapy problems).[25] Gourley and colleagues developed and validated the Pharmaceutical Care Satisfaction Questionnaire (PCSQ), a 30-item instrument measuring consumer satisfaction with pharmacy services.[23] Table 1 provides applications of these instruments.

That many patient satisfaction instruments have been developed so quickly underscores the importance of properly measuring all the components in patient satisfaction with pharmacist services. These also reflect the expansion of the role of the pharmacist, who is currently gravitating towards a primary care role in the outpatient setting where medication therapy management (MTM) and disease state management (DSM) programs will need evaluations of clinical and patient-reported outcomes. A review of patient satisfaction instruments for pharmacist services in health and disease management (HDM) reflects that, with the exception of the 2 mentioned above, each of these instruments has been developed and used for specific health conditions in specific settings, and rarely validated or replicated.

## Emergence of Patient Satisfaction as an Objective Measurement of Quality Health Care

Objective measurements of the quality of health care should encompass the ECHO model in a health care intervention or service. As part of the humanistic outcomes, patient satisfaction represents the patient's perceived quality of health care received. Patient satisfaction emerged as an objective measurement to assess the value of an intervention, to identify patient characteristics that appear to influence quality assessment, and for health plans and hospitals to assess the satisfaction of their members or patients with their services. Reports on patient satisfaction can be used to monitor and improve service in order to maintain patient enrollment.

But, more importantly, patient satisfaction reporting can provide a way for patients and other key players to compare grades between health plans. For example, the Center for Medicare & Medicaid Services has provided patients with the ability to compare hospitals based on the experiences of former patients using a standardized instrument.[30] The Hospital Compare Website can be accessed through the Department of Health and Human Services and has information on former patients' experiences with different aspects of the hospital where they were treated.[30] This provides some transparency between different hospitals that are reported by the actual end users of the system.

Patients or consumers of the system are provided access to patient satisfaction scores, which provide comparative assessments between hospitals that can be used to assist with their decision making. Hence, hospitals must address the perceptions of their patients to be competitive in a market that is patient focused. The emergence of patient satisfaction as an objective measurement has transformed health care into a value-based system where patients compare and evaluate their experiences with various hospitals, resulting in quality improvement and accountability.

## 5. Relationship between Patient Satisfaction and Clinical Outcomes

Exploration into patient satisfaction occurred as early as the 1950s and 1960s and has evolved into a major component of the patient's overall care.[31,32] Initially, researchers could not find sufficient evidence to demonstrate a direct relationship between patient satisfaction and clinical efficacy. Edwards and colleagues reported no association between satisfaction and success of treatment.[33] Furthermore, Francis and colleagues reported that patients' rating of their satisfaction was not related to a therapist's ratings of success.[34]

The most recent evidence suggests that increased patient satisfaction is strongly associated with increased adherence to therapy and treatment regimens.[35-38] Patients who have higher satisfaction have an increased potential to be more adherent with their medication(s). Although Edwards and colleagues demonstrated that providers and patients do not view health care in the same way, it leaves open the possibility that patient satisfaction is a component of health care quality despite this disparity in the patient and physician viewpoints.[33] According to Press, patient satisfaction is not only a component of quality of care, but also an indicator that should be a measured.[39] As confirmation, Tan and colleagues found a relationship between patient satisfaction and treatment outcome measures.[40]

A study by Willson and McNamara demonstrated that patients based their satisfaction on physician courtesy and competency, which in turn, affected their compliance.[37] Satisfaction was strongly correlated with perceived courtesy of the physician, moderately associated with perceived competence of the physician, and slightly related to compliance.[8] Patients who disagreed with their providers were more likely to be noncompliant and several studies have shown that decreased adherence is associated with worsening of clinical outcomes.[41-43] This relationship between adherence/compliance and clinical outcomes is dependent on patient satisfaction. Clinical outcomes are in part dependent on compliance which, in turn, is dependent on patient satisfaction. As a result, increasing or maintaining patient satisfaction is important to achieving positive clinical outcomes.

## 6. Patient Satisfaction Measurement in Health and Disease Management

Health care plans initially developed HDM programs to control costs while maintaining quality; however Bodenheimer warns that HDM programs operated by pharmaceutical companies may lead to increased overall total direct costs due to the obvious bias associated with such sponsors.[44] To maintain impartiality, HDM programs should operate without the influence of external factors that may potentially contribute to the final treatment decision.

Although clinical and economic outcomes take precedence in evaluations of HDM programs, patient satisfaction has become an important secondary end point for much HDM program research. However, there are no validated instruments to measure patient satisfaction in disease-specific HDM programs, with the exception of diabetes. Moreover, the lack of instruments to measure patient satisfaction in HDM programs makes it difficult to evaluate these programs for patients.

In a study by Sen and colleagues, HDM programs that use patient satisfaction instruments find them to be of value; 47% of respondents reported that it was very important and 31% of respondents reported that it was important.[45] However, 22% of respondents reported that it was very unimportant in regard to the long-term success of these programs.[45] Greater emphasis on patient satisfaction is needed to measure the patient perception of care they receive from the HDM programs but, more importantly, patient satisfaction should be an outcome that decision makers weigh along with clinical and economic outcomes when deciding whether or not to fund or continue HDM programs. Ignoring this critical component of health care quality would eventually lead to an HDM program whose interest is in saving money rather than improving a patient's perception of their care—which is not always concordant with what their providers believe.[33]

A limitation of using patient satisfaction as an outcome measure in HDM programs is the paucity of validated instruments available for specific chronic diseases. The literature currently has validated patient satisfaction instruments for only diabetes;[46-48] very little is available for other chronic conditions. Likewise, the pharmacy literature has various instances of short patient satisfaction surveys developed specifically for a clinic that are generally not validated beyond the study and hence not commonly used.[49-51]

Most of the instruments used in the literature appear to be basic, mailed surveys that vary in their questions and response categories. In addition, a literature review conducted in 2004 found that "with the exception of diabetes disease management, there are no prevalent, systematic, or statistically validated approaches for measuring patient satisfaction within the disease management industry."[45] Discussion about developing a standardized patient satisfaction instrument for HDM programs proved unfruitful because of the subjectivity of the concept and uniqueness of different chronic conditions.

One of the challenges with patient satisfaction research is the limited exposure it has garnered in the development of HDM programs. As mentioned before, clinical and economic consequences are valued moreso than patient perspectives because newly developed programs are often funded with temporary funding limited to a specific timeline or set of outcomes. Notable outcomes include: reduction in blood pressure, decrease in glycosylated hemoglobin (HbA1c), prevention of a myocardial infarction, or reduction in mortality rates. Other outcomes include the measurement of benefit usually in the form of a cost-benefit analysis in which benefits are represented as monetary units. Attention to patient satisfaction is neglected, because the outcomes reported are unintuitive to decision makers. For example, the true meaning of an overall patient satisfaction score of 80% is unknown. Moreover, the lack of standardization across different instruments prevents HDM programs from using patient satisfaction score as a benchmark, making it difficult to compare and determine health care quality.

In the future, HDM programs should establish a standardized patient satisfaction instrument for different programs with different diseases to capture this integral element of Donabedian's framework. The absence of one of these elements will only explain a part of health care quality and will prevent us from progressing into a more global evaluation of HDM programs. The CAHPS is nearly a standardized patient satisfaction instrument. However, its primary limitations are related to one of its primary advantages—it is general and may not capture the nuances of specific diseases.

## 7. Conclusion

The conceptualization of patient satisfaction in health care has moved from a previous business model borrowed from consumer behavior literature to one based on a patient-focused model. Patient satisfaction in HDM programs is critical to overall health care quality but is limited by its availability and interest. There has not been a generally accepted conceptualization, and subsequently, a review of literature on patient satisfaction in health care indicates a need for a standardized instrument that can be used across settings, diseases, and providers.[52]

Current patient satisfaction instruments are mostly not validated or standardized. Furthermore, there are recommendations that patient satisfaction should be conceptualized as a method to improve compliance, which in turn can improve medical outcomes, in addition to being viewed as an outcome by itself.[45] The lack of standardization makes it difficult to compare the health care quality of HDM programs and limits the value of these patient satisfaction instruments in HDM evaluation. Developing standardized instruments should be an important goal for the future.

## References:

1. Mahar M. *Money-Driven Medicine: The Real Reason Health Care Costs So Much*. New York, NY: HarperCollins; 2006.
2. Donabedian A. The quality of care: how can it be assessed? *JAMA*. 1988;260:1743-1748.
3. Zastowny TR, Roghman KJ, Hengst A. Satisfaction with medical care: replications and theoretic reevaluation. *Med Care*. 1983;21:294-322.
4. Cleary PD, McNeil BJ. Patient satisfaction as an indicator of quality care. *Inquiry*. 1988;25:25-36.
5. Schulman KA, Johnson AE, Rathore SS. The use of satisfaction measures in oncology. In: Perry MC, ed. *Educational Book*. Denver, CO: American Society of Clinical Oncology; 1997: 337-341.
6. Epstein AM. The outcomes movement—will it get us where we want to go? *N Engl J Med*. 1990;323:266-270.
7. Pascoe GC. Patient satisfaction in primary care: a literature review and analysis. *Eval Prog Plan*. 1983;6:185-210.
8. Willson P, McNamara JR. How perceptions of a simulated physician-patient interaction influence intended satisfaction and compliance. *Soc Sci Med*. 1982;16:1699-1704.
9. Huag M, Lavin B. Practioner or patient—who's in charge? *J Health Soc Behav*. 1981;22:212-229.
10. Hillman AL, Goldfard N. Exemplary quality improvement programs in HMOs. *J Qual Improv*. 1995;21:457-464.
11. Bolus R, Pitts J. Patient satisfaction: the indispensible outcome. *Managed Care*. 1999: 8:24-28.
12. Ware JE, Davies AR. Behavioral consequences of consumer dissatisfaction with medical care. *Eval Program Plann*. 1983;6:291-297.
13. Spranca M, Kanouse DE, Elliott M, Short PF, Farley DO, Hays RD. Do consumer reports of health plan quality affect health plan selection? *Health Serv Res*. 2000;35(5 pt 1):933-947.
14. Chernew M, Gowrisankaran G, McLaughlin C, Gibson T. Quality and employers' choice of health plans. *J Health Econ*. 2004;23:471-492.
15. Agency for Healthcare Research and Quality (AHRQ). CAHPS: Assessing HealthCare Quality from the Patient's Perspective program brief. Washington, DC: AHRQ Publication No. 08-PB015; October2008.
16. Morales LS, Elliot M, Brown J, Rahn C, Hays RD. The applicability of the Consumer Assessments of Health Plans Survey (CAHPS) to preferred provider organizations in the United States: a discussion of industry concerns. *Int J Qual Health Care*. 2004;16(3):219-227.
17. Donabedian A. Evaluating the quality of medical care. *Milbank Mem Fund Q*. 1966;44:166-206.
18. Kozma CM, Reeder CE, Schulz RM. Economic, clinical, and humanistic outcomes: a planning model for pharmacoeconomic research. *Clin Ther*. 1993;16(6):1121-1132.
19. Kamins MA, Assael H. Moderating disconfirmation of expectations through the use of two-sided appeals: a longitudinal approach. *J Econ Psychol*. 1987;8:237-253.

20. Larson LN, MacKeigan LD. Further validation of an instrument to measure patient satisfaction with pharmacy services. *J Pharm Market Manage*. 1994;8:125-139.
21. Ware JE Jr, Snyder MK, Wright WR, Davies AR. Defining and measuring patient satisfaction with medical care. *Eval Program Plann*. 1983;6:247-263.
22. Johnson CL, Cooper PK. Patient-focused care: what is it? *Holist Nurs Pract*. 1997;11:1-7.
23. Gourley GK, Gourley DR, La Monica Rigolosi E, Reed P, Solomon DK, Washington E. Development and validation of the pharmaceutical care satisfaction questionnaire. *Am J Manag Care*. 2001;7:461-466.
24. MacKeigan LD, Larson LN. Development and validation of an instrument to measure patient satisfaction with pharmacy services. *Med Care*. 1989;27:522-536.
25. Larson LN, Rovers JP, MacKeigan LD. Patient satisfaction with pharmaceutical care: update of a validated instrument. *J Am Pharm Assoc* (Wash). 2002;42:44-50.
26. Ware JE Jr, Snyder MK. Dimensions of patient attitudes regarding doctors and medical care services. *Med Care*. 1975;13(8):669-682.
27. Grogan S, Conner M, Willits D, Norman P. Development of a questionnaire to measure patients' satisfaction with general practitioners' services. *Br J Gen Pract*. 1995;45:525-529.
28. Grogan S, Conner M, Norman P, Willits D, Porter I. Validation of a questionnaire measuring patient satisfaction with general practitioner services. *Qual HealthCare*. 2000;9:210-215.
29. Druss BG, Rosecheck RA, Stolar M. Patient satisfaction and administrative measures as indicators of the quality of mental health care. *Psychiatr Serv*. 1999;50(8):1053-1058.
30. United States Department of Health and Human Services. Hospital Compare website tool. Available at: http://www.hospitalcompare.hhs.gov. Accessed July 8, 2009.
31. Parsons T. *The Social System*. Glencoe, IL: Free Press; 1951.
32. Szasz T, Hollender M. A contribution to the philosophy of medicine: the basic model of doctor-patient relationship. *Arch Intern Med*. 1956;97:585.
33. Edwards DW, Yarvis RM, Mueller DP, Langsley DG. Does patient satisfaction correlate with success? *Hosp Community Psychiatry*. March 1978;29:188-190.
34. Francis V, Korsch B, Morris M. Gaps in doctor-patient communication. *N Engl J Med*. 1969;280:535-540.
35. Aharony L, Strasser S. Patient satisfaction: what we know about and what we still need to explore. *Med Care Res Rev*. 1993;50:49-79.
36. Gu NY, Gai Y, Hay JW. The effect of patient satisfaction with pharmacist consultation on medication adherence: an instrumental variable approach. *Pharmacy Practice* 2008;6:201-210. http://redalyc.uaemex.mx/pdf/690/69011553006.pdf; Accessed February 7. 2009.
37. Willson P, McNamara JR. How perceptions of a simulated physician-patient interaction influence intended satisfaction and compliance. *Soc Sci Med*. 1982;16:1699-1704.
38. Hardy GE, West MA, Hill F. Components and predictors of patient satisfaction. *Bt J Health Psychol*. 1996;1:65-85.
39. Press I. *Patient Satisfaction: Understanding and Managing the Experience of Care*. 2nd ed. Chicago, IL: Health Administration Press; 2006.
40. Tan G, Jensen MP, Thornby JI, Anderson KO. Are patient ratings of chronic pain services related to treatment outcome? *J Rehabil Res Dev*. 2006;43:451-460.
41. Cole JA, Norman H, Weatherby LB, Walker AM. Drug copayment and adherence in chronic heart failure: effect on cost and outcomes. *Pharmacotherapy*. 2006;26:1157-1164.
42. Schultz JS, O'Donnell C, McDonough KL, Sasane R, Meyer J. Determinants of compliance with statin therapy and low-density lipoprotein cholesterol goal attainment in a managed care population. *Am J Manag Care*. 2005;11:306-321.
43. Cherry SB, Benner JS, Hussein MA, Tang SSK, Nichol MB. The clinical and economic burden on nonadherence with antihypertensive and lipid-lowering therapy in hypertensive patients. *Value Health*. 2009;12:489-497.
44. Bodenheimer T. Disease management-promises and pitfalls. *N Engl J Med*. 1999;340:1202-1205.
45. Sen S, Fawson P, Cherrington G, et al. Patient satisfaction measurement in the disease management industry. *Dis Manag*. 2005;8:288-300.

46. Krass I, Delaney C, Glaubitz S, Kanjanarach T. Measuring patient satisfaction with diabetes disease state management services in community pharmacy. *Res Social Adm Pharm.* 2009;5:31-39.
47. Ahlgren SS, Shultz JA, Massey LK, Hicks BC, Wysham C. Development of a preliminary diabetes dietary satisfaction and outcomes measure for patients with type 2 diabetes. *Qual Life Res.* 2004;13:819-832.
48. Charron-Prochownik D, Zgibor JC, Peyrot M, et al. The Diabetes Self-management Assessment Report Tool (D-SMART): process evaluation and patient satisfaction. *AADE/UPMC Diabetes Education Outcomes Project Diabetes Educ.* 2007;33:833-838.
49. Shibley MC, Pugh CB. Implementation of pharmaceutical care services for patients with hyperlipidemias by independent community pharmacy practitioners. *Ann Pharmacother.* 1997;31:713-719.
50. Stergachis A, Gardner JS, Anderson MT, Sullivan SD. Improving pediatric asthma outcomes in the community setting: does pharmaceutical care make a difference? *J Am Pharm Assoc* (Wash). 2002;42:743-752.
51. Moultry AM, Poon IO. Perceived value of a home-based medication therapy management program for the elderly. *Consult Pharm.* 2008;23:877-885.
52. Fitzner K, Fox K, Schmidt J, Roberts M, Rindress D, Hay J. Implementation and outcomes of commercial disease management programs in the United States: the disease management outcomes consolidation survey. *Dis Manag.* 2005;8:253-264.

Part 3: Patient-Reported Outcomes

**TABLE 1.** Patient Satisfaction Instruments for Different Services in Health Care

| | Citation | Service specialty | Instrument type | Description |
|---|---|---|---|---|
| Physicians | Van der Feltz-Cornelis CM, Van Oppen P, Van Marwijk HW, De Beurs E, Van Dyck R. A patient-doctor relationship questionnaire (PDRQ-9) in primary care: development and psychometric evaluation. *Gen Hosp Psychiatry* 2004;26(2):115-20. | Patient-doctor relationship | PDRQ-9 | 2 factors (9 items):<br>1. Doctor<br>2. Medical symptoms of patient |
| | Marcinowicz L, Chlabicz S, Grebowski R. Patient satisfaction with health care provided by family doctors: primary dimensions and an attempt at typology. *BMC Health Serv Res* 2009 16;9:6. | Family doctors | Qualitative study to identify dimensions of patient satisfaction. | 5 dimensions:<br>1. Assessment of personality features<br>2. Assessment of competences<br>3. Assessment of doctor-patient interactions<br>4. Contextual factors<br>5. General assessment |
| | Ware JE Jr, Snyder MK. Dimensions of patient attitudes regarding doctors and medical care services. *Med Care.* August 1975;13(8):669-682. | Doctors and Medical Care Services | 80-item instrument | 4 factors (80 items):<br>1. Physician conduct (humanness and quality)<br>2. Availability of services<br>3. Continuity/Convenience of care<br>4. Access mechanisms (cost, payment mechanisms, and ease of emergency care) |
| | Grogan S, Conner M, Willits D, Norman P. Development of a questionnaire to measure patients' satisfaction with general practitioners' services. *Br J Gen Pract.* 1995;45:525-529. | General Practitioners | 148-item instrument | The results of the principal component analysis resulted in an instrument with 40 items total with good factor loading in 5 factors:<br>1. Doctors<br>2. Access<br>3. Nurses<br>4. Appointments<br>5. Facilities |

*continued >*

< continued from previous page

**TABLE 1.** Patient Satisfaction Instruments for Different Services in Health Care

| | Citation | Service specialty | Instrument type | Description |
|---|---|---|---|---|
| Physicians | Grogan S, Conner M, Norman P, Willits D, Porter I. Validation of a questionnaire measuring patient satisfaction with general practitioner services. *Qual HealthCare.* 2000;9:210-215. | General Practitioners | Patient Satisfaction Questionnaire (PSQ) | 5 factors (40 items):<br>1. Doctors<br>2. Access<br>3. Nurses<br>4. Appointments<br>5. Facilities |
| Pharmacists | Gourley GK, Gourley DR, La Monica Rigolosi E, Reed P, Solomon DK, Washington E. Development and validation of the pharmaceutical care satisfaction questionnaire. *Am J Manag Care.* 2001;7:461-466. | Pharmacy Services | Pharmaceutical Care Satisfaction Questionnaire (PCSQ) | 4 subscales (20 items):<br>1. Patient understanding<br>2. Provision of pharmaceutical care<br>3. Patient empowerment<br>4. Pharmacist-Patient relations |
| | MacKeigan LD, Larson LN. Development and validation of an instrument to measure patient satisfaction with pharmacy services. *Med Care.* 1989;27:522-536. | Pharmacy Services | Patient Satisfaction with Pharmacy Services Questionnaire (PSPSQ) | 10 scales (40 items):<br>1. Explanation<br>2. Consideration<br>3. Technical competence<br>4. Financial aspects<br>5. Accessibility<br>6. Efficacy of medications<br>7. OTC availability<br>8. Drug quality<br>9. General satisfaction<br>10. Continuity with the pharmacy |
| | Larson LN, Rovers JP, MacKeigan LD. Patient satisfaction with pharmaceutical care: update of a validated instrument. *J Am Pharm Assoc* (Wash). 2002;42:44-50. | Pharmacy Services | 20-item instrument | 2 dimensions (20 items):<br>1. Friendly explanation<br>2. Managed therapy |

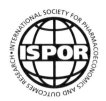

# PART 4

## Alternative, Population-Based Data Sources

CHAPTER 18  Introduction to Alternative, Population-Based Data Sources... 223

CHAPTER 19  Medical Expenditure Panel Survey Data from the Agency for Healthcare Research and Quality ................... 225

CHAPTER 20  Survey Data Sources from the National Center for Health Statistics ............................................................. 239

CHAPTER 21  Healthcare Cost and Utilization Project (HCUP) ..................... 255

CHAPTER 22  Medicare Databases ................................................................. 281

CHAPTER 23  Veterans Health Administration ........................................... 290

CHAPTER 24  The Role of Patient Registries ............................................... 298

CHAPTER 25  Randomized Controlled Trial Data ........................................ 315

CHAPTER 26  Genetics Databases ................................................................. 323

CHAPTER 18

# Introduction to Alternative, Population-Based Data Sources

Christopher R. Frei, PharmD, MSc

Complementing and supplementing the sources of data presented in Parts 1 through 3, alternative, population-based data sources provide rich information that can be used to help plan and evaluate health and disease management programs. This section characterizes several common, population-based data sources from health insurance payers, national surveys, and direct study of patients to provide basic information regarding the utility of each for health and disease management. Each chapter provides an overview, description, and purpose for each data source, and assists the reader in understanding the complexity of these data sources and how the individual components are interrelated. Moreover, the authors provide examples of how these data can be used for health and disease management. Data sources are grouped into 4 primary categories: payers, surveys, patients, and other (see Figure 1).

**Figure 1.** Alternative, Population-Based Data Sources Available for Health and Disease Management*

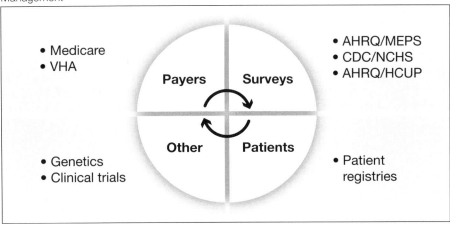

*VHA, Veterans Health Administration; AHRQ, Agency for Healthcare Research and Quality; MEPS, Medical Expenditure Panel Survey; CDC, Centers for Disease Control and Prevention; NCHS, National Center for Health Statistics; HCUP, Healthcare Cost and Utilization Project.

Chapters 19, 20, and 21 describe national surveys conducted by the United States government through its Agency for Healthcare Research and Quality (AHRQ) and Centers for Disease Control and Prevention (CDC), and how they may provide in-

## Part 4: Alternative, Population-Based Data Sources

formation for the study of health and disease management. These national surveys contain data from a variety of health care settings including outpatient physicians' office visits and inpatient hospital stays. Health care encounters are generally eligible for survey inclusion regardless of disease state or health care payer. The chapters further highlight surveys that contain information about medication use and dispensing.

Chapters 22 and 23 describe data obtained from public health care payers in the United States. Data that can be publicly accessed from the Centers for Medicare & Medicaid Services (CMS) and Veterans Health Administration (VHA) programs are described, as are the implications for external validity when data from these programs are used to extrapolate findings to other populations. Each of these programs maintains multiple data sources that can be integrated to provide a relatively comprehensive description of the care and outcomes experienced by the patients covered by each system.

Chapter 24 describes the use of data obtained directly from patients through patient registry studies in evaluating health and disease management. The authors concentrate on the most common type of registries, those established to monitor product safety and, more recently, to examine comparative-effectiveness of health care interventions. The authors provide guidance for registry development and health and disease applications of patient registry data.

The last 2 chapters describe the utility of data obtained from randomized controlled trials (RCT) (Chapter 25) and those procured through databases that contain genetic information (Chapter 26). The RCT chapter discusses the need for additional outcomes measurement in RCTs to better inform studies of health outcomes and disease management. The authors debate the strengths and limitations of such data as compared to observational data. The genetics chapter highlights the application of databases from the SNP Health Association Resource (SHARe) Project, a major epidemiological genetics initiative by the US National Institutes of Health (NIH). Current perspectives and future challenges for genetics databases that are to be used for health and disease management are discussed in this chapter.

CHAPTER 19

# Medical Expenditure Panel Survey Data from the Agency for Healthcare Research and Quality

Jayashri Sankaranarayanan, MPharm, PhD; Mariam K. Hassan, BPharm, PhD; and Teresa Hartman, MLS

Important goals of the United States' health care system are to achieve and maintain an efficient system that provides high quality care while keeping costs of care low and maintaining access to care.[1] To understand the impact of health and disease management programs that balance access, cost and quality, researchers and policy makers need accurate, nationally representative data on health care use, expenditures, insurance coverage and access to health care. One existing organization that meets the need for such data is the Agency for Healthcare Research and Quality (AHRQ), which sponsors a series of national medical expenditure surveys.[2]

This chapter provides a brief description of AHRQ and its databases with a specific focus on the Medical Expenditure Panel Survey (MEPS)—a national survey and a comprehensive resource on health care use, spending (cost), insurance coverage, and accessibility of care. MEPS components, sampling, survey design and data collection procedures yield reliable and nationally representative data for researchers and policy makers involved in developing and evaluating health and disease management programs. Since year 2003, AHRQ and the Department of Health and Human Services (HHS) have produced the National Health Quality Report (NHQR) and the National Health Disparities Report (NHDR) yearly using data that include the MEPS data[2-6] to inform stakeholders about quality of care and disparities in health and disease management.

This chapter begins with a description of the AHRQ and its databases. After that, we describe the 4 major components (household, insurance, medical provider, nursing home) of MEPS data. Next, data availability and examples of published studies are discussed to show how MEPS data can be used to inform evaluations of health and disease management programs. Finally, strengths and limitations of using MEPS data for health and disease management research are reviewed. Because information on these databases is updated periodically, we suggest readers refer to www.meps.ahrq.gov for additional details.

## 1. The Agency for Healthcare Research and Quality

AHRQ is one of 12 agencies within the Department of Health and Human Services (HHS) in the US. Its goal is to improve all aspects and outcomes of care in clinical practice through use of evidence-based medicine, health information technology and comparative effectiveness research. Specifically, AHRQ strives to use research to document quality, safety, and efficiency to improve the cost-effectiveness and efficiency of delivering health care. The research supported and sponsored by AHRQ focuses on the organization and delivery of care, use of health care resources, health care costs and financing, and public health readiness within the health care system.[7]

To implement its mission, AHRQ carries out and supports health services research within the agency as well as in external settings across the US, including leading academic institutions, hospitals, doctors' offices, and health care systems at the national, state, and local market levels. AHRQ-sponsored research provides evidence-based information on health care access, use, costs, outcomes, and quality. The resulting information aids health care decision makers—patients and clinicians, health system leaders, purchasers, and policy makers—make more informed decisions toward supporting the stated mission and underlying goals.[7]

## 2. Agency for Healthcare Research and Quality Databases

AHRQ sponsors 4 databases: the Healthcare Cost and Utilization Project (HCUP), HIV and AIDS Costs and Use, US Health Information Knowledgebase (USHIK) and MEPS.[8] Chapter 21 provides details of HCUP, which is a longitudinal database on hospital care in US. The HIV and AIDS Costs and Use database consists of patient interview and medical records data from the AIDS Cost and Services Utilization Survey (ACSUS), a longitudinal study of HIV and AIDS patients.[8] The USHIK database consists of definitions of data elements and other information needed for cataloging and sharing information across databases and organizations.[8] The MEPS database is sponsored by AHRQ along with the National Center for Health Statistics (NCHS) and is discussed in detail in this chapter. Federal, state, and local health care decision makers often use evidence from the national survey databases of AHRQ—MEPS and HCUP, in particular—to benchmark cost, quality and access to care in the delivery of health and disease management in the US.[6,8]

### Historical Background of Earlier Surveys and Medical Expenditure Panel Survey

The impetus for the launch of MEPS in the 1990s began in the 1970s when the characteristics of the US population and the structure and delivery of health care services, private insurance, and federal health care programs started changing. During this time, several surveys were launched to collect data on medical spending. In 1977, the National Center for Health Services Research conducted the National Medical Care Expenditure Survey (NMCES). The NMCES consisted of a household survey, a physician survey, and an employer health insurance survey. In 1987, the NMCES had about 16,000 respondents, including those from American Indian and Alaskan Native households. In addition to household information, a survey of medical and health insurance providers used by the household respondents was added to the household information. The MEPS database was launched in its current form by AHRQ in 1996.

## Major Medical Expenditure Panel Survey Components

MEPS are a set of publicly available, ongoing, large-scale national surveys of families and individuals from a nationally representative sample of US households, their medical providers (doctors, hospitals, pharmacies, and other providers), and employers. MEPS surveys Americans on the costs (including that of health insurance), use frequency, and method of payment for coverage of health care services.[5]

MEPS consist of 4 surveys: the Household Component (HC), the Medical Provider Component (MPC), the Insurance Component (IC) and the Nursing Home Component (NHC). Table 1 summarizes key information from the various components of MEPS data. To appreciate how AHRQ ensures reliability, national representativeness, and high survey response rates in MEPS data, the steps taken by AHRQ to choose sample and design the survey components as well as the sample sizes of and response rates of each MEPS component are described below.

### Medical Expenditure Panel Survey Household Component

*Sample*

The MEPS-HC survey collects data from a sample of households that took part in the previous year's National Health Interview Survey (NHIS) conducted by the NCHS, which is a part of Centers for Disease Control and Prevention. The NHIS monitors the progress of the US in achieving health goals by tracking health care status and access to care.[9] The MEPS-HC survey sample aims to be representative of the nation, which enables national and regional estimates of health service use outcomes that can be generalized to the broader US population. Families and individuals in MEPS-HC participate voluntarily through 5 rounds of telephone interviews that use computer-assisted personal interviewing technology and self-administered mail surveys to collect information.[2]

To encourage high response rates to the interviews and surveys, a respondent receives an incentive for participating in and completing each of the 5 rounds of interviews. The HC sample size included upwards of 15,000 families and 35,000 individuals in 2008. To permit analysis of policy-relevant groups that may be underrepresented in the sample, the MEPS-HC panel explicitly oversamples respondents from Hispanic, African American, Asian, and low income households so that they are represented in the data. Another subgroup that is oversampled is that most likely to incur high medical spending, as determined based on their characteristics in the previous year as measured in the NHIS.[2]

## Part 4: Alternative, Population-Based Data Sources

*Survey Design*

MEPS-HC uses a panel design of sample households scientifically selected to join the study over time. To provide overlapping panels of survey data, each year MEPS-HC selects a new panel or sample of US households that took part in the previous year's NHIS. The smallest sampling unit of MEPS is the household from which all individuals are surveyed. Each individual household, once included in the survey, remains in the survey for up to 2 years.

*Data Collected*

The careful sampling and survey design gave an overall response rate for MEPS-HC of about 78% in 1996, 64% in 2008 and 59% in 2010.[2,10] MEPS response rate is considered conditional for each round because the rate applies to the set of households, known as residential units (RUs), that qualifies for MEPS for that round. Therefore, the response rate is conditional, and calculated with the number of RUs that responded in the earlier round as the denominator, and is not the overall response rate. Response rates for rounds 2 to 5 have been over 90% conditional on participation in earlier rounds.

For the MEPS-HC, household members are interviewed about their employment, income, health-related status, conditions, access to care, and satisfaction with care (Table 1). The survey is made up of 49 sections including sections on access to care, preventive care, caregiver information, child preventive health, health status, and medical provider visits.[11] The access to health care section of the survey lends itself to policy discussions in health and disease management. This survey section tracks individuals' information on primary language, identification and satisfaction with health care providers, and reasons why usual providers or access to treatments were not available. Further, to collect information on assessments of patient experiences with quality of health care received from a patient's perspective, the MEPS-HC in 2000 included the self-administered questionnaire (SAQ).[12]

For this purpose, the SAQ consists of quality of care measures present in the Consumer Assessments of Health Plans (CAHPS®). The CAHPS is an AHRQ-sponsored instrument that includes questions on smoking and blood pressure as well as experiences with getting an appointment.[13] To improve the survey's capacity to measure health status, the MEPS-HC also includes a series of questions from the SF-12 (Short Form with 12 items), a generic quality-of-life survey covering the physical and mental health status domains and the EQ-5D (European Health Related Quality of Life with 5 dimensions, also known as the EuroQol) health preference measure.[14] Another series of questions about specific health conditions is designed to identify treatment prescribed and whether or not it followed practice guidelines.[14]

## Medical Expenditure Panel Survey Insurance Component

In 1994, the National Employer Health Insurance Survey (NEHIS) was carried out by the NCHS and was the impetus for the MEPS-IC. The NEHIS was designed to estimate the state- and national-level costs and coverage of health insurance paid for employees by employers. The MEPS-IC (recognized as the Health Insurance Cost Study) began surveying employers about their health insurance offerings in 1997.[15,16]

*Sample and Survey Design*

The MEPS-IC is an annual panel survey of private and public sector employers, the self-employed with no employees, unions, and other sources. It was designed to collect data on employer-based health insurance information.[2] The MEPS-IC sample could include more than one establishment from the same firm. MEPS defines an *establishment* as "a particular workplace or location and a firm as a business entity consisting of one or more business establishments under common ownership or control."[2] A nationally representative sample of employers from private and government sectors developed from the Census Bureau list is used for the IC survey and tables of estimates.

*Data Collected*

For the IC, the US Census Bureau collects data from the sampled organizations. To ensure high responses to the data collection efforts within budgeted costs, first each organization is contacted through a telephone interview, then mailed a survey, and followed up with if they do not respond. The response rates of private and state (and local) governmental establishments from 1996 to 2009 were 67-88% and 81-82%, respectively.[2] The high response rates indicate that the survey data are representative of the noninstitutionalized US population. The IC represents national and state data on the various health insurance plans available from employers. For this purpose, the IC data for every organization include characteristics of employer, employee eligibility criteria, number and type of available private insurance plans, premiums, amounts paid by employers and employees, and benefits of these plans.[2]

## Medical Expenditure Panel Survey Medical Provider Component

The accuracy of medical expenditure estimates from MEPS data could be biased by self-reports by household member respondents. Therefore, MPC data are collected from surveys of medical and health insurance providers. For this purpose, HC respondents identify a sample of providers from pharmacies, hospitals, and home health care and allow that they be contacted by the MPC. The MPC then collects information from the sample of providers via telephone.

Further, the MPC data collect dates of visit, diagnosis and payment information for medical care events to correct inaccurate information in HC. To correct inaccurate data in HC, the pharmacy component of MPC collects medication information such as name, date filled, and payment sources. As such, expenditure information and medical care event and medication information collected in the MPC validates, supplements and/or replaces data in MEPS-HC from households for selected persons (like Medicaid recipients) and for physician charges associated with medical events that are not billed by a hospital.

Because of inconsistencies in reporting the same medical events between the HC and MPC, medical events from the 2 sources must be linked and then used as the primary source of data for spending estimates. If the data from both sources (HC and MPC) are available, the provider-reported data are considered to be more accurate than household-reported data, so the MPC data are used for calculating the MEPS expenditure variables.[17] Response rates for the MPC are high, ranging from about 69% for pharmacies to more than 89% for hospitals in 2009.[6]

## Nursing Home Component

The NHC follows people beginning in 1996 as they moved from one nursing home to another; collecting patient data on history of their residence and health care use, including prescribed medications, expenses, and health episodes. The NHC was a yearlong panel survey only for calendar year 1996; therefore, only estimates for 1996 are available.[18]

### Sample and Survey Design

The NHC survey sample is selected using a multistage stratified probability design. Thus, the NHC sample included facilities based on number of beds in the first stage of selection and residents in the last stage of selection. The sample frame for facilities was selected from the National Health Provider Inventory, which is updated occasionally by NCHS. All Medicare or Medicaid skilled nursing facility-certified units of licensed hospitals, long-term care nursing units of retirement communities and of Department of Veterans Affairs (VA) are eligible for the sample. Data from selected residents are collected in person using computer-assisted survey interviewing (CASI) technique. Data from the community are collected via telephone using computer-assisted personal interviewing (CAPI) technology.

### Data Collected

From a national sample of nursing homes and residents, the NHC collected information on the characteristics of the facilities and services available; and characteristics of deidentified residents, including functional status, cognitive functioning, age, income, expenditures and sources of payment, and health insurance coverage.

## Data Availability

The MEPS data and its components are available to researchers in various forms ranging from brief reports, data files, and tables.[6] The HC data consist of tables, and files (sorted by individual, job, health condition, or health event), and are also available as cost projections that are aligned with the 2002 National Health Expenditure Accounts (NHEA), which gives information on the total and per capita spending of the nation.[19] In addition, full-year consolidated files are also available on the website with related documentation, and codebooks that give information on ICD-9-CM codes, variables, as well as details on weighting procedures to extrapolate results to the general US population. These are available free to the public and for download on the Internet.[6,15]

MPC data are only available as part of the MEPS-HC, as their main use is to be compared with the medical cost data acquired during the MEPS-HC. Because the IC data collected by the Census Bureau are protected under constraints of confidentiality, not all the IC data are available to the general public. Therefore, IC data are disseminated publicly only through the MEPS website as summary data estimate tables posted on a yearly schedule for national, state, and metropolitan areas.[6] In addition, reports from IC data and interactive data tools are provided on the MEPS website.[6] The IC data that are not available for public release maintain survey respondents' confidentiality but are available at the Census Bureau Research Data Center, as well as an AHRQ data center located in Rockville, Maryland, which welcomes researchers to access the files in person.

In addition to the above, users can examine MEPS (HC and IC) data in real time using a menu-driven environment in MEPSnet—a collection of online, interactive, statistical and analytical tools that can produce statistics from public use HC and IC data.[20] These analytical tools can connect researchers to data and help generate statistics on data gathered by the HC and IC surveys on health insurance coverage, costs and trends.

## Data Analysis Considerations

The full-year consolidated household component files consist of variables referring to survey administration, demographics, employment, health status, disability days, quality of care, patient satisfaction, health insurance, health service use, and health expenditures.[6] For example, the data file for the 2008 survey contains 1,155 variables associated with patient demographics, health and employment status, patient satisfaction, health insurance information, and survey administration. This full-year file can be linked with the medical condition file and other individual event files (one each for prescribed medications, hospitalization, office-based physician visits, emergency room visits, home health visits, dental visits, and hospital outpatient visits) for more detailed analyses of health service use.

As MEPS data collected represents a small sample of the entire US population, weight and variance estimation variables are available to generate national estimates. For example, 2008 MEPS data include approximately 33,000 persons.[21] To produce national estimates of health care use and spending that represent the overall civilian noninstitutionalized US population, responses from surveyed individuals are weighted by applying the appropriate weight variables to the data. The weighting is done with sampling weights that adjust for survey nonresponse and for population totals from the Current Population Survey. All weights are available in the MEPS file and do not have to be computed by analysts. The MEPS online workbook has details of the weighting method and how weights need to be applied.[22]

Because MEPS uses a complex sampling design and not simple random sampling, it is important to know that the accuracy of calculated estimates (size of standard errors) declines when MEPS data are analyzed. Statistical software programs such as SAS, SUDAAN, STATA, and SPSS can adjust for the complex design of MEPS and estimate robust standard errors. The MEPS website has details on how to compute standard errors for MEPS data.[23] Because smaller racial and ethnic groups like American Indians and Alaska Natives represent few records in MEPS data; multiple years of data can be combined to increase the sample size. At least 100 unweighted cases are needed to produce national estimates.[24] MEPS and NHIS data can be linked to provide a year period of longitudinal analysis on individuals, households, and patient encounters.[25]

## 3. Utility of Medical Expenditure Panel Survey Data for Designing and Evaluating Health and Disease Management Programs

In order to understand how MEPS can be used to design and evaluate health and disease management programs, it is important to understand who is using MEPS data and for what purpose. Governmental and health care researchers, along with universities and health policy institutes, use the MEPS data to conduct research relating to the access, use and costs of health care.[2] Further, the data can be used to explore alternative health care delivery proposals using microsimulation model analyses.[26] The federal government uses MEPS data to evaluate the extent, availability, and cost, of private and public health insurance coverage and potential benefits for the US population and for subgroups. Similarly, state governments can study health insurance coverage and various choices of expanding health insurance coverage by using state-level data from the MEPS-IC.[27]

MEPS data could help in the design of health and disease management priorities nationally as well locally and regionally. For example, AHRQ's yearly reports since 2003 (the National Healthcare Quality Reports (NHQR) and the National Healthcare Disparities Reports (NHDR)) use data that include MEPS. The reports provide continued focus and public reporting on the quality of health care and health care disparities in US. The reports identified the need for health and disease management to improve preventive care, chronic disease management, patient safety and health care-associated infections (HAIs).[4]

The NHDR uses the MEPS data to give a comprehensive review of disadvantaged racial, ethnic, and socioeconomic groups including the uninsured, children, and the elderly who may not get recommended health care because of deficiencies in accessing care.[5] The NHQR uses MEPS data and gives important insights into measures, and evaluations of quality and access in various care settings and populations that can inform stakeholders involved in health and disease management initiatives. The NHQR focuses on the following quality measures: "effectiveness, patient safety, timeliness, and patient centeredness."[3] The quality measures represent 4 states of care from maintaining health, improving health, living with sickness or disability, and coping at the end of life. Since 2009, the NHQR and NHDR have also included measures to assess efficiency and access to health care in the US. As the goal of disease management programs is associated with these stages of care, the NHQR report can provide useful information to assess the need for and design of these programs as well as to determine standards and measures for evaluating health and disease management programs.

Previous studies by researchers and policy makers using MEPS data can also provide valuable insights into designing and evaluating health and disease management programs based on the changing needs of the populations. Researchers of health services in public and private health care systems have used MEPS data to inform health and disease management in the US, including health care disparities, direct and indirect medical costs, health insurance, health care use and spending, and patient-reported outcomes. Studies using MEPS data have reported racial and ethnic disparities in children's access to care[28] and in receiving preventive services under managed care[29] and barriers to care under managed care.[30] Other studies with MEPS data include those on disparities in colorectal cancer screening based on patients spending enough time with their health care provider,[31] in receiving blood pressure and cholesterol management,[32] and in preventive health examinations across urban metropolitan counties that differ by size, and nonmetropolitan (rural) counties that differ by level of urbanization and nearness to metropolitan counties.[33]

MEPS data has also been used to evaluate several health care topics including: the economic costs of influenza-related work absenteeism,[34] health insurance and absenteeism,[35] continuity of antidepressant treatment,[36] worker insurance choices,[37] preventive services in Medicare beneficiaries,[38] health status and cost of expanding insurance coverage,[39] potentially inappropriate medication use in the elderly and health-related quality of life,[40] out-of-pocket spending in chronic medical conditions,[41] prescription drug spending by Medicaid enrollees,[42] benefits of newer drugs in reducing nondrug spending,[43] and dissatisfaction with usual source of care associated with nonurgent emergency department visits.[44] One study used MEPS data to produce a "national catalog of preference based scores for chronic conditions in the U.S. populations"[45] that could be used in cost-effective evaluations of new drugs or health and disease management programs. Thus, MEPS data are frequently used to aid in the development of new policies for health care in the US.

The data can help identify the populations in need of specific health care interventions and can help develop appropriate health and disease management programs depending upon the regional need. MEPS data can provide estimates for the quality and access measures by specific subpopulations at the national level[2] and track changes in these measures across time. To improve quality of care in the US, outcomes of local and regional health and disease management programs can be compared with estimates of health service use and spending outcomes from MEPS data.

## Strengths of Medical Expenditure Panel Survey Data

MEPS data have several strengths that make them useful as a standard for comparison with health and disease management programs. One strength of MEPS is that it provides reliable and comprehensive data to produce national estimates of the level and distribution of health care use and expenditures, insurance coverage, and sources of payment for the US civilian noninstitutionalized population.[2] Reports of household condition in MEPS are most accurate for highly prevalent diseases like heart conditions, diabetes, cancer, trauma-related disorders, mental disorders, and asthma, because they involve continuing treatment, prescribed medications, or lifestyle changes. Thus, MEPS can support analyses on many types of conditions. A second strength is that when MEPS data are aligned and reconciled to the NHEA, it further improves estimates of the costs of illness.[2,19]

Third, MEPS provide data from the patient perspective by collecting information from key household respondents about the health experience of all household members. Further, because of the panel design, 2 years of MEPS data can be linked with earlier year's NHIS data to give a third time point of observations and help in conducting longitudinal studies. This design allows analysis of change over time to study the effect of changes in the sources of payment and insurance coverage on different racial/ethnic populations of interest or to study the effect of an intervention or treatment trends on health status that are available in MEPS.

A fourth strength of using MEPS data is its data quality. AHRQ builds in "validity, reliability, and consistency of its data products, including MEPS, by conducting various "standardized quality assurance procedures."[46] These procedures are available on the MEPS website.[46] Specifically, for the data it collects, MEPS assures quality of information by confirming interviewers' output and by conducting quality control tests on groups of analytic variables. Furthermore, MEPS benchmarks its data by comparing with data from earlier years and other similar sources such as the Current Population Survey of the US Census Bureau and the NHIS.[46]

A fifth strength of MEPS data is that they can be linked to specific survey respondents and their families and analyzed. Beyond producing national and regional estimates of health care use and spending, these data allow researchers to study how individual and family characteristics such as their health insurance may impact medical care use and spending.[47] This makes it possible for researchers and policy makers to evaluate potential relationships between insurance coverage, health and employment statuses, income levels with costs or payment for health care services.

Further, MEPS data can be analyzed on multiple levels not found in other databases: at the person level, the event level, the family level, or the health insurance unit level. The final strength of using MEPS is that it provides information on both charges and actual payment, and on portions shared by each payer type. Thus, MEPS is the only source containing actual data on payments and amounts paid including an individual's out-of-pocket spending for health care visits that are often used for inputs in cost-effectiveness analyses[2,24] of health interventions including health and disease management programs.

## Limitations of Medical Expenditure Panel Survey Data

Although MEPS data are unique in breadth and depth of information on individuals' insurance coverage, they have some limitations. First, the survey is limited to the US civilian, noninstitutionalized population. The MEPS data exclude individuals in military or longer-stay institutions, such as nursing homes. As a result, the survey excludes some high-cost populations and prevents studies of transitions between acute and long-term care. Therefore, spending estimates from MEPS tend to be underestimates as they do not include the spending of these high-cost individuals.

MEPS data can be used as a standard against which to compare the health care use, spending, and quality outcomes of local and regional health and disease management programs. However, one limitation of the MEPS data is that they were not developed to give state-level estimates.[2] Though total estimates for a selected number of large states may be possible, small sample sizes may add variations to estimates, reducing reliability. Therefore, some of the state-level estimates vary widely from one year to the next. Specifically, the MEPS-IC survey has a large national sample of establishments. However, state-level estimates are produced from generally smaller samples.

Therefore, to help researchers understand the variability in resulting data, all MEPS-IC estimates are published with standard errors. To discover if the changes in state-level estimates are statistically significant, suitable statistical tests for the difference between the 2 estimates of interest are needed. Researchers should note that MEPS data can be inappropriate to use for all types of analysis, due to small sample sizes. For example, because of small sample sizes, state estimates of the racial/ethnic populations are not possible, though annual estimates are possible.[48] All of these limitations may restrict researchers from comparing regional estimates of health use and spending outcomes from MEPS data with those of regional health and disease management programs.

When evaluating health and disease management programs for rare conditions, MEPS data pose additional limitations. The MEPS data cannot be used to study all conditions because the small sample sizes do not support research to evaluate health care use and spending in rare conditions. Also, the designated household respondent in MEPS data may not have reported all conditions. A household member may not know or recall or report all health services that were used by other individuals in the same household and might underreport the conditions.[2] Furthermore, if the information reported is not confirmed by medical record, misreporting of medical conditions is possible. In addition, due to confidentiality concerns, medical conditions are reported at a 3-digit level of specificity, rather than the full 5-digit level in public use files. This leads to a lack of specificity in the information collected.[2]

## 4. Summary and Conclusions

MEPS data are designed for policy-relevant research on health care use, spending, insurance coverage, and access across diverse American households that helps policy makers make informed decisions. Thus, the MEPS data produce key inputs to help develop, implement, and evaluate policies and practices of health care in the US. Despite the limitations, the strengths of MEPS data from AHRQ make them useful in developing and tracking quality and access measures for the American population as a whole and for specific vulnerable subpopulations (for example, racial and ethnic minorities, children, elderly).[2]

Although there is a paucity of information on such comparisons, local and regional health and disease management programs can greatly benefit by designing initiatives based on national needs emerging from MEPS data. Further, by evaluating themselves with national quality improvement standards from the MEPS data on standardized core measures, local and regional health and disease management program initiatives can document their value in improving quality of and access to care in the US.

## References

1. Docteur E, Berenson RA. How Does the Quality of U.S. Health Care Compare Internationally? Washington, DC :The Urban Institute; 2009. Available at: http://www.rwjf.org/content/dam/web-assets/2009/08/how-does-the-quality-of-u-s--health-care-compare-internationally. Accessed March 7, 2010.
2. Cohen JW, Cohen SB, Banthin JS. The medical expenditure panel survey: a national information resource to support healthcare cost research and inform policy and practice. *Med Care*. 2009;47:S44-S50.
3. Agency for Healthcare Research and Quality. *2011 National Healthcare Quality & Disparities Reports*. http://www.ahrq.gov/qual/qrdr11.htm. Accessed October 17, 2012.
4. Agency for Healthcare Research and Quality. *AHRQ Annual Highlights, 2007*. http://www.ahrq.gov/about/highlt07.htm Accessed August 25, 2008.
5. Agency for Healthcare Research and Quality. *National Healthcare Disparities Report, 2011*. Available at: http://www.ahrq.gov/qual/nhdr11/nhdr11.pdf. Accessed October 17, 2012.
6. Agency for Healthcare Research and Quality. *Medical Expenditure Panel Survey*. http://www.meps.ahrq.gov. Accessed March 7, 2010.
7. Agency for Healthcare Research and Quality. *AHRQ Profile: Advancing Excellence in Health Care* .AHRQ Publication No. 12-P014-EF, September 2012. Available at: http://www.ahrq.gov/about/profile.htm. Accessed October 17, 2012.
8. Agency for Healthcare Research and Quality. *Data Sources Available from AHRQ*. Available at: http://www.ahrq.gov/data/dataresources.htm. Accessed March 7, 2010.

9. Centers for Disease Control and Prevention (CDC); National Center for Health Statistics (NCHS). *National Health Interview Survey*. http://www.cdc.gov/nhis/. Accessed June 15, 2010.
10. Agency for Healthcare Research and Quality. *MEPS-HC Response Rates by Panel*. http://www.meps.ahrq.gov/mepsweb/survey_comp/hc_response_rate.jsp. Accessed March 12, 2010.
11. Agency for Healthcare Research and Quality. *Questionnaire Sections for Rounds 1-5*. http://www.meps.ahrq.gov/survey_comp/hc_ques_sections.jsp. Accessed June 15, 2010.
12. Agency for Healthcare Research and Quality. *MEPS Topics: Access to Health Care*. http://www.meps.ahrq.gov/mepsweb/data_stats/MEPS_topics.jsp?topicid=1Z-1. Accessed March 7, 2010.
13. Agency for Healthcare Research and Quality. *MEPS Topics: Quality of Health Care*. http://www.meps.ahrq.gov/mepsweb/data_stats/MEPS_topics.jsp?topicid=16Z-1. Accessed March 7, 2010.
14. Fleishman JA. *Methodology Report #15: Demographic and Clinical Variations in Health Status*. January 2005. Agency for Healthcare Research and Quality, Rockville, MD. Available at: http://meps.ahrq.gov/mepsweb/data_files/publications/mr15/mr15.pdf Accessed October 17, 2012.
15. Cohen SB. Design strategies and innovations in the medical expenditure panel survey. *Med Care*. 2003;41:III5-III12.
16. Agency for Healthcare Research and Quality. *MEPS-IC Sample Design and Data Collection Process*. http://www.meps.ahrq.gov/mepsweb/survey_comp/ic_data_collection.jsp Accessed June 15, 2010.
17. Agency for Healthcare Research and Quality. *Methodology Report #23: Design, Methods, and Field Reports of the Medical Expenditure Panel Survey Medical Provider Component (MEPS MPC): 2006 Calendar Year Data*. http://www.meps.ahrq.gov/mepsweb/data_files/publications/mr23/mr23.pdf#xml=http://meps.ahrq.gov/cgi-bin/texis/webinator/search/pdfhi.txt?query=MPC&pr=MEPSFULLSITE&prox=page&rorder=500&rprox=500&rdfreq=500&rwfreq=500&rlead=500&sufs=0&order=r&cq=&id=4c28d24c12c. Accessed June 15, 2010.
18. Potter DEB. *Design and Methods of the 1996 Medical Expenditure Panel Survey, Nursing Home Component*. Rockville, MD: U.S. Dept. of Health and Human Services, Public Health Service, Agency for Health Care Policy and Research; 1998. Available at: http://www.meps.ahrq.gov/mepsweb/data_files/publications/mr3/mr3.shtml. Accessed March 7, 2010.
19. Agency for Healthcare Research and Quality. *NHEA-Aligned MEPS: Projected Expenditure Data Files: 2002-2016*. http://www.meps.ahrq.gov/mepsweb/data_stats/download_data_files_detail.jsp?cboPufNumber=NHEA-Aligned MEPS. Accessed March 7, 2010.
20. Agency for Healthcare Research and Quality. *MEPSnet Query Tools*. http://www.meps.ahrq.gov/mepsweb/data_stats/meps_query.jsp. Accessed March 7, 2010.
21. Agency for Healthcare Research and Quality. *Medical Expenditure Panel Survey: MEPS-HC Sample Sizes*. http://meps.ahrq.gov/survey_comp/hc_sample_size.jsp. Accessed March 12, 2010.
22. Agency for Healthcare Research and Quality. *Medical Expenditure Panel Survey HC-036:1996-2009 Pooled Linkage Variance Estimation File, December 2011*. http://meps.ahrq.gov/mepsweb/data_stats/download_data/pufs/h36/h36u09doc.pdf. Accessed October 17, 2012.
23. Machlin S, Yu W, Zodet M. *Computing Standard Errors for MEPS Estimates*. Rockville, MD: Agency for Healthcare Research and Quality. http://www.meps.ahrq.gov/mepsweb/survey_comp/standard_errors.jsp. Published January 2005. Accessed March 12, 2010.
24. Office of the Assistant Secretary for Planning and Evaluation, *US Department of Health & Human Services. Medical Expenditure Panel Survey* (MEPS). http://aspe.hhs.gov/hsp/06/Catalog-AI-AN-NA/MEPS.htm. Accessed August 25, 2008.
25. Morgan PA, Strand J, Ostbye T, et al. Missing in action: care by physician assistants and nurse practitioners in national health surveys. *Health Serv Res*. 2007;42:2022-2037.
26. Agency for Healthcare Research and Quality. *Medical Expenditure Panel Survey Researcher Information*. http://www.meps.ahrq.gov/mepsweb/about_meps/index_researcher.jsp. Accessed August 25, 2008.
27. Agency for Healthcare Research and Quality. *Medical Expenditure Panel Survey Policymaker Information*. http://www.meps.ahrq.gov/mepsweb/about_meps/index_policymaker.jsp. Accessed August 25, 2008.

## Part 4: Alternative, Population-Based Data Sources

28. Weinick RM, Krauss NA. Racial/Ethnic differences in children's access to care. *Am J Public Health.* 2000;90:1771-1774.
29. Haas JS, Phillips KA, Sonneborn D, et al. Effect of managed care insurance on the use of preventive care for specific ethnic groups in the United States. *Med Care.* 2002;40:743-751.
30. Phillips KA, Mayer ML, Aday LA. Barriers to care among racial/ethnic groups under managed care. *Health Aff* (Millwood). 2000;19:65-75.
31. Carcaise-Edinboro P, Bradley CJ. Influence of patient-provider communication on colorectal cancer screening. *Med Care.* 2008;46:738-745.
32. Stewart SH, Silverstein MD. Racial and ethnic disparity in blood pressure and cholesterol measurement. *J Gen Intern Med.* 2002;17:405-411.
33. Larson S, Correa-de-Araujo R. Preventive health examinations: a comparison along the rural-urban continuum. *Womens Health Issues.* 2006;16:80-88.
34. Akazawa M, Sindelar JL, Paltiel AD. Economic costs of influenza-related work absenteeism. *Value Health.* 2003;6:107-115.
35. Lofland JH, Frick KD. Workplace absenteeism and aspects of access to health care for individuals with migraine headache. *Headache.* 2006;46:563-576.
36. Olfson M, Marcus SC, Tedeschi M, et al. Continuity of antidepressant treatment for adults with depression in the United States. *Am J Psychiatry.* 2006;163:101-108.
37. Blumberg LJ, Nichols LM, Banthin JS. Worker decisions to purchase health insurance. *Int J Health Care Finance Econ.* 2001;1:305-325.
38. Carrasquillo O, Lantigua RA, Shea S. Preventive services among Medicare beneficiaries with supplemental coverage versus HMO enrollees, medicaid recipients, and elders with no additional coverage. *Med Care.* 2001;39:616-626.
39. Holahan J. Health status and the cost of expanding insurance coverage. *Health Aff* (Millwood) 2001;20:279-286.
40. Franic DM, Jiang JZ. Potentially inappropriate drug use and health-related quality of life in the elderly. *Pharmacotherapy.* 2006;26:768-778.
41. Hwang W, Weller W, Ireys H, et al. Out-of-pocket medical spending for care of chronic conditions. *Health Aff* (Millwood). 2001;20:267-278.
42. Banthin JS, Miller GE. Trends in prescription drug expenditures by Medicaid enrollees. *Med Care.* 2006;44:I27-I35.
43. Lichtenberg FR. Are the benefits of newer drugs worth their cost? Evidence from the 1996 MEPS. *Health Aff* (Millwood). 2001;20:241-251.
44. Sarver JH, Cydulka RK, Baker DW. Usual source of care and nonurgent emergency department use. *Acad Emerg Med.* 2002;9:916-923.
45. Sullivan PW, Lawrence WF, Ghushchyan V. A national catalog of preference-based scores for chronic conditions in the United States. *Med Care.* 2005;43:736-749.
46. US Health and Human Services. *Guidelines for Ensuring the Quality of Information Disseminated to the Public - Agency for Healthcare Research and Quality.* http://aspe.hhs.gov/infoQuality/Guidelines/AHRQinfo.shtml. Accessed March 12, 2010.
47. Cohen JW, Monheit AC, Beauregard KM, et al. The Medical Expenditure Panel Survey: a national health information resource. *Inquiry.* 1996;33:373-389.
48. Agency for Healthcare Research and Quality. *Medical Expenditure Panel Survey: FAQs - Answers.* http://www.meps.ahrq.gov/mepsweb/about_meps/faq_answers.jsp?FAQID=55&ChooseCategory=-1&keyword=standard+errors. Accessed March 12, 2010.

CHAPTER 20

# Survey Data Sources from the National Center for Health Statistics

Jayashri Sankaranarayanan, MPharm, PhD; Mariam K. Hassan, BPharm, PhD; Yaozhu J. Chen, MPA; and Teresa Hartman, MLS

The primary aim of this chapter is to familiarize the reader with the publicly available, national survey databases maintained by the Centers for Disease Control and Prevention (CDC), Division of Health Care Statistics. The chapter begins with an introduction to 2 National Center for Health Statistics (NCHS) databases: the National Ambulatory Medical Care Survey (NAMCS) and the National Hospital Ambulatory Medical Care Survey (NHAMCS). Subsequent sections describe the information contained in the NAMCS and NHAMCS databases in more detail and introduce the reader to additional NCHS data sources. The next section provides details on how to access the NAMCS and NHAMCS databases, confidentiality concerns of which to be aware, and analysis considerations. Lastly, how NAMCS and NHAMCS databases can be used to inform health and disease management is discussed followed by strengths and limitations of these data sources. In addition, one should periodically refer to http://www.cdc.gov/nchs/ahcd.htm to ensure the most up-to-date information on these databases.

The NCHS is a division of the CDC that compiles information to identify critical health problems and to guide actions and policies for improving public health in the United States. The mission of the NCHS is to provide accurate, relevant, and timely statistical information on the use of health care services at the regional and national levels. To carry out this mission, the NCHS works with partners throughout the health care community and compiles information from various sources such as interviews, surveys, and records of birth, medical and death data.[1]

The NCHS website (http://www.cdc.gov/nchs/)[2] provides information on data collection efforts and quality, data findings, special activities and initiatives, links to other sources, and directions on how to submit electronically queries to obtain answers to specific health statistics questions. Information derived from the NCHS databases help to describe, monitor, and identify health problems and disparities in the population and in the use of health care services. These data can be stratified by subgroups defined by race or ethnicity, socioeconomic status, and region, thus making the NCHS an important public resource for health information that can help inform changes to public policies and programs to impact the quality and delivery of care in health and disease management programs in the US.[1]

To fulfill its mission of providing surveillance information, the NCHS conducts several national surveys.[2] These surveys inform federal, state, and local health care decision makers on health and disease management of various medical conditions. The current NCHS[2] national surveys and data collection systems are summarized in Table 1.

The NAMCS and NHAMCS provide objective and reliable sources of information on how medical care services are provided and used in various ambulatory settings such as doctor visits, hospital outpatient department (OPD) visits, and emergency department (ED) visits in the US. The NAMCS, NHAMCS, and National Nursing Home Survey (NNHS) report on medication dispensing, which can be used for studying drug utilization across various ambulatory medical care settings.[3]

This chapter provides an overview of the publicly available national survey databases conducted by the CDC Division of Health Care Statistics. We discuss the usefulness of the national survey data in benchmarking quality and effectiveness in the delivery of ambulatory health care, which is the principal method of providing health care services in the US. Additionally, the strengths and limitations of commonly used survey sources (NAMCS and NHAMCS databases that report medication use in ambulatory care) are also discussed.

## 1. National Ambulatory Medical Care Survey

NAMCS is a collection of data related to the use of ambulatory medical services in the US. The unit for sampling in NAMCS is the patient visit to the physician. NAMCS collects visit-level data for patients from physicians or physician office staff. These data are extrapolated to provide national estimates of medication dispensing and other health services' use. The NAMCS was carried out each year from 1973 to 1981 and again in 1985; it has continued to be conducted annually since 1989.[4]

### National Ambulatory Medical Care Survey Sampling Procedure

NAMCS includes office visits to physicians who are not federally employed and provide office-based patient care. NAMCS excludes physicians whose primary role is teaching, research, administration, or hospital-based care, and those who are unclassified as to their principal activity or those in specified specialties (for example, anesthesiology, pathology, and radiology). NAMCS further excludes telephone visits, house calls, visits to hospitals or institutions such as nursing homes, and visits specifically to settle bills or collect insurance documents. However, since 2006, NAMCS data include health providers identified as doctors, physician assistants, nurse practitioners, and nurse midwives from community health centers.

The NAMCS sample consists of "primary sampling units (PSUs), physician practices within PSUs, and patient visits within practices."[4] Through a multistage probability design, NAMCS in the first stage, selects a sample of approximately 100 PSUs that "are geographic segments composed of counties, groups of counties, county equivalents (such as parishes or independent cities), towns, townships, and minor civil divisions (for some PSUs in New England) within the 50 states and the District of Columbia."[4] In the second stage, a probability sample of practicing doctors from the American Medical Association and the American Osteopathic Association's master files are selected within each PSU. In the final stage, a random sample of patient visits to each subsample of the practicing doctors is selected.[4]

## Data Collection

Before the physicians take part in the survey, interviewers make visits to supply them with materials for the survey and to train them on how to fill out the surveys correctly. A 1-week reporting period is randomly assigned to collect data from each physician office or site. During this period, the participating physician or office staff record information for a systematic random sample of patient visits on an encounter form provided by NAMCS. The survey data include provider specialty, patient characteristics (for example, age, race, sex, insurance payer), and visit characteristics. Examples of visit characteristics are reason for visit, diagnoses, referral, time spent with physician, patient seen before, physician specialty, and services provided including diagnostic procedures, patient management, medications ordered or provided, and planned future treatment.

## 2. National Hospital Ambulatory Medical Care Survey

Initiated in 1992, NHAMCS data provide estimates of medication use in hospital ambulatory care services such as emergency departments (ED) and outpatient department (OPD) clinics; NHAMCS data do not contain the same information collected in NAMCS. Thus, NHAMCS provides data to fill critical gaps in the NAMCS data by collecting hospital ED and OPD visit information that represent a proportion of total ambulatory medical care representing a spectrum of patient demographics based on visit site.[5]

## National Hospital Ambulatory Medical Care Survey Sampling Procedure

Similar to NAMCS, the basic sampling unit of the NHAMCS is the patient visit to ED or OPD at nonfederal, short-stay (average length of stay of fewer than 30 days), general hospitals (medical or surgical), or children's general hospitals that were not ineligible due to closing or other reasons.[5] NHAMCS excludes federal hospitals, hospital units of institutions, and hospitals with fewer than 6 beds.

To sample patient visits, the NHAMCS uses a 4-stage probability design. In the first stage, PSUs defined geographically based on counties or metropolitan statistical areas of the 1980 Census classification are selected. Next, approximately 600 hospitals within these PSUs are selected. Care is taken to select hospitals so that each hospital is chosen only once to avoid multiple inclusions of very large hospitals. To exclude hospitals from participating during the same time period each year, the sample of 600 hospitals is randomly divided into 16 subsets of roughly equivalent size and is allocated 1 data reporting week that rotates across each survey year and each hospital is included approximately 1 time in a 15-month period.[5] Third, OPD clinics or emergency service areas (ESAs) within EDs from the sampled hospitals are selected. In the fourth and final stage, patient visits within OPD clinics or ESAs are systematically selected over a randomly assigned 4-week reporting period.[4] More details of the sampling procedures are available on the NHAMCS website.[5]

A patient visit in NHAMCS data is defined as a direct, personal exchange between a patient seeking care and a physician rendering health services, or a staff member acting under a physician's direction. Similar to the NAMCS, administrative visits are not captured in NHAMCS data if no medical care was provided at the time of contact (eg, bill paid, insurance form picked up). The NHAMCS data in 2007 were estimated based on approximately 35,490 visits to roughly 400 participating EDs and approximately 35,000 visits to 250 participating OPDs.[5] These data represent more than 500 noninstitutional, general, short-stay hospitals and can be used to extrapolate to national estimates of patient characteristics, medication use, and other health service utilization. Starting in 2009, Patient Record Forms (PRFs) from 100 visits to hospital-based ambulatory surgery centers were also completed.[4]

## Data Collection

Similar to NAMCS, before data collection is initiated for the NHAMCS, interviewers visit the selected hospitals to explain the survey procedures. These interviewers verify eligibility, develop a sampling plan, and train hospital staff in data collection procedures. The visit-level data for each patient are collected from hospital staff using the PRFs.[5] There are 2 versions of the PRF; one for use in OPDs and another for use in EDs.[6] The interviewers train hospital staff to complete the proper PRF for a systematic random sample of patient visits during a randomly assigned 4-week reporting period. Survey data collected on the PRF include payment source, reason for visit, diagnoses, diagnostic/screening services, medication name, injury or adverse events, provider type or hospital ownership type.

## 3. Other National Center for Health Statistics Databases

Table 1 summarizes a few commonly used NCHS surveys and data systems besides the NAMCS and NHAMCS. The National Survey of Ambulatory Surgery (NSAS) is a national survey conducted by NCHS which provides insight on surgery in ambulatory care services. NCHS also maintains the National Nursing Home Survey (NNHS), a continuing series of national sample surveys of nursing homes, their residents, and their staffs that were conducted in the years of 1973-1974, 1977, 1985, 1995, 1997, 1999 and 2004.[7] In addition, NCHS conducts the National Health and Nutrition Examination Survey (NHANES) and National Health Interview Survey (NHIS), which collect self-reported medication, vaccines, and immunization data.[2] However, this type of medication information is limited in both depth and breadth because of the nature of self-reported data. One strength of the NHANES data is that they are collected from interviews, examinations, and laboratory tests through blood and urine samples over several decades from 1971 to 2012.[2] This allows users to access comprehensive patient-level examination or lab test results such as blood pressure, serum cholesterol, and hemoglobin A1c that are not widely available from claims data.

## 4. Availability, Confidentiality, and Access to the National Ambulatory Medical Care Survey and the National Hospital Ambulatory Medical Care Survey Data

### Availability

The NCHS website has public-use NAMCS and NHAMCS data files for all years with related documentation and yearly survey questionnaires instruments as well as related SAS input statements, variable labels, value labels, and format assignments (see http://www.cdc.gov/nchs/ahcd/ahcd_questionnaires.htm).[6,8]

### Confidentiality and Privacy issues

Patient privacy and confidentiality are important when using publicly available data and NCHS takes several steps to safeguard this information. Under the Public Health Service Act (Section 308 (d)), the NCHS data may be used to analyze and report health statistics, however, steps that identify a patient or doctor or hospital are prohibited by this law. To protect the disclosure of subjects' identity, NCHS omits all identifiers and characteristics that might lead to identification of individuals or facilities in the datasets.[9]

### Access Considerations

Public-use files can be downloaded directly from the NCHS website for research. Accessing additional restricted data not available in public use files is possible through the Research Data Center (RDC) that provides masked variables and confidential data items. However, linking information (for example, based on race/ethnicity, country of birth, geographic codes of state, county or census tract) between NCHS databases or linking NCHS data to non-NCHS data collected by researchers or private institutions with geographic codes could compromise the confidentiality of survey respondents or institutions, or may be sensitive by nature. Therefore, the NCHS RDC allows researchers meeting certain qualifications to access confidential statistical microdata files under strict supervision.[10] To qualify, researchers must submit a proposal for review and approval. Upon approval, the RDC can merge the survey with contextual variables from other NCHS databases like National Health Interview Survey (NHIS) and National Hospital Discharge Survey (NHDS). The RDC also can use its record linkage program[11] to merge the survey with non-NCHS data sources.

## 5. Analysis and Other Considerations

It is useful to consider several aspects of the NAMCS and NHAMCS datasets when analyzing and interpreting the data, and when designing survey evaluations of health and disease management programs. First, survey participation by physician offices and hospital OPDs and EDs is voluntary.[9] While the response rates are high for NHAMCS (hospitals), between 85 and 95% response rate during the period from 1992 to 2004,[12] this is not the case with physicians. Health surveys targeting physicians historically have been lower for NAMCS (physician office-based surveys). The response rate was between 65 % and 75% during the survey period of 1989 to 2004. Therefore, to decrease nonresponse bias and to consistently increase response rates to 70%, other strategies have been used. NAMCS addresses survey nonresponse by using a weighted method that considers the physician specialty, geographic region, and metropolitan statistical area (MSA) status.[12]

Second, NCHS carries out quality control checks and edit checks to ensure that the data quality is robust. Similarly, when evaluating health and disease management programs such quality checks of data collected can improve the quality of data collected. Third, since 2005, the characteristics in the ambulatory care databases for NAMCS and NHAMCS include chronic disease checklists, status of medication new or continued, nonmedication treatment, and whether or not the patient is enrolled in a disease management program. Some of these variables can also be adapted for use in designing evaluations of health and disease management programs.

Fourth, from 2005 forward, researchers can use provider weights, available in the NAMCS (physician level) and NHAMCS (ED and OPD levels) files, to make estimates at the level of the provider setting.[13] Understanding this process can give insight into how estimates from health and disease management programs can also be made at the provider (physician office or hospital) practice level. Fifth, the NCHS website provides information on the validity of the information collected in the national surveys.[14] For example, the NAMCS and NHAMCS are completed by medical care providers shortly after patient encounters. Therefore, accuracy and validity of the collected information is likely to be high for the information that requires expertise of medical providers such as diagnoses, therapies, and types of provider seen at the patient visit.[15] Thus, when designing evaluations of health and disease management programs, such provider-level data may be collected to ensure accuracy of findings.

Sixth, health and disease management program evaluations can draw ideas from how NCHS defines standards to measure reliability of estimates and how NCHS improves reliability of estimates from its data. Because the NAMCS and NHAMCS are sample surveys, smaller estimates can be unreliable. Therefore, the NCHS defines the standard error of an estimate "as a measure of the sampling variability that occurs by chance, because only a sample rather than the entire universe is surveyed."[16] Furthermore, the NCHS "considers an estimate to be reliable if it has a relative standard error of 30 percent or less (that is, the standard error is no more than 30 percent of the estimate)" and if the estimates are based on more than 30 records.[16] In addition, to improve the reliability of estimates, NCHS recommends that multiple years of NAMCS and NHAMCS data be combined to obtain reliable estimates on medication use and other health services like psychotherapy, counseling, and cancer screenings.

Understanding how NCHS uses data can help health and disease management programs use similar measures to evaluate their programs with national estimates from NCHS data. For example, NCHS uses various measures such as patient-reported reason for visit, ICD-9-CM codes for diagnoses and procedures, drug entry list and generic ingredient list, and the National Drug Code (NDC) directory. Physicians enter "drug mentions" information on the PRF referring to drugs provided, prescribed or continued at the ambulatory care visit.[17] Drugs may be entered as either brand or generic name and given by any route of administration—for prevention, diagnosis, or treatment.[18]

Drug data are classified as new or continued in NAMCS and in NHAMCS OPD databases; data are given in ED/Rx at discharge in the NHAMCS ED database. Visits with one or more drug mentions are called *drug visits*. The NCHS defines a rate for drug mentions as "the number of mentions for a particular drug code per 10,000 ambulatory medical care visits in any year."[18] Drug mention rates are available online in the Ambulatory Care Drug Database System (http://www2.cdc.gov/drugs/).[18]

When planning data collection on medication use for health and disease management programs, one can consider how NCHS collects, codes and estimates drug information. From 1973 to 1979, NAMCS collected drug information as checks for prescription or nonprescription. From 1980, NAMCS surveys included an open-ended write-in item so that physicians can record up to 8 medications provided to the patient at a given visit. However, NAMCS collected data from 1985 to 1994 on up to 5 medications, from 1995 to 2002 on up to 6 medications and from 2003 to present on up to 8 drugs.[17-19] Combining several years of NAMCS and NHAMCS data with several drug mentions to get reliable estimates have not been reported to bias national estimates of medication use.

## 6. NAMCS and NHAMCS Data for Informing Health and Disease Management Practices

In general, the NCHS databases can provide information on Americans' health care profiles in various ways. First, health problems, disparities in health status, and use of health care are identified and documented by race/ethnicity, socioeconomic status, region, and other population characteristics. Second, national trends are monitored in health status and health care delivery. Third, cross-sectional data are provided over time to allow evaluation and to provide information for making changes in public policies and local or regional health and disease management programs.

## Part 4: Alternative, Population-Based Data Sources

For informing health and disease management, both NAMCS and NHAMCS data have been used to document national estimates of quality of care in various disease states such as diabetes, hypertension, depression, bipolar disorders, schizophrenia and psychotic disorders. Furthermore, national estimates of health service that use outcomes, including medication use, have also been studied with these databases. Studies included real-world prescribing practice patterns of medications such as antibiotics,[20-26] cyclooxygenase inhibitors,[27] selective serotonin reuptake inhibitors,[28] aspirin,[29] and antipsychotics.[30] Others report increased antidepressant prescribing by office-based physicians for less severe psychiatric disorders,[31,32] inappropriate[33-37] or decreased[38] medication use in the elderly, poisoning-related ED visits to inform effective poison prevention programs,[39] prevalent variations in psychotropic drug prescribing in children[40] and in youth,[41] national trends in attention deficit hyperactivity disorder and its treatment in children[42] and in adults,[43] characteristics of preventable ED visits for gynecological disorders[44] and characteristics of antipsychotic-associated ED visits.[45]

Moreover, the survey data have been used to evaluate disparities in health management by studying the provision of preventive services like smoking cessation,[46] preventive counseling in cardiovascular disease,[47] breast cancer screening,[48] skin cancer screening and prevention,[49] and diet and physical activity counseling.[50] Another study reported on the inefficiency of primary care providers as gatekeeper, as evidenced by high rates of referrals to specialists for skin disorders.[51] Insurance disparities in pediatric ED visits for nonurgent care have also been reported.[52]

Use of these databases has also shown differences in practice styles by physician specialty, which has implications for training health professionals and distribution of health care resources.[53] NAMCS data are also used to compare other ambulatory data available. For example, the Ambulatory Sentinel Practice Network (ASPN) is a family medicine network that provides care for about a half million patients and currently consists of 125 practices of about 750 clinicians from 38 states and 6 Canadian provinces. ASPN data differed from NAMCS data on patient demographic characteristics, but were similar to NAMCS for information on problems, diagnoses, services, disposition, and time spent with patients.[54]

One study showed that although visits for skin conditions increased, the demand for dermatology services reduced.[55] Another study evaluated the quality and the temporal trends of US outpatient care[56] by examining 23 measures of racial/ethnic disparities. The study found that there was "greater angiotensin-converting enzyme inhibitor use for congestive heart failure among blacks and less unnecessary antibiotic use for uncomplicated upper respiratory tract infections among whites."[56]

In summary, the NCHS survey data (NAMCS and NHAMCS, in particular) have been used extensively to benchmark national patterns of medication use and identify gaps in quality of care that can improve the delivery of preventive services and treatment in health and disease management. Thus, the studies using NCHS data can inform health and disease management practices as well as inform the design and evaluations of health and disease management programs. The findings can be used specifically by localized health care systems to compare the quality of care of their health and disease management programs with those from these national survey databases.

## 7. Strengths

The NAMCS and NHAMCS surveys have several strengths that can inform the design and evaluations of health and disease management programs. First, the NAMCS and NHAMCS surveys are 2 of the largest publicly available databases in the US used by policy makers and researchers. They are designed in a cross-sectional framework and obtain a cross-section of information over time on patient ambulatory care services from health care providers. Thus, the NAMCS/NHAMCS national surveys provide estimates that may be generalized to the ambulatory visits made by the American population.[15] Users can analyze NAMCS and NHAMCS data to estimate each year's pattern separately, which helps to infer year-by-year trends of medication use. Several NCHS surveys provide information on duration of services: NHDS informs hospital inpatient days, NAMCS informs length of time (in minutes) patients spent with physicians, and NHAMCS informs duration of visit (in minutes).

Second, the validity of ICD-9-CM codes and miscoding has not been a problem with NAMCS and NHAMCS data. For items requiring medical coding, discrepancy rates are generally under 2%. Third, NCHS makes the NAMCS and NHAMCS data available and gives recommendations on how to combine and use the data for analyses. Researchers can download and use the microlevel data files of NAMCS and NHAMCS, documentation, and programming statements in SAS,® SPSS® and Stata® for each year from the NCHS website.[57] For cross-sectional analyses of larger datasets of NAMCS or NHAMCS ED, or NHAMCS OPD, NCHS recommends combining survey years with the same PRF (survey instrument), and years when the same question of interest is asked.

Furthermore, NCHS also recommends that within each year, the 3 care settings (NAMCS, NHAMCS ED, and NHAMCS OPD) should be combined because they have different sampling frames.[9] Thus, the information in the national databases can be combined over several years to create larger datasets to facilitate study of trends in medication use across these years and to increase sample size to produce reliable estimates. Finally, the nature of the cross-sectional survey design allows for the study of the potential associations of patient and visit characteristics of interest.

## 8. Limitations

The NAMCS and NHAMCS data have several limitations that need to be considered when designing and evaluating health and disease management programs. First, a major limitation of NCHS survey data is the lack of information collected on outcomes, such as duration (especially number of days of treatment) and intensity of health service use (for example, dose and duration of medication use, hospitalizations and readmissions) and the associated costs. Second, while the National Nursing Home Survey provides information on medication use and economic data such as charges and payment, economic and patient-reported outcomes are not collected in NAMCS and NHAMCS. Third, studies on the appropriateness of therapy are limited because reasons that influenced prescribing decisions are not obtained in these databases.

Fourth, neither NAMCS nor NHAMCS can be linked across multiple years to get longitudinal information on patient visits. Therefore, NAMCS and NHAMCS data users cannot link multiple years of data to do longitudinal analysis on same subjects. Fifth, both the NAMCS and NHAMCS are visit-record-based surveys and not population-based surveys. Because the surveys are based on a sample of *visits* and not of *people*, the estimates obtained from these data are representative of *visits* made by people and *not of people* themselves. Therefore, the survey data cannot be used to find out how many people have a certain diagnosis or treatment.

However, the data can be used to find out how many ambulatory care visits were made for a certain diagnosis to get the rate of visits for a diagnosis of interest (that is, number of visits divided by the population of interest). Nonetheless, because they are not population-based surveys, researchers and policy makers need to be aware that they cannot calculate incidence or prevalence rates of health conditions or diseases from the estimates.[9]

Sixth, nonurgent ED visits, (that is, those in which the patient does not require attention immediately or within a few hours, when frequent, are commonly more expensive than alternative modes of care resulting in avoidable health care waste. While NHAMCS data have been used to study these nonurgent ED visits, NHAMCS data have been reported to have inherent methodological problems arising from retrospective coding by hospital staff and the inconsistency in geographic coding.[58]

Seventh, because NAMCS samples physicians only, rather than all providers, the results cannot be generalized to other providers, like the national PA (Physician Assistant) and NP (Nurse Practitioner) office-based practices.[15] However, because the NHAMCS-ED and the NHAMCS-OPD sample institutions (rather than physicians), the estimates from these data could be generalized nationally to PAs and NPs who practice in nonfederal hospital outpatient and emergency departments. Finally, nonsampling errors are possible in the estimates from NAMCS and NHAMCS data and could arise from issues in reporting and processing of the surveys as well as bias from nonresponse or incomplete responses to the surveys.

## 9. Conclusions

In summary, this chapter provides a brief introduction to NAMCS and NHAMCS databases and how they are used to inform health and disease management. Using various methods, the NCHS efficiently obtains information from the health community partners and provider sources that are most able to provide information in interview surveys. The NCHS databases are publicly available to decision makers and researchers to get and compare national estimates with estimates from local and regional health and disease management programs. Despite their limitations, the national survey databases from NCHS provide robust evidence to help decision makers understand and guide policies on designing and monitoring the real-world health and disease management programs to ultimately improve the quality of care in the US.

## Part 4: Alternative, Population-Based Data Sources

**TABLE 1:** Commonly Used Current and Completed NCHS Surveys and Data Systems

| No. | Name and Planned Sample | Data Source/Methods | Selected Applications of Data Produced | Race/Ethnicity, Socioeconomic, Drug, Data Frequency* |
|---|---|---|---|---|
| | **Population surveys** | | | |
| 1 | National Health and Nutrition Examination Survey (NHANES) ~5,000 persons per year, all ages, oversamples 60+, blacks and Hispanics | Personal interview, physical examination, laboratory tests, nutritional assessment, DNA repository | Total prevalence of disease or conditions (heart disease, diabetes, etc.) including those unrecognized or undetected | Income and poverty index, education, occupation, type of living quarters, all years |
| 2 | National Health Interview Survey (NHIS) ~35,000 to 51,000 households including 87,500 persons; from 2006 oversamples blacks, Hispanics, and Asians, and these minorities if 65+ | Personal interviews provide sampling frame for Medical Expenditure Panel Survey | Health status and limitations, functioning, utilization of health care, family resources, health insurance, access to care, health behaviors, HIV/AIDS testing, injuries, immunizations | OMB Race and Ethnic Standards-based categories,** Hispanic groups, family and individual, income, poverty level, education and occupation, type of living quarters, language spoken during interview, birthplace, citizenship status, annual with capability for longitudinal follow-up |
| | **Vital records** | | | |
| 3 | National Death Index (NDI) All deaths, and most NCHS surveys can be linked to NDI | State registration area-death certificates | Facilitates epidemiological follow-up studies, verification of death for individuals under study | Same race groups as VSCP, annual |
| | **Provider surveys** | | | |
| 4 | National Hospital Discharge Survey (NHDS) 239 non-federal short-stay hospitals, 150,000 inpatient discharges | Hospital records, computerized data sources | Demographics, diagnosis, procedures, length of stay | 1965-2008 |

*Survey Data Sources from the National Center for Health Statistics*

**TABLE 1:** Commonly Used Current and Completed NCHS Surveys and Data Systems

| No. | Name and Planned Sample | Data Source/Methods | Selected Applications of Data Produced | Race/Ethnicity, Socioeconomic, Drug, Data Frequency* |
|---|---|---|---|---|
| 5 | National Ambulatory Medical Care Survey (NAMCS) 180,000 patient visits, 15,726 physicians in office-based practices, 6,024 physicians or mid-level providers from 2,008 community health centers | Review medical records for patient visits, interview physicians, encounter forms completed by office-based physicians and other staff | Characteristics of patients' visits and practices, diagnoses and treatment, prescribing patterns, provider/clinician characteristics (specialty, practice size, ownership), use of electronic medical records | OMB categories,** drug data (1980 onwards), annual (1973-1981, 1985, 1989-current) |
| 6 | National Hospital Ambulatory Medical Care Survey (NHAMCS) 600 hospitals, 100,000 patient visits, 480 hospitals with EDs, outpatient departments, or ambulatory surgery centers (200 free standing) | Review medical records for patient visits, interview hospital administrators, encounter forms completed by physicians and other hospital facility staff | Characteristics of patients' visits to OPD and ED, diagnoses/treatment prescribing patterns, facility characteristics (specialty, volume), use of electronic medical records | OMB categories,** drug data (1992 onwards), annual (1992-current) |
| 7 | National Nursing Home Survey (NNHS) 1,174 facilities, 13,670 current residents, 3,017 nursing assistants | Facility/Medical records, long-term care providers, interviews with facility administrators and staff familiar with residents, and resident-level facility/medical records | Facility-level practices and staffing characteristics, resident-level health status (functional status), diagnoses medications, ED visits, hospitalizations | OMB categories,** drug data (2004), periodically (1973-74,1977,1985, 1995,1997,1999), and last conducted in 2004 |

Adapted from Summary of Current Surveys and data collection systems, NCHS, May-June 2012.[59]

OMB – Office of Management and Budget; OPD - hospital outpatient departments; ED - emergency departments; VSCP – Vital Statistics Cooperative Program

*drug data when collected.

**OMB categories include white, black or African American, Asian, Native Hawaiian and other Pacific Islanders, American Indian or Alaska Native. Hispanic origin is asked as a separate question.

Other NCHS surveys are – population surveys (National Survey of Family Growth); provider surveys (National Home and Hospice Care Survey, National Home Health Aide Survey, and National Survey of Residential Care Facilities); vital records (National Vital Statistics Systems (including data systems for births, deaths, marriage and divorce)); telephone surveys (National Immunization Survey, National Survey of Children with Special Health Care Needs)

Part 4: Alternative, Population-Based Data Sources

# References

1. Centers for Disease Control and Prevention. *About the National Center for Health Statistics.* http://www.cdc.gov/nchs/about.htm. Accessed March 7, 2010.
2. Centers for Disease Control (CDC). *National Center for Health Statistics – Monitoring the Nation's Health.* http://www.cdc.gov/nchs. Accessed March 7, 2010.
3. Schappert SM, Rechtsteiner EA. Ambulatory medical care utilization estimates for 2006. *Natl Health Stat Report.* 2008;(8):1-29.
4. National Center for Health Statistics. *NAMCS/NHAMCS Scope and Sample Design.* http://www.cdc.gov/nchs/ahcd/ahcd_scope.htm. Accessed March 12, 2010.
5. Ambulatory and Hospital Care Statistics Branch, National Center for Health Statistics. *2007 NHAMCS Micro-Data File Documentation.* Hyattsville, MD: United States Centers for Disease Control and Prevention; 2009. Available at: ftp://ftp.cdc.gov/pub/Health_Statistics/NCHS/Dataset_Documentation/NHAMCS/doc07.pdf. Accessed March 12, 2010.
6. National Center for Health Statistics. *Questionnaires, Datasets and Related Documentation.* http://www.cdc.gov/nchs/ahcd/ahcd_questionnaires.htm. Accessed March 12, 2010.
7. Long Term Care Statistics Branch Division of Health Care Statistics, National Center for Health Statistics. *Survey Methodology, Documentation, and Data Files Survey from the National Nursing Home Survey.* http://www.cdc.gov/nchs/nnhs/nnhs_questionnaires.htm. Accessed October 17, 2012.
8. National Center for Health Statistics. *Survey Content for the National Ambulatory Medical Care Survey and National Hospital Ambulatory Medical Care Survey.* Hyattsville, MD: United States Centers for Disease Control and Prevention, Department of Health and Human Services.; 2006. Available at: http://www.cdc.gov/nchs/data/ahcd/body_NAMCSOPD_072406.pdf. Accessed March 20, 2010.
9. National Center for Health Statistics. *Ambulatory Health Care Data - Frequently Asked Questions* (FAQs). http://www.cdc.gov/nchs/ahcd/ahcd_faq.htm. Accessed October 17, 2012.
10. National Center for Health Statistics. *Research Data Center - Restricted Data.* http://www.cdc.gov/rdc/B1DataType/Dt100.htm. Accessed October 17, 2012.
11. National Center for Health Statistics. *NCHS Data Linkage Activities.* http://www.cdc.gov/nchs/data_access/data_linkage_activities.htm. Accessed March 12, 2010.
12. Burt CW, Woodwell DA. *Physician Survey Response Methods Research.* ASA Proceedings of the Section on Survey Research Methods. 2006. Available at: http://www.amstat.org/Sections/Srms/Proceedings/y2006/Files/JSM2006-000198.pdf. Accessed April 7, 2013.
13. National Center for Health Statistics. *SAS Code to Produce Aggregated Visit Statistics at the Physician or Facility Level.* Rockville, MD: Centers for Disease Control and Prevention Available at: http://www.cdc.gov/nchs/data/ahcd/provider-visit-code.pdf. Accessed March 12, 2010.
14. Burt CW. *Use of Geographic Contextual Variables in Examining Survey Item Validity.* Proceedings from the Seventh Conference on Health Survey Research Methods. 2001:194. Available at: http://www.cdc.gov/nchs/data/slaits/conf07.pdf. Accessed March 12, 2010.
15. Morgan PA, Strand J, Ostbye T, et al. Missing in action: care by physician assistants and nurse practitioners in national health surveys. *Health Serv Res.* 2007;42:2022-2037.
16. National Center for Health Statistics. *Ambulatory Health Care Data - Reliability of Estimates.* http://www.cdc.gov/nchs/ahcd/ahcd_estimation_reliability.htm. Accessed March 12, 2010.
17. Schappert SM, Rechtsteiner EA. *Using NAMCS and NHAMCS Drug Data: A Hands-on Workshop.* Available at: www.cdc.gov/nchs/ppt/ahcd/Schappert_48.ppt. Accessed March 12, 2010.
18. National Center for Health Statistics, Division of Health Care Statistics. *Ambulatory Care Drug Database System.* http://www2.cdc.gov/drugs/. Accessed March 7, 2010.
19. National Center for Health Statistics. *Ambulatory Health Care Data: Trend Analysis Using NAMCS and NHAMCS Drug Data.* http://www.cdc.gov/nchs/ahcd/trend_analysis.htm#more_info. Accessed March 12, 2010.
20. Gonzales R, Steiner JF, Sande MA. Antibiotic prescribing for adults with colds, upper respiratory tract infections, and bronchitis by ambulatory care physicians. *JAMA.* 1997;278:901-904.

21. Gonzales R, Malone DC, Maselli JH, et al. Excessive antibiotic use for acute respiratory infections in the United States. *Clin Infect Dis*. 2001;33:757-762.
22. Nyquist AC, Gonzales R, Steiner JF, et al. Antibiotic prescribing for children with colds, upper respiratory tract infections, and bronchitis. *JAMA*. 1998;279:875-877.
23. Stone S, Gonzales R, Maselli J, et al. Antibiotic prescribing for patients with colds, upper respiratory tract infections, and bronchitis: a national study of hospital-based emergency departments. *Ann Emerg Med*. 2000;36:320-327.
24. Linder JA, Stafford RS. Antibiotic treatment of adults with sore throat by community primary care physicians: a national survey, 1989-1999. *JAMA*. 2001;286:1181-1186.
25. Cantrell R, Young AF, Martin BC. Antibiotic prescribing in ambulatory care settings for adults with colds, upper respiratory tract infections, and bronchitis. *Clin Ther*. 2002;24:170-182.
26. McCaig LF, Besser RE, Hughes JM. Trends in antimicrobial prescribing rates for children and adolescents. *JAMA*. 2002;287:3096-3102.
27. Dai C, Stafford RS, Alexander GC. National trends in cyclooxygenase-2 inhibitor use since market release: nonselective diffusion of a selectively cost-effective innovation. *Arch Intern Med*. 2005;165:171-177.
28. Pirraglia PA, Stafford RS, Singer DE. Trends in prescribing of selective serotonin reuptake inhibitors and other newer antidepressant agents in adult primary care. *Prim Care Companion J Clin Psychiatry*. 2003;5:153-157.
29. Stafford RS, Monti V, Ma J. Underutilization of aspirin persists in US ambulatory care for the secondary and primary prevention of cardiovascular disease. *PLoS Med*. 2005;2:e353.
30. Sankaranarayanan J, Puumala SE. Antipsychotic use at adult ambulatory care visits by patients with mental health disorders in the United States, 1996-2003: national estimates and associated factors. *Clin Ther*. 2007;29:723-741.
31. Olfson M, Marcus SC, Pincus HA, et al. Antidepressant prescribing practices of outpatient psychiatrists. *Arch Gen Psychiatry*. 1998;55:310-316.
32. Skaer TL, Sclar DA, Robison LM, et al. Trends in the rate of depressive illness and use of antidepressant pharmacotherapy by ethnicity/race: an assessment of office-based visits in the United States, 1992-1997. *Clin Ther*. 2000;22:1575-1589.
33. Aparasu RR, Fliginger SE. Inappropriate medication prescribing for the elderly by office-based physicians. *Ann Pharmacother*. 1997;31:823-829.
34. Aparasu RR, Mort JR, Sitzman S. Psychotropic prescribing for the elderly in office-based practice. *Clin Ther*. 1998;20:603-616.
35. Mort JR, Aparasu RR. Prescribing potentially inappropriate psychotropic medications to the ambulatory elderly. *Arch Intern Med*. 2000;160:2825-2831.
36. Zhan C, Sangl J, Bierman AS, et al. Potentially inappropriate medication use in the community-dwelling elderly: findings from the 1996 Medical Expenditure Panel Survey. *JAMA*. 2001;286:2823-2829.
37. Zhan C, Correa-de-Araujo R, Bierman AS, et al. Suboptimal prescribing in elderly outpatients: potentially harmful drug-drug and drug-disease combinations. *J Am Geriatr Soc*. 2005;53:262-267.
38. Rathore SS, Mehta SS, Boyko WL Jr, et al. Prescription medication use in older Americans: a national report card on prescribing. *Fam Med*. 1998;30:733-739.
39. McCaig LF, Burt CW. Poisoning-related visits to emergency departments in the United States, 1993-1996. *J Toxicol Clin Toxicol*. 1999;37:817-826.
40. Zito JM, Safer DJ, Riddle MA, et al. Prevalence variations in psychotropic treatment of children. *J Child Adolesc Psychopharmacol*. 1998;8:99-105.
41. Goodwin R, Gould MS, Blanco C, et al. Prescription of psychotropic medications to youths in office-based practice. *Psychiatr Serv*. 2001;52:1081-1087.
42. Robison LM, Sclar DA, Skaer TL, et al. National trends in the prevalence of attention-deficit/hyperactivity disorder and the prescribing of methylphenidate among school-age children: 1990-1995. *Clin Pediatr* (Phila). 1999;38:209-217.

**Part 4: Alternative, Population-Based Data Sources**

43. Sankaranarayanan J, Puumala SE, Kratochvil CJ. Diagnosis and treatment of adult attention-deficit/hyperactivity disorder at US ambulatory care visits from 1996 to 2003. *Curr Med Res Opin.* 2006;22:1475-1491.
44. Curtis KM, Hillis SD, Kieke BA Jr, et al. Visits to emergency departments for gynecologic disorders in the United States, 1992-1994. *Obstet Gynecol.* 1998;91:1007-1012.
45. Sankaranarayanan J, Puumala SE. Epidemiology and characteristics of emergency departments visits by US adults with psychiatric disorder and antipsychotic mention from 2000 to 2004. *Curr Med Res Opin.* 2007;23:1375-1385.
46. Jaen CR, Stange KC, Tumiel LM, et al. Missed opportunities for prevention: smoking cessation counseling and the competing demands of practice. *J Fam Pract.* 1997;45:348-354.
47. Centers for Disease Control and Prevention (CDC). Missed opportunities in preventive counseling for cardiovascular disease—United States, 1995. *MMWR Morb Mortal Wkly Rep.* 1998;47:91-95.
48. Wallace AE, MacKenzie TA, Weeks WB. Women's primary care providers and breast cancer screening: who's following the guidelines? *Am J Obstet Gynecol.* 2006;194:744-748.
49. Oliveria SA, Christos PJ, Marghoob AA, et al. Skin cancer screening and prevention in the primary care setting: national ambulatory medical care survey 1997. *J Gen Intern Med.* 2001;16:297-301.
50. Ma J, Urizar GG Jr, Alehegn T, et al. Diet and physical activity counseling during ambulatory care visits in the United States. *Prev Med.* 2004;39:815-822.
51. Feldman SR, Fleischer AB Jr, Chen JG. The gatekeeper model is inefficient for the delivery of dermatologic services. *J Am Acad Dermatol.* 1999;40:426-432.
52. Fong C. The influence of insurance status on nonurgent pediatric visits to the emergency department. *Acad Emerg Med.* 1999;6:744-748.
53. Conry CM, Pace WD, Main DS. Practice style differences between family physicians and internists. *J Am Board Fam Pract.* 1991;4:399-406.
54. Green LA, Miller RS, Reed FM, et al. How representative of typical practice are practice-based research networks? A report from the Ambulatory Sentinel Practice Network Inc (ASPN). *Arch Fam Med.* 1993;2:939-949.
55. Feldman SR, Williford PM, Fleischer AB Jr. Lower utilization of dermatologists in managed care: despite growth in managed care, visits to dermatologists did not decrease: an analysis of National Ambulatory Medical Care Survey data, 1990-1992. *J Invest Dermatol.* 1996;107:860-864.
56. Ma J, Stafford RS. Quality of US outpatient care: temporal changes and racial/ethnic disparities. *Arch Intern Med.* 2005;165:1354-1361.
57. National Center for Health Statistics. *NAMCS/NHAMCS Data Collection and Processing.* http://www.cdc.gov/nchs/ahcd/ahcd_data_collection.htm. Accessed March 12, 2010.
58. Liu T, Sayre MR, Carleton SC. Emergency medical care: types, trends, and factors related to nonurgent visits. *Acad Emerg Med.* 1999;6:1147-1152.
59. National Center for Health Statistics. *Summary of NCHS Surveys and Data Collection Systems.* http://www.cdc.gov/nchs/data/factsheets/factsheet_summary.htm. Accessed October 18, 2012.

CHAPTER 21

# Healthcare Cost and Utilization Project (HCUP)

Frank R. Ernst, RPh, PharmD, MS

This chapter on the Healthcare Cost and Utilization Project (HCUP) will introduce the HCUP databases and orient the researcher to the available data, online query tools, and software support provided by HCUP. The chapter will discuss specific elements and uses for each of the available datasets, as well as the strengths and limitations. Since HCUP provides hospital data, this chapter compares HCUP data other federal and nonfederal inpatient and outpatient hospital databases. Rationale is given for determining which of the HCUP data may be appropriate for particular research topics, populations, and questions. Practical aspects of using HCUP data including contact sources and pricing will be covered as well. Much of the information contained herein is available and was drawn from HCUP sources online, to which links and references are provided. Other information such as peer-reviewed journal references was found via Medline searches, personal experience, and holdings of the chapter's author.

The implementation of electronic medical records and the improved access to administrative health care databases have increased the popularity of pharmacoepidemiology and outcomes research studies. The basic principles of research are the same regardless of the data source, but there are a few special considerations. A summary report on the value of hospital discharge databases,[1,2] for example, begins with the fact that most states in the United States already collect hospital discharge data in one form or another. These data are relatively inexpensive to obtain and use compared to similar data from surveys and abstracted medical records. They are often more reliable than patient- or physician-reported data and more inclusive than data from third-party insurers since they include patients without insurance. In addition, they can often be employed for research on rare conditions or population subgroups when they capture large, geographically and demographically diverse populations of patients.

When using secondary data for research purposes, an appropriate data source must be selected to ensure that relevant information is available to answer the research question at hand.[3] Although not prospectively collecting data may save time, the process of manipulating the data for analysis in secondary databases can be complex. For example, estimating a treatment effect using secondary sources may require special statistical procedures to overcome the lack of randomization to treatment. By becoming familiar with available data sources and special issues relevant to the chosen data source, practitioners can conduct studies that make valuable contributions to the improvement of patient care. Discharge data are used

### Part 4: Alternative, Population-Based Data Sources

by a variety of researchers in a wide range of studies, including those involving public health, health outcomes, health care quality and health technology, health and disease management, and policy.

A continuing desire to improve outcomes and control public and private costs has stimulated greater interest in assessments of population health and factors involved with disease management. The application of health outcomes research principles and methods, which incorporates aspects of epidemiology and pharmacoepidemiology, health service utilization research, health economics, and psychometric evaluations, has prompted the implementation of disease management programs and subsequent assessments of their effectiveness and cost. These programs are based on appropriate, systematic, population-based approaches to identify persons at risk for health-related problems, to intervene with specific programs of care, and to measure outcomes of these interventions. Highly supportive in the efforts to understand and manage health and disease effectively, HCUP databases contain extensive clinical and economic information on medical, surgical, and pharmaceutical care received by the patients each covers. This makes the data highly useful for research related to assessments of health and disease management. The linkage of records by patient number in HCUP allows researchers to perform longitudinal studies. Also, depending on the disease area being evaluated and patient selection criteria, patients can be identified using International Classification of Diseases, 9th Revision, Clinical Modification (ICD-9-CM) codes for inpatient diagnoses and Current Procedural Terminology (CPT)-4 for outpatient procedures; demographic information and outcomes assessments can be analyzed at various levels.

Data on various outcomes such as hospitalizations and readmissions, length of stay, outpatient visits, inpatient and outpatient procedure utilizations and costs can be studied, depending on the selection of suitable variables and analytic methods. Inpatient and outpatient data can be used to study patterns of medication use and costs, medication adherence, and treatment/prescribing behaviors. Where feasible, the linking of medical files to external mortality information sources facilitates studies of diagnoses and treatments looking at mortality as an outcome. HCUP datasets can provide comprehensive information on inpatient, outpatient and pharmacy services at national, regional, and state levels.

A limitation of HCUP, however, is the potential for selection bias, because factors that influenced prescribing decisions are not directly available; however, this concern is not unique to HCUP and can apply in all large databases. Prospective research of patient outcomes is not feasible with HCUP data since HCUP does not permit the re-identification of patients from deidentified records. Additionally, analyses are vulnerable to certain coding errors or restrictions known to be at issue among hospital databases in general.

# 1. The Healthcare Cost and Utilization Project Family of Databases

The HCUP represents a group of 3 national-level and 3 state-level longitudinal health care databases, related software tools, and products sponsored by the Agency for Healthcare Research and Quality (AHRQ) and developed through a partnership between the federal government, state governments, and industry. The objectives of HCUP are to obtain data from statewide information sources, to design and develop multistate health care databases for health services research and health policy analysis, and to make these data available to a broad set of public and private users for various decision-making purposes and health care policy testing and implementation.

Data from the 3 state-level databases described below are also available from many contributing states. The latter are separate databases with some common data elements that may be combined to form custom multistate datasets of interest. Some of the state-level data can be linked at the patient level using an encrypted patient identifier for certain states. At the hospital level, it is also possible to link the HCUP databases to external data sources such as the American Hospital Association (AHA) Annual Survey and to county-level data from the Area Resource File.

The data contained in HCUP begin in 1988, with a lag of about 2 years, and are collected to the present. The uniformity and multistate reach of these data facilitate comparative studies of various aspects of health care including the cost and quality of hospital care, medical practice variation, relative effectiveness of medical treatment and technologies, and health care service utilization among special populations of interest. The privacy of patients in the databases is protected in compliance with Health Insurance Portability and Accountability Act of 1996 (HIPAA) regulations, though access to the limited dataset is widely available. Database users must agree to use each database only for research and statistical purposes and also agree not to attempt to identify individuals whose data are contained therein by using patient data in deidentified and aggregate manner.

# 2. Data Captured by Healthcare Cost and Utilization Project Databases

While some of the HCUP databases focus solely on inpatient stays, others include only ambulatory or outpatient data. Many of the data elements in HCUP databases are based on elements found on the Uniform Billing Form (UB-92 or UB-04) used by hospitals for reimbursement purposes. Hospitals create discharge abstracts for every patient for the purposes of billing and reimbursement. When these abstracts are compiled from administrative hospital records they include deidentified patient demographic details such as age or date of birth, gender, race/ethnicity, and diagnoses. They also include masked hospital information such as urban/rural designation, teaching/nonteaching status, number of beds, US census region and/or state. A limited number of diagnosis and procedure codes are also available (ICD-9-CM). Individual abstracts are stored electronically (computerized). State regulatory agencies require all hospitals to submit all discharge abstracts regularly; these are routinely audited and subject to penalties if hospitals do not comply. The latter step helps ensure a degree of quality, accuracy, and standardization within the abstracted record.

The data are captured for different time frames within each individual database, as well. Data from State Inpatient Databases (SID) are typically made available for all years starting in the 1990s, either for individual years or in aggregate. However, limited data (only 8 states) in the Nationwide Inpatient Sample (NIS) are available for 1988-1989; furthermore, data start from 1997 in the Kids' Inpatient Database (KID) and the State Emergency Department Databases (SEDD), from 1999 in the State Ambulatory Surgery Databases (SASD), and from 2006 in the Nationwide Emergency Department Sample (NEDS), as detailed in subsequent sections. In all cases, the data capture is described by HCUP as a federal-state-industry cooperative effort with implied high quality and standards in its ties to AHRQ.[4]

## 3. National Healthcare Cost and Utilization Project Hospital Inpatient and Outpatient Data

### Nationwide Inpatient Sample

The 2007 release of the Nationwide Inpatient Sample (NIS)[5] represented some 5 to 8 million hospital stays annually from a stratified sample of 1,045 hospitals from the majority (n=40) of US states; NIS data date back to 1988, although only 8 states reported data in this year. This approximates a 20% stratified sample of community hospitals for any given year. The NIS excludes short-term rehabilitation hospitals, long-term hospitals, psychiatric hospitals, and alcoholism and chemical dependency treatment centers. A large sample size in the NIS facilitates the analysis of rare conditions like congenital abnormalities[6] and rare treatments like organ transplantation.[7]

The NIS patient-level data format is derived from the State Inpatient Database (SID). As with a typical inpatient discharge abstract, it captures more than 100 core data elements for each hospitalization, including:

- patient demographics such as age, gender, race/ethnicity, and others;

- principal and secondary ICD-9-CM coded diagnoses and procedures;

- admission source and type;

- discharge disposition;

- payer type including Medicare, Medicaid, private/commercial, self-pay, and others;

- hospital characteristics such as bed size, teaching/nonteaching status, urban/rural status, region, and ownership type;

- total charges; and
- length of stay.

A complete list of variables in the NIS and their descriptions is available online from AHRQ.[8]

National- and regional-level hospitalization rates can be calculated using weights applied to NIS discharges. Also, with data releases from 2002 forward, case severity can be adjusted using All Patient Refined Diagnosis Related Groups (APR-DRGs),[9] All Payer Severity-adjusted (APS)-DRGs,[10] disease staging, and AHRQ comorbidity indicators. Beginning with the 2005 release, diagnosis and procedure group files are available, which contain elements adaptable to HCUP data.

Provider (that is, hospital) identities are available for a limited subset of institutions that already make their information public or agree to its release. However, data users must complete a training course and submit a Data Use Agreement and agree to data privacy terms. Additional provider data may be used to link the NIS to data from the Annual Survey of the AHA Annual Survey Database[11] and to county-level data from the Area Resource File,[12] a database available from the Health Resources and Services Administration comprising information on health facilities, health professions, measures of resource scarcity, health status, economic activity, health training programs, and socioeconomic and environmental characteristics. The NIS may be used to conduct research on topics as wide ranging as access to care,[13,14] quality of care,[15] medical treatment practice variation and effectiveness,[5,16] use of hospital services, cost of those services, and impact of changes in policy or practice,[17,18] and use of hospital services by special populations.[19-22]

NIS Trends Supplemental[23] files are available to assist with analyses that are designed to track patients across time frames and hospital settings. The utility of these files stems from changes to the NIS that have occurred over time; for instance, the data elements and their definitions and sampling and weighting strategies. Two advantages of the NIS supplemental files are that that they contain revised trend weights and that data elements have consistent definitions across multiple years.

Numerous published peer-reviewed journal articles have resulted from analyses conducted with the NIS. Topics of those articles include stroke,[24-26] Guillain-Barré Syndrome,[27,28] hospital resource utilization and mortality,[15] traumatic injury and fractures,[17,18] diabetes,[19] bleeding,[29] coronary artery bypass,[16] organ transplantation,[7] catheterization and other procedures,[13,14] hospitalization costs involving various disease states and subpopulations,[20-22] and numerous others.

## Kids' Inpatient Database

The Kids' Inpatient Database (KID)[30] is the only inpatient data source specifically for the hospital care of children and adolescents to include all payer types. Like the NIS, the KID is also derived from the SID as a stratified sample of SID discharges; however, whereas the NIS contains a proportion of patients age 20 or younger, the

KID contains *only* young patients and therefore a much larger sample of them. The KID is produced every 3 years. Data are available starting from 1997 forward, though the states and discharge counts vary by year. The 2003 KID sample contained approximately 3 million discharges for children 20 years or younger from more than 3,000 hospitals.

The KID is created by sampling 1 of every 10 noncomplicated hospital births and 8 out of every 10 other cases (complicated births or pediatric nonbirths) cases involving children. Data elements are similar to those shared by the NIS and SID; in addition, the KID contains variables applicable to research on children, such as age in days and in months, birth weight, discharge weight, neonatal/maternal diagnosis or procedure flag, complicated/uncomplicated birth flag, and KID-specific patient strata. A complete list of variables and their descriptions is available.[31]

The KID facilitates national- and regional-level studies owing to its multistate coverage. A number of published journal articles have come from analyses of the KID. Topics of those articles include hospital mortality and complications following hematopoietic stem cell transplantation,[32] pediatric injuries and fractures,[33-38] pediatric sepsis,[39] meningitis,[40] other infectious disease,[41] pediatric spinal cord injury,[42] rheumatic fever,[43] HIV,[7] congenital heart disease,[44] and many more.

## National Emergency Department Sample

The National Emergency Department Sample (NEDS)[45] captures a 20% stratified sample of hospital-based emergency department (ED) visits from about 1,000 hospital-based EDs. These data became available in early 2009, covering years 2006-2007 from 24 and 27 states, respectively, and now includes 29 states. The NEDS has been built from more than 25 million unweighted records in the HCUP State Emergency Department Databases (SEDD) and the State Inpatient Databases (SID; See Figure 1). This makes the NEDS the largest all-payer ED database in the US. Because the ED is both a point of entry for many hospital inpatient admissions and a health care treatment setting for treat-and-release outpatient (nonadmitted) ED visits, the NEDS is designed to provide national estimates of ED visits and to facilitate analyses of ED utilization patterns.

The NEDS data permit research concerning patients presenting to the ED, capturing patient and hospital characteristics and clinical conditions associated with ED visits. The NEDS includes ED visits not resulting in admission, whereas patients admitted through the ED as inpatients are found in the NIS. The NEDS data can produce nationally weighted or projected estimates. Data elements are similar to many of those in the NIS and SID, including principal and secondary ICD-9 diagnoses and procedures, CPT-4 procedures,[46] patient status at the time of discharge from the ED, total ED charges, and total hospital charges in cases of post-ED inpatient admission. No state identifiers are present in the NEDS, nor does it contain the same hospitals as the NIS. A complete list of variables and their descriptions is available.[47]

# 4. State-Level Healthcare Cost and Utilization Project Hospital Inpatient and Outpatient Data

## State Inpatient Database

The State Inpatient Database (SID)[48] covers inpatient hospitalizations from 1990 forward in community hospitals in most states. This repository of state data reportedly encompasses more than 90% of community hospital discharges in the United States.[4] Prior to 1994, the SID data were only obtained from community hospitals; since 1994, however, data from psychiatric hospitals, alcohol and drug dependency facilities, ambulatory surgery facilities, and state, federal, and veterans hospitals are available from self-selected states. The common format of the database makes the SID useful for comparing data across or between multiple states or regions of the country, as well as within single states. Indeed, this format was used to derive the NIS data format. And lacking the standardized format applied within the SID, each individual state may have its own NIS data format that may not be as easy to use.

As with the NIS, the SID includes more than 100 data elements for each hospitalization. These contain a core set of clinical and nonclinical details as well as resource utilization information. The core set of variables provides patient demographics such as age and gender, principal and secondary ICD-9 diagnosis codes, principal and secondary ICD-9 procedure codes, admission and discharge status, total charges, total hospital length-of-stay, anticipated payment source (for example, Medicare, Medicaid, private/commercial insurance, self-pay, and in some states managed care and other discrete payer types).[49]

Some states also include other elements such as race/ethnicity and hospital and county identifiers to facilitate linking to the AHA provider information. One may find each state's list of SID variables via the HCUP SID website.[48] The SID does not include data elements that can directly or indirectly identify individual patients or physicians, in compliance with HIPAA privacy regulations. The SID, like all HCUP datasets, does not contain medication information.

As with the NIS, there are many examples of published peer-reviewed journal articles that have employed data from the SID. Topics of those articles include patient safety measurement,[50] hospitalizations for poisoning,[51] sepsis,[52,53] Kawasaki syndrome,[54] men's health quality,[55] and others. These studies have used volume of procedures as proxy measures of quality, relying on secondary evidence that increased volume in certain surgical procedures may be associated with better outcomes. Other studies have studied the mortality variance across hospitals as a measure of quality, or utilization (overuse, underuse, and misuse).

## State Ambulatory Surgery Databases

The State Ambulatory Surgery Databases (SASD)[56] contain sets of data available from 28 states. These databases capture ambulatory patient, also called hospital

Part 4: Alternative, Population-Based Data Sources

outpatient, encounters occurring at both hospital-affiliated and free-standing (in some cases) ambulatory surgery sites. These data are available for years beginning in 1999 and facilitate the study of statewide trends in the volume and types of ambulatory surgery procedures being performed, access, charges, and outcomes, as well as similar clinical markets across state-defined regions of the country. These data also permit policy-related research concerning associations between insurance coverage and inpatient-versus-outpatient procedure utilization and teaching-versus-nonteaching hospital types, among others.

Data elements are similar to those in the SID and the NIS. A complete list of variables and their descriptions by year is available.[57] Analyses of the SASD have produced a number of published articles in peer-reviewed journals. Topics of those articles include, among others, hospitalizations for poisoning,[51] HIV,[58] and cholangiopancreatography, which involves a radiologic examination of the bile ducts and pancreas.[59]

### State Emergency Department Databases

The State Emergency Department Databases (SEDD)[60] are available from EDs associated with hospitals in a number of states. In the most recent databases available from HCUP, the SEDD captures ED visits that do not result in an inpatient stay. These data are available for years beginning in 1997 and data elements are in many ways similar to those shared by the SID and the NIS. A complete list of variables and their descriptions by year is available.[61]

The value of these data is in their utility to address research topics such as injury surveillance, emergent infectious diseases, nonfatal preventable illnesses, health care market access, ED-based care, and potential health care environment issues including the uninsured population who may use the emergency room for primary access. The state-specific nature of the data facilitates the study of statewide trends in ED use, access, charges, and outcomes, which can focus on a single state or on multiple states when procured from each separately, Topics of published papers that used this database include hospitalizations for poisoning,[51] injury,[62] and others.

## 5. Comparisons of Healthcare Cost and Utilization Project Databases to Other Hospital Data Sources

Naturally, aspects of certain hospital databases are sure to appeal differently to different researchers under different conditions. Where it may be important to compare the HCUP databases[63] to other hospital data sources, there are some key noteworthy differences. Each HCUP database has its own strengths and limitations. Once a researcher has gained experience with one HCUP database or a non-HCUP database with similar structure, that knowledge can be applied to other databases in the HCUP family. This is a major benefit to using the family of HCUP databases.

For the inpatient setting, the SID contains the population of *all* hospitalizations in the given states, whereas the National Hospital Discharge Survey (NHDS)[64] data represent a smaller, probabilistic sample of nonfederal US acute care (short stay) inpatient hospital stays (1965 and later, compared to 1998 and later for HCUP databases). The NIS, KID, and NEDS are like the NHDS in that they too are samples of the larger population of discharges. The latter and the SID from which they come are limited to data from self-selecting US states; thus the coverage of certain areas of the US is limited.

Databases from the HCUP family are also constrained by the absence of medication data in terms of the research questions that may be asked. By contrast, certain proprietary, nationally representative, hospital databases such as those from the Premier Health Care Alliance (Premier Inc., Charlotte, North Carolina),[65] Truven Health Analytics (Ann Arbor, Michigan) (formerly Thomson Reuters),[66] and Cerner Corporation (Kansas City, Missouri)[67] contain fine details about medication use, such as day/time of use, dose, quantity, and cost. Some of these latter named databases also contain date- or time-stamped clinical and resource utilization details within the hospital stay that enable the researcher to analyze patient location and treatment flow. Some contain direct quality measures and others contain information that may be used to infer indirectly quality of care in other ways such as how often treatment modalities are used in agreement with clinical guidelines.

In addition, parts of the hospital discharge abstracts are contained within each of the proprietary databases mentioned. They provide certain elements similar to HCUP databases. It should be noted that the HCUP and proprietary databases may differ in their coverage of population and geographic regions as well as in breadth and depth of detail.

For the outpatient or ambulatory setting, there are some important databases to consider and to compare with HCUP. One of the most prominent of these is the National Ambulatory Medical Care Survey (NAMCS),[68] a nationwide sample based on physician office visits. Another is the National Hospital Ambulatory Medical Care Survey (NHAMCS),[69] which captures data from emergency rooms and acute care facility-associated outpatient departments other than those in Veterans Health Administration, military and federal facilities. The NHAMCS captures patient complaints also and began collecting data in 1992 over 4-week periods for random samples of patients; the HCUP data do not capture measures of the patient experience.

Because nonhospital outpatient visits, such as physician office visits, are absent from HCUP databases, a proprietary claims database may be a better choice for studies of those encounters. Examples include the OptumInsights (formerly Ingenix i3) InVision™ Data Mart (OptumInsights, Eden Prairie, MN),[70] the Truven MarketScan® database,[66] or linked hospital and claims databases such as one available from Premier and Optum.[65,70] The first of these primarily represents the inpatient and outpatient medical claims from a commercially insured population covered by a single payer group in the US, and the second consists of health care insurance claims of patients insured with a variety of commercial health plans, many of which are self-insured employers, and both would be more suitable for physician visit research than most hospital-based databases. The linked database contains elements of both hospital administrative data and adjudicated insurance claims data.

Much as with the inpatient databases, the HCUP ambulatory and ED databases contain parts of the hospital discharge abstracts found within other databases detailed in other chapters of this book. These aforementioned alternative databases provide certain elements similar to HCUP at the same time as they contain, by design, different populations that differ in the breadth and depth of detail compared to HCUP. To help potential users gain a better understanding of the populations covered and the research topics that may be explored, HCUP publishes a large number of methodological white papers, statistical reports and report generators online.[71-78]

## 6. Using Healthcare Cost and Utilization Project Data

The HCUP data are readily accessible to researchers with the appropriate credentials and funding. Available in ASCII format, the SID, NIS, KID, NEDS, SASD, and SEDD data can be analyzed on desktop computers with CD-ROM capability using statistical software such as SAS (SAS Institute, Cary, NC), SPSS (SPSS Inc., Chicago, Illinois), or Stata (StataCorp LP, College Station, Texas). SAS and SPSS users will find helpful programs included with the purchased data that will convert ASCII files to acceptable formats. Because resources are available to explain the data elements for each database the researcher may be considering, and because many of the data elements are common across the HCUP databases, past experience can be readily transferred to new projects.

### Choosing the Appropriate Data Source

Choosing the data source for the researcher's requirements involves both understanding the differences between the datasets and determining which suits the types of analyses to be conducted. Table 1 shows some of the primary features of each HCUP database. The SID is useful for comparing data within 40 single states or across or between several states, perhaps in certain regions of the country. The NIS draws from the SID and may be used to conduct research on a wide range of topics at national and regional levels, and may be linked to the Annual Survey of the AHA Annual Survey Database[11] or to county-level data from the Area Resource File[12] as mentioned above.

The KID, which draws from the SID and is specifically focused on pediatric patients, contains variables applicable to research on children, such as age in days and in months, birth weight, discharge weight, neonatal/maternal diagnosis/procedure flags, complicated/uncomplicated birth flags, and KID-specific strata, The NEDS draws from the SID and the SEDD and concentrates on details of care received during ED visits. The SASD draw from the SID and are state-level sets of data available from 28 states that capture ambulatory patient encounters. Finally, as one of the most recent HCUP databases, the SEDD draw for the SID and contain data specific to EDs associated with hospitals.

## Available Software, Reports, and Support

Specific comorbidity software programs and documentation are available to researchers from HCUP, as are other software, tools, reports, and general support.

### Software

Software available from HCUP helps to identify comorbid medical conditions, clinical classifications, procedure classes, ratios of costs to charges, quality indicators (inpatient care, prevention, pediatrics, patient safety), and chronic conditions.

#### Comorbidity Software

The comorbidity software is constructed around the work by Elixhauser and colleagues[79] and is available free of charge. The algorithms may be applied to all of the HCUP databases. Moreover, its use is supported and available without restriction or fee for application to other similarly structured, nongovernmental and proprietary databases that contain ICD-9 diagnosis and procedure coding. It assigns variables to identify comorbidities in discharge records using ICD-9-CM diagnosis coding, and is updated annually; thus it can currently be applied both to the older DRG system and to the newer Medicare Severity Diagnosis Related Groups (MS-DRG) system.[80] Detailed documentation is available for the data elements requiring user-defined programming considerations, SAS programs for its use, and SAS programming instructions. A large number of peer-reviewed publications have used and described the HCUP Comorbidity Algorithm, applied to topics such as risk adjustment and mortality prediction,[81-85] fractures and injury,[86,87] mental disorders,[88] infection and related topics,[89,90] and others.

#### Clinical Classifications Software

The HCUP Clinical Classifications Software (CCS)[91] for ICD-9 is a diagnosis and procedure categorization scheme that can be employed in many types of projects. The ICD-9 codes are rolled into clinically meaningful categories that are sometimes more useful for presenting descriptive statistics than are individual ICD-9-CM codes. Electronic files are in ASCII format containing the translation of ICD-9-CM diagnosis and procedure codes into CCS categories. CCS categories are used in HCUP's electronic query tool, HCUPnet. In addition, CCS has been used in a number of published articles.[92-95]

## Part 4: Alternative, Population-Based Data Sources

### Procedure Classes Software

The Procedure Classes[96] were specifically created so that the researcher can readily determine if an ICD-9 coded procedure is diagnostic or therapeutic and is minor or major in terms of invasiveness and/or resource use:

- Minor Diagnostic: Nonoperating room procedures that are diagnostic
- Minor Therapeutic: Nonoperating room procedures that are therapeutic
- Major Diagnostic: All procedures considered valid operating room procedures by the Diagnosis-Related Group (DRG) grouper and that are performed for diagnostic reasons
- Major Therapeutic: All procedures considered valid operating room procedures by the Diagnosis-Related Group (DRG) grouper and that are performed for therapeutic reasons

Since ICD-9 codes are revised every October for the following fiscal year (October 1-September 30), the 4 Procedure Class categories are revised annually to reflect those changes.

Therefore, researchers are well advised to take the following actions when using the Procedure Classes:

- Alphanumeric procedure codes must be left-justified.
- One space must always follow a 3-character procedure code.
- Trailing blanks should never be zero-padded (ie, blank spaces following a 3-character procedure code should not be filled with zeroes).
- Leading zeroes must be preserved; they are significant.

### Inpatient Quality Indicators

The HCUP Inpatient Quality Indicators (IQI)[97] are a set of measures released in 2002, including a free software tool, which provides perspective on hospital quality of care using hospital administrative data. These indicators reflect quality of care inside hospitals and include inpatient mortality for certain procedures and medical conditions; utilization of procedures for which there are questions of overuse, underuse, and misuse; and volume of procedures for which there is some evidence that a higher volume of procedures is associated with lower mortality.

Development of quality indicators involves challenges such as defining indicators using administrative data, establishing validity and reliability, detecting bias and designing appropriate risk adjustment, and overcoming challenges of implementation and use. The IQI software programs can be applied to any hospital inpatient administrative data. The IQIs include mortality rates for medical conditions (7 indicators), mortality rates for surgical procedures (8 indicators), hospital-level procedure utilization rates (7 indicators), area-level utilization rates (4 indicators), and volume of procedures measures (6 indicators)

## Prevention Quality Indicators

The HCUP Prevention Quality Indicators (PQI)[98] are a set of measures released in late 2001 that can be used with hospital inpatient discharge data to identify quality of care for *ambulatory care-sensitive conditions*. These are conditions for which good outpatient care can potentially prevent the need for hospitalization or for which early intervention can prevent complications or more severe disease.

The PQIs are a software tool distributed free by AHRQ. The software can be used to help hospitals identify quality-of-care events that might need further study. The PQI software programs can be applied to any hospital inpatient administrative data. These data are readily available and relatively inexpensive to use.

Even though these indicators are based on hospital inpatient data, they provide insight into the community health care system or services outside the hospital setting. For example, patients may be hospitalized for complications of an underlying disease. The Prevention Quality Indicators represent hospital admission rates for the following ambulatory care-sensitive conditions, including diabetes, short-term complications, perforated appendicitis, diabetes, long-term complications, chronic obstructive pulmonary disease, hypertension, congestive heart failure, low-birth weight, dehydration, bacterial pneumonia, urinary infections, angina without procedure, uncontrolled diabetes, adult asthma, and lower extremity amputations among patients with diabetes.

## Pediatric Quality Indicators

The HCUP Pediatric Quality Indicators (PDI)[99] are a set of measures that can be used with hospital inpatient discharge data to provide a perspective on the quality of pediatric health care. Development of quality indicators for the pediatric population involves many of the same challenges associated with the development of quality indicators for the adult population. Four additional challenges that involve differentiating child health care visits from adult visits, children's dependency status, demographics, and development make it difficult to apply adult indicators to younger age ranges. Therefore, PDIs focus on potentially preventable complications and iatrogenic events for pediatric patients treated in hospitals, and on preventable pediatric hospitalizations.

The PDIs include 13 provider-level indicators, such as accidental puncture or laceration; iatrogenic pneumothorax—the presence of air or gas in the pleural cavity outside the lungs as a result of a therapeutic intervention like mechanical ventilation or tracheostomy tube placement, in neonates or non-neonates at risk; pediatric heart surgery mortality and volume; and postoperative hemorrhage or hematoma, respiratory failure, sepsis, or wound dehiscence. The PDIs also include 5 area-level indicators that describe the admission rates for asthma, diabetes, short-term complications, gastroenteritis, perforated appendix, and urinary tract infection.

## Patient Safety Indicators

The Patient Safety Indicators (PSI)[100] are a set of indicators in the form of a free software tool released in 2003 that provides information on potential in-hospital complications and adverse events following surgeries, procedures, and childbirth. The PSIs were developed after a comprehensive literature review, analysis of ICD-9 codes, review by a clinician panel, implementation of risk adjustment, and empirical analyses. The PSI software programs can be applied to any hospital inpatient administrative data.

The PSIs provide a perspective on patient safety events including the following hospital-level patient safety indicators:

- Complications of anesthesia
- Death in low-mortality DRGs
- Decubitus ulcer
- Failure to rescue
- Foreign body left in during procedure
- Iatrogenic pneumothorax
- Selected infections due to medical care
- Postoperative hip fracture
- Postoperative hemorrhage or hematoma
- Postoperative physiologic and metabolic derangements
- Postoperative respiratory failure
- Postoperative pulmonary embolism or deep vein thrombosis
- Postoperative sepsis
- Postoperative wound dehiscence in abdominopelvic surgeries
- Accidental puncture and laceration
- Transfusion reaction
- Birth trauma, injury to neonate
- Obstetric trauma, vaginal delivery with instrument
- Obstetric trauma, vaginal delivery without instrument
- Obstetric trauma, cesarean delivery

The PSIs provide a perspective on patient safety events including the following area-level patient safety indicators:

- Foreign body left in during procedure
- Iatrogenic pneumothorax
- Selected infections due to medical care
- Postoperative wound dehiscence in abdominopelvic surgeries
- Accidental puncture and laceration

- Transfusion reaction
- Postoperative hemorrhage or hematoma

*Chronic Condition Indicator*

The HCUP Chronic Condition Indicator (CCI)[101] provides a method to categorize ICD-9 diagnosis codes into chronic or not chronic categories. The CCI is updated each year, the current version based on ICD-9 diagnosis codes that are valid for January 1, 1980, through September 30, 2010. A *chronic condition* is defined as a condition that lasts 12 months or longer and either places limitations on self-care, independent living, and social interactions, or results in the need for ongoing intervention with medical products, services, and special equipment.[102,103]

Since ICD-9 codes are revised every October for the following fiscal year (October 1-September 30), the 4 Procedure Class categories are revised annually to reflect those changes.

Therefore, researchers are well advised to take the following actions when using the Procedure Classes:

- Alphanumeric procedure codes must be left-justified.
- One space must always follow a 3-character procedure code.
- Trailing blanks should never be zero-padded (ie, blank spaces following a 3-character procedure code should not be filled with zeroes).
- Leading zeroes must be preserved; they are significant.

## Reports

Readily available reports derived from HCUP databases are available online.[104] With national statistics, for example, HCUP Facts and Figures[105] is one set of reports that provides national statistics on hospital stays for 2007 and trends from 1993. At least 10 HCUP Fact Books provide summary details and comparative analyses related to topics such as hospitalizations and procedures in specific years (Fact Books 1, 2, 5, 6, 7, 9) and for specific patient populations such as women, children, and the uninsured (Fact Books 3, 4, 8). Fact Book 10[106] studies persons with mental health and substance abuse disorders.

Like the Facts and Figures reports, the HCUP Statistical Briefs provide descriptive statistics, the latter on a variety of specific, focused topics.[107] These include but are not limited to medical diagnoses and procedures (birth defects, cancer, diabetes, injury, pregnancy/childbirth, and more), patient populations (death, elderly, low income, men's and women's health, and more), hospital costs and charges, hospital characteristics, insurance type, EDs, and hospital quality and preventable hospitalizations. Technical HCUP reports include reports about each HCUP database, as well as reports on HCUP methods and spotlighted examples of peer-reviewed journal articles involving HCUP data, software, tools, and other products.

Part 4: Alternative, Population-Based Data Sources

*US Congress-Mandated Reports*

The National Healthcare Quality Report (NHQR),[108] a US Congress-mandated report in its fifth year (2007 data) will have provided more than 50,000 data points about health care quality in the United States. The fifth report summarizes the progress that has been made and the remaining challenges to improve health care quality in this nation, built on more than 200 measures categorized across 4 dimensions of quality—effectiveness, patient safety, timeliness, and patient centeredness. This year's report focuses on the state of health care quality for a group of 41 core report measures that represent the most important and scientifically credible measures of quality for the nation, as selected by the HHS Interagency Work Group. The National Healthcare Disparities Report (NHDR),[109] another US Congress-mandated report in its fifth year (2007 data) provides an overview of disparities in health care among racial, ethnic, and socioeconomic groups in the general US population and within specific priority populations, and it tracks the progress of activities to reduce disparities. The NHDR tracks disparities related to the quality of and access to health care. Both the NHQR and the NHDR measure health care quality and track changes over time.

## Healthcare Cost and Utilization Project Supplemental Files

*Cost-to-Charge Ratios*

The HCUP Cost-to-Charge Ratio (CCR) Files[110] are hospital-level files designed to supplement the data elements in the NIS (2001-2006), KID (2003 and 2006), and SID (2001-2006) databases. These databases contain data on total charges for each hospital in the databases. This charge information represents the amount that hospitals billed for services, but does not reflect how much hospital services actually cost or the specific amounts that hospitals received in payment. In some cases, users may be interested in seeing how hospital charges translate into actual costs and CCR Files contain hospital-specific cost-to-charge ratios based on all-payer inpatient cost for nearly every hospital in the corresponding databases.

Cost information is obtained from the hospital accounting reports collected by the Centers for Medicare & Medicaid Services (CMS). HCUP Cost-to-Charge Ratio Files are designed to be used exclusively with the HCUP NIS, SID, or KID; they should not be used for other databases. Users can merge the data elements on the appropriate file to the corresponding NIS, SID, or KID databases by the data element hospital identification number. Multiplying total charges with the appropriate cost-to-charge ratio yields the estimated hospital total cost. Finally, user guides for the CCR Files for each database are available. They contain detailed descriptions of the files, key variables and internal validation methods; linking instructions; and indications of which states participate each year.

## Supplemental Files for Revisit Analyses

The HCUP Supplemental Files for Revisit Analyses[111] are designed for analyses that track patients within a state and across time and hospital settings (inpatient, ED, and ambulatory surgery). While doing so, the privacy guidelines that apply to all HCUP databases are strictly retained. The Supplemental Files for Revisit Analyses may be used with the HCUP state-level databases: SID, SASD, and SEDD; however, there are no such files available for the HCUP nationwide databases: NIS, KID, and NEDS. The Supplemental Files for Revisit Analyses are available free of charge.

## American Hospital Association Linkage Files

The HCUP AHA Linkage Files[112] contain a small number of hospital-level data elements that allow researchers to supplement the HCUP SID, SASD, and SEDD with information from the AHA Annual Survey Databases.[11] Data elements from the AHA Annual Survey Databases can be linked to the HCUP AHA Linkage Files and then to the SID, SASD, and SEDD by using the encrypted hospital identification number. Separate linkage files are applied at the state and year levels.

## Nationwide Inpatient Sample and Kids' Inpatient Database Trend Files

The NIS Trends Files[113] and KID Trends Files[114] are discharge-level files that provide NIS and KID data users, respectively, with consistently defined trend weights and data elements for available years of the data. Both sets of files are available free of charge. Their purpose is to facilitate analyses that span multiple years and account for sample design changes. There is one NIS-Trends data file for each year from 1988 to 2002, and one KID-Trends data file for 1997 designed to match the weighting method used in subsequent years of the KID database.

# HCUPnet Online Healthcare Cost and Utilization Project Database Query System

An online HCUP database query system, HCUPnet (www.hcupnet.ahrq.gov/)[64] is available at no cost to users. This provides access to health information across the capabilities of the various HCUP databases. Researchers may explore national statistics on all hospital stays based on the NIS, mental health hospitalizations based on NIS, and state-level hospitalizations based on SID. Preformatted statistics may be found via the HCUPnet tool regarding state-level statistics, in addition to the custom research queries. Also accessible are ED statistics based on SEDD data, statistics on peer hospital types (hospitals with combinations of user-selectable characteristics), and AHRQ quality indicator information based on NIS.

## 7. Discussion and Summary

The HCUP longitudinal health care databases, related software tools, and products span from 1988 to only a few years in the immediate past. The uniform, multistate reach of these data facilitate comparative studies of the cost and quality of hospital care, medical practice variation, relative effectiveness of medical treatment and technologies, and health care service utilization among special populations, while holding to strict HIPAA protections of these private health care data. This chapter compared HCUP databases including the SID, the NIS, the KID, the new NEDS, the SASD, and the SEDD, to each other and to similarly intended federal and nonfederal inpatient and outpatient hospital databases. The chapter discussed ways to determine which of the HCUP data may help with analysis of particular topics, populations, and research questions. Each database in the family of HCUP databases, while similar to the others, is unique in its application.

Any summary of the value of hospital discharge databases such as HCUP starts with the fact that most states in the US already collect hospital discharge data in one form or another. Uses include public health and population-based applications, as well as quality assessment, informed purchasing, strategic planning, and policy making. Strategies to enhance the utility of discharge data include improving the quality of existing data elements and adding new data elements that will support more advanced analyses, improving linkages with data from nonhospital settings and databases outside health care, and developing a technical assistance network to support statewide data organizations in their efforts to collect and analyze discharge data. As our nation moves toward universal electronic medical records, it will be important to keep in mind the many uses of discharge data in order to maintain the data capacity to fill these needs.

## References

1. Schoenman JA, Sutton JP, Kintala S, Love D, Maw R. The value of hospital databases: final report. May 2005. Available at: www.hcup-us.ahrq.gov/reports/final_report.pdf. Accessed October 22, 2012.
2. Schoenman JA, Sutton JP, Elixhauser A, Love D. Understanding and enhancing the value of hospital discharge data. *Med Care Res Rev.* 2007;64:449-468.
3. Harpe SE. Using secondary data sources for pharmacoepidemiology and outcomes research. *Pharmacotherapy.* 2009;29:138-153.
4. Databases and Related Tools from the Healthcare Cost and Utilization Project (HCUP). Fact Sheet. AHRQ Publication No. 10-P009-EF, March 2011. Agency for Healthcare Research and Quality, Rockville, MD. Available at://www.ahrq.gov/data/hcup/datahcup.htm. Accessed October 25, 2012.
5. HCUP NIS Description of Data Elements. Healthcare Cost and Utilization Project (HCUP). May 2012. Agency for Healthcare Research and Quality, Rockville, MD. Available at: www.hcup-us.ahrq.gov/db/nation/nis/nisdde.jsp. Accessed October 25, 2012.
6. Robbins JM, Tilford JM, Bird TM, et al. Hospitalizations of newborns with folate-sensitive birth defects before and after fortification of foods with folic acid. *Pediatrics.* 2006;118:906-915.

7. Kourtis AP, Bansil P, Posner SF, et al. Trends in hospitalizations of HIV-infected children and adolescents in the United States: analysis of data from the 1994-2003 Nationwide Inpatient Sample. *Pediatrics*. 2007;120:e236-e243.
8. HCUP NIS Description of Data Elements. Healthcare Cost and Utilization Project (HCUP). May 2012. Agency for Healthcare Research and Quality, Rockville, MD. Available at: www.hcup-us.ahrq.gov/db/nation/nis/nisdde.jsp. Accessed October 25, 2012.
9. Averill R, Goldfield N, Hughes J, et al. What are APR-DRGs? *An introduction to severity of illness and risk of mortality adjustment methodology*. [white paper] Salt Lake City, UT: 3M™Health Information Systems; 2003. Available at: http://solutions.3m.com/3MContentRetrievalAPI/BlobServlet?locale=it_IT&lmd=1218718280000&assetId=1180603360910&assetType=MMM_Image&blobAttribute=ImageFile. Accessed October 25, 2012.
10. All Payer Severity-adjusted-DRGs Definitions Manual. Healthcare Cost and Utilization Project (HCUP). 2000-2003. Rockville, MD: Agency for Healthcare Research and Quality. Available at: www.hcup-us.ahrq.gov/db/nation/nis/APS-DRGsV20DefinitionsManual.pdf. Accessed October 25, 2012.
11. Annual Survey of the American Hospital Association (AHA) Annual Survey Database. Chicago, IL: Health Forum, LLC; 2007. www.healthforum.com/healthforum/html/pubs/pubs_ahapress.html. Accessed October 25, 2012.
12. Area Resource File (ARF) Overview. Health Resources and Services Administration. US Department of Health and Human Services; 2012. Available from Fairfax, VA: Quality Resource Systems, Inc.: http://arf.hrsa.gov/overview.htm. Accessed October 25, 2012.
13. Wiener RS, Welch HG. Trends in the use of the pulmonary artery catheter in the United States, 1993-2004. *JAMA*. 2007;298:423-429.
14. Neighbors CJ, Rogers ML, Shenassa ED, et al. Ethnic/racial disparities in hospital procedure volume for lung resection for lung cancer. *Med Care*. 2007;45:655-663.
15. Zilberberg MD, Luippold RS, Sulsky S, Shorr AF. Prolonged acute mechanical ventilation, hospital resource utilization, and mortality in the United States. *Crit Care Med*. 2008;36:724-730.
16. Swaminathan M, Shaw AD, Phillips-Bute BG, et al. Trends in acute renal failure associated with coronary artery bypass graft surgery in the United States. *Crit Care Med*. 2007;35: 2286-2291.
17. Phillips B, Clark DE, Nathens AB, et al. Comparison of injury patient information from hospitals with records in both national trauma data bank and the nationwide inpatient sample. *J Trauma*. 2008;64:768-779.
18. Daniels AH, Arthur M, Hart RA. Variability in rates of arthrodesis for patients with thoracolumbar spine fractures with and without associated neurologic injury. *Spine*. 2007;32: 2334-2338.
19. Cook C, Tackett S, Shah A, et al. Diabetes and perioperative outcomes following cervical fusion in patients with myelopathy. *Spine*. 2008;33:E254-E260.
20. Russell RB, Green NS, Steiner CA, et al. Cost of hospitalization for preterm and low birth weight infants in the United States. *Pediatrics*. 2007;120:e1-e9.
21. Qureshi AI, Suri MF, Nasar A, et al. Changes in cost and outcome among US patients with stroke hospitalized in 1990 to 1991 and those hospitalized in 2000 to 2001. *Stroke*. 2007;38:2180-2184.
22. Dombrovskiy VY, Martin AA, Sunderram J, Paz HL. Rapid increase in hospitalization and mortality rates for severe sepsis in the United States: a trend analysis from 1993 to 2003. *Crit Care Med*. 2007;35:1244-1250.
23. HCUP NIS Trends Supplemental Files. Healthcare Cost and Utilization Project (HCUP). May 2008. Rockville, MD: Agency for Healthcare Research and Quality. www.hcup-us.ahrq.gov/db/nation/nis/nistrends.jsp. Accessed October 25, 2012.
24. Bateman BT, Schumacher HC, Boden-Albala B, et al. Factors associated with in-hospital mortality after administration of thrombolysis in acute ischemic stroke patients: an analysis of the nationwide inpatient sample 1999 to 2002. *Stroke*. 2006;37:440-446.

25. Choi JH, Bateman BT, Mangla S, et al. Endovascular recanalization therapy in acute ischemic stroke. *Stroke*. 2006;37:419-424.
26. Janjua N, Nasar A, Lynch JK, Qureshi AI. Thrombolysis for ischemic stroke in children: data from the nationwide inpatient sample. *Stroke*. 2007;38:1850-1854.
27. Frenzen PD. Economic cost of Guillain-Barré syndrome in the United States. *Neurology*. 2008; 71:21-27.
28. Alshekhlee A, Hussain Z, Sultan B, Katirji B. Immunotherapy for Guillain-Barré syndrome in the US hospitals. *J Clin Neuromuscul Dis*. 2008;10:4-10.
29. Shea AM, Reed SD, Curtis LH, et al. Characteristics of nontraumatic subarachnoid hemorrhage in the United States in 2003. *Neurosurgery*. 2007;61:1131-1137.
30. HCUP Databases. Healthcare Cost and Utilization Project (HCUP). November 2011. Agency for Healthcare Research and Quality, Rockville, MD. Available at: www.hcup-us.ahrq.gov/kidoverview.jsp. Accessed October 25, 2012.
31. HCUP KID Description of Data Elements. Healthcare Cost and Utilization Project (HCUP). June 2011. Agency for Healthcare Research and Quality, Rockville, MD. www.hcup-us.ahrq.gov/db/nation/kid/kiddde.jsp. Accessed October 25, 2012.
32. Bratton SL, Van Duker H, Statler KD, et al. Lower hospital mortality and complications after pediatric hematopoietic stem cell transplantation. *Crit Care Med*. 2008;36:923-927.
33. Guice KS, Cassidy LD, Oldham KT. Traumatic injury and children: a national assessment. *J Trauma*. 2007;63(suppl 6):S68-S80.
34. Pressley JC, Trieu L, Kendig T, Barlow B. National injury-related hospitalizations in children: public versus private expenditures across preventable injury mechanisms. *J Trauma*. 2007;63(3 suppl):S10-S19.
35. Loder RT, O'Donnell PW, Feinberg JR. Epidemiology and mechanisms of femur fractures in children. *J Pediatr Orthop*. 2006;26:561-566.
36. Mooney DP, Rothstein DH, Forbes PW. Variation in the management of pediatric splenic injuries in the United States. *J Trauma*. 2006;61:330-333.
37. Schneier AJ, Shields BJ, Hostetler SG, et al. Incidence of pediatric traumatic brain injury and associated hospital resource utilization in the United States. *Pediatrics*. 2006; 118:483-492.
38. Brophy M, Sinclair SA, Hostetler SG, Xiang H. Pediatric eye injury-related hospitalizations in the United States. *Pediatrics*. 2006;117:e1263-e1271.
39. Odetola FO, Gebremariam A, Freed GL. Patient and hospital correlates of clinical outcomes and resource utilization in severe pediatric sepsis. *Pediatrics*. 2007;119:487-494.
40. Odetola FO, Tilford JM, Davis MM. Variation in the use of intracranial-pressure monitoring and mortality in critically ill children with meningitis in the United States. *Pediatrics*. 2006;117: 1893-1900.
41. Malek MA, Curns AT, Holman RC, et al. Diarrhea- and rotavirus-associated hospitalizations among children less than 5 years of age: United States, 1997 and 2000. *Pediatrics*. 2006;117: 1887-1892.
42. Vitale MG, Goss JM, Matsumoto H, Roye DP Jr. Epidemiology of pediatric spinal cord injury in the United States: years 1997 and 2000. *J Pediatr Orthop*. 2006;26:745-749.
43. Miyake CY, Gauvreau K, Tani LY, et al. Characteristics of children discharged from hospitals in the United States in 2000 with the diagnosis of acute rheumatic fever. *Pediatrics*. 2007;120:503-508.
44. Connor JA, Gauvreau K, Jenkins KJ. Factors associated with increased resource utilization for congenital heart disease. *Pediatrics*. 2005;116:689-695.
45. HCUP-US NEDS Overview. Healthcare Cost and Utilization Project (HCUP). November 2011. Agency for Healthcare Research and Quality, Rockville, MD. Available at: www.hcup-us.ahrq.gov/nedsoverview.jsp. Accessed October 25, 2012.
46. Current Procedural Coding (CPT©). American Medical Association (Chicago, IL). Available at: www.ama-assn.org/ama/pub/physician-resources/solutions-managing-your-practice/coding-billing-insurance/cpt.page. Accessed October 25, 2012.

47. HCUP NEDS Description of Data Elements. Healthcare Cost and Utilization Project (HCUP). September 2011. Agency for Healthcare Research and Quality, Rockville, MD. Available at: www.hcup-us.ahrq.gov/db/nation/neds/nedsdde.jsp. Accessed October 25, 2012.
48. HCUP Databases. Healthcare Cost and Utilization Project (HCUP). October 2012. Agency for Healthcare Research and Quality, Rockville, MD. Available at: www.hcup-us.ahrq.gov/sidoverview.jsp. Accessed October 25, 2012.
49. HCUP Central Distributor SID Description of Data Elements - Multiple Variables for All States Healthcare Cost and Utilization Project (HCUP). April 2008. Agency for Healthcare Research and Quality, Rockville, MD. Available at: www.hcup-us.ahrq.gov/db/state/siddist/sid_multivar.jsp. Accessed October 25, 2012.
50. Glance LG, Li Y, Osler TM, et al. Impact of date stamping on patient safety measurement in patients undergoing CABG: experience with the AHRQ Patient Safety Indicators. *BMC Health Serv Res*. 2008;8:176.
51. Zaloshnja E, Miller T, Jones P, et al. The potential impact of poison control centers on rural hospitalization rates for poisoning. *Pediatrics*. 2006;118:2094-2100.
52. Dombrovskiy VY, Martin AA, Sunderram J, Paz HL. Facing the challenge: decreasing case fatality rates in severe sepsis despite increasing hospitalizations. *Crit Care Med*. 2005;33: 2700-2701.
53. Dombrovskiy VY, Martin AA, Sunderram J, Paz HL. Occurrence and outcomes of sepsis: influence of race. *Crit Care Med*. 2007;35:763-768.
54. Holman RC, Curns AT, Belay ED, et al. Kawasaki syndrome in Hawaii. *Pediatr Infect Dis J*. 2005;24:429-433.
55. Felix-Aaron K, Moy E, Kang M, et al. Variation in quality of men's health care by race/ethnicity and social class. *Med Care*. 2005;43(3 suppl):I72-I81.
56. HCUP Databases. Healthcare Cost and Utilization Project (HCUP). January 2012. Agency for Healthcare Research and Quality, Rockville, MD. Available at: www.hcup-us.ahrq.gov/sasdoverview.jsp. Accessed October 25, 2012.
57. HCUP Central Distributor SASD Availability of Data Elements by Year. Healthcare Cost and Utilization Project (HCUP). September 2012. Agency for Healthcare Research and Quality, Rockville, MD. Available at: www.hcup-us.ahrq.gov/db/state/sasddist/sasddist_ddeavail-byyear.jsp. Accessed October 25, 2012.
58. Kourtis AP, Paramsothy P, Posner SF, et al. National estimates of hospital use by children with HIV infection in the United States: analysis of data from the 2000 KIDS Inpatient Database. *Pediatrics*. 2006;118:e167-e173.
59. Mazen Jamal M, Yoon EJ, Saadi A, et al. Trends in the utilization of endoscopic retrograde cholangiopancreatography (ERCP) in the United States. *Am J Gastroenterol*. 2007;102: 966-975.
60. HCUP Databases. Healthcare Cost and Utilization Project (HCUP). August 2012. Agency for Healthcare Research and Quality, Rockville, MD. Available at: www.hcup-us.ahrq.gov/seddoverview.jsp. Accessed October 25, 2012.
61. HCUP Central Distributor SEDD Availability of Data Elements by Year. Healthcare Cost and Utilization Project (HCUP). August 2012. Agency for Healthcare Research and Quality, Rockville, MD. Available at: www.hcup-us.ahrq.gov/db/state/sedddist/sedddist_ddeavail-byyear.jsp. Accessed October 25, 2012.
62. Coben JH, Steiner CA, Barrett M, et al. Completeness of cause of injury coding in healthcare administrative databases in the United States, 2001. *Inj Prev*. 2006;12:199-201.
63. HCUP Databases. Healthcare Cost and Utilization Project (HCUP). September 2012. Agency for Healthcare Research and Quality, Rockville, MD. Available at: www.hcup-us.ahrq.gov/databases.jsp. Accessed October 25, 2012.
64. National Hospital Discharge Survey (NHDS). Atlanta, GA: Centers for Disease Control and Prevention. Available at: www.cdc.gov/nchs/nhds.htm. Accessed October 25, 2012.
65. Premier Database. Charlotte, NC: Premier Inc. Available at: www.premierinc.com/quality-safety/tools-services/prs/data/perspective.jsp. Accessed October 25, 2012.

## Part 4: Alternative, Population-Based Data Sources

66. Truven Health Analytics. Ann Arbor, MI: Truven Health Analytics. Available at: http://www.truvenhealth.com/your_healthcare_focus/pharmaceutical_and_medical_device/. Accessed October 25, 2012.
67. Cerner Corporation. Kansas City, MOAvailable at: www.cerner.com. Accessed October 25, 2012.
68. Centers for Disease Control and Prevention. National Ambulatory Medical Care Survey (NAMCS). Available at: www.cdc.gov/nchs/ahcd.htm. Accessed October 25, 2012.
69. Centers for Disease Control and Prevention. National Hospital Ambulatory Medical Care Survey (NHAMCS). Available at: www.cdc.gov/nchs/ahcd.htm. Accessed October 25, 2012.
70. OptumInsight™. Eden Prairie, MN: OptumInsight. Available at: www.OptumInsight.com Accessed October 25, 2012.
71. HCUPnet. Healthcare Cost and Utilization Project (HCUP). Rockville, MD: Agency for Healthcare Research and Quality. Available at: hcupnet.ahrq.gov/. Accessed October 25, 2012.
72. HCUP Procedure Classes 2013. Healthcare Cost and Utilization Project (HCUP). Rockville, MD: Agency for Healthcare Research and Quality. Available at: www.hcup-us.ahrq.gov/toolssoftware/procedure/procedure.jsp. Accessed October 25, 2012.
73. HCUP Comorbidity Software, Version 3.7. Healthcare Cost and Utilization Project (HCUP). 2000. Rockville, MD: Agency for Healthcare Research and Quality. Available at: www.hcup-us.ahrq.gov/toolssoftware/comorbidity/comorbidity.jsp. Accessed October 25, 2012.
74. HCUP Cost-to-Charge Ratio Files (CCR). Healthcare Cost and Utilization Project (HCUP). September 2012. Rockville, MD: Agency for Healthcare Research and Quality. Available at: www.hcup-us.ahrq.gov/db/state/costtocharge.jsp. Accessed October 25, 2012.
75. HCUP MHSA. Healthcare Cost and Utilization Project (HCUP). January 2012. Agency for Healthcare Research and Quality, Rockville, MD. Available at: www.hcup-us.ahrq.gov/toolssoftware/mhsa/mhsa.jsp. Accessed October 25, 2012.
76. HCUP CCS-Services and Procedures. Healthcare Cost and Utilization Project (HCUP). April 2012. Agency for Healthcare Research and Quality, Rockville, MD. www.hcup-us.ahrq.gov/toolssoftware/ccs_svcsproc/ccssvcproc.jsp. Accessed October 25, 2012.
77. HCUP Clinical Classifications Software (CCS) for ICD-10. Healthcare Cost and Utilization Project (HCUP). January 2012. Rockville, MD: Agency for Healthcare Research and Quality. Available at: www.hcup-us.ahrq.gov/toolssoftware/icd_10/ccs_icd_10.jsp. Accessed October 25, 2012.
78. HCUP CCS. Healthcare Cost and Utilization Project (HCUP). August 2012. Agency for Healthcare Research and Quality, Rockville, MD. Available at: www.hcup-us.ahrq.gov/toolssoftware/ccs/ccs.jsp. Accessed October 25, 2012.
79. Elixhauser A, Steiner C, Harris DR, Coffey RM. Comorbidity measures for use with administrative data. *Med Care.* 1998;36:8-27.
80. Centers for Medicare & Medicaid Services. Acute Inpatient PPS. Available at: http://www.cms.gov/Medicare/Medicare-Fee-for-Service-Payment/AcuteInpatientPPS/index.html. Accessed October 25, 2012.
81. Li B, Evans D, Faris P, et al. Risk adjustment performance of Charlson and Elixhauser comorbidities in ICD-9 and ICD-10 administrative databases. *BMC Health Serv Res.* 2008;8:12.
82. Bass E, French DD, Bradham DD, Rubenstein LZ. Risk-adjusted mortality rates of elderly veterans with hip fractures. *Ann Epidemiol.* 2007;17:514-519.
83. Livingston EH. Development of bariatric surgery-specific risk assessment tool. *Surg Obes Relat Dis.* 2007;3:14-20.
84. Southern DA, Quan H, Ghali WA. Comparison of the Elixhauser and Charlson/Deyo methods of comorbidity measurement in administrative data. *Med Care.* 2004;42:355-360.
85. Johnston JA, Wagner DP, Timmons S, et al. Impact of different measures of comorbid disease on predicted mortality of intensive care unit patients. *Med Care.* 2002;40:929-940.
86. French DD, Bass E, Bradham DD, et al. Rehospitalization after hip fracture: predictors and prognosis from a national veterans study. *J Am Geriatr Soc.* 2008;56:705-710.
87. Thombs BD, Singh VA, Halonen J, et al. The effects of preexisting medical comorbidities on mortality and length of hospital stay in acute burn injury: evidence from a national sample of 31,338 adult patients. *Ann Surg.* 2007;245:629-634.

88. Carney CP, Jones L, Woolson RF. Medical comorbidity in women and men with schizophrenia: a population-based controlled study. *J Gen Intern Med*. 2006;21:1133-1137.
89. Baldwin LM, Klabunde CN, Green P, et al. In search of the perfect comorbidity measure for use in administrative claims data: does it exist? *Med Care*. 2006;44:745-753.
90. Brasel KJ, Guse CE, Layde P, Weigelt JA. Rib fractures: relationship with pneumonia and mortality. *Crit Care Med*. 2006;34:1642-1646.
91. HCUP Clinical Classifications Software (CCS) for ICD-9-CM. Healthcare Cost and Utilization Project (HCUP). August 2012. Rockville, MD: Agency for Healthcare Research and Quality. Available at: www.hcup-us.ahrq.gov/toolssoftware/ccs/ccs.jsp. Accessed October 25, 2012.
92. Ash AS, Posner MA, Speckman J, et al. Using claims data to examine mortality trends following hospitalization for heart attack in Medicare. *Health Serv Res*. 2003;38:1253-1262.
93. Bao Y, Sturm R. How do trends for behavioral health inpatient care differ from medical inpatient care in U.S. community hospitals? *J Ment Health Policy Econ*. 2001;4:55-63.
94. Cook CB, Tsui C, Ziemer DC, et al. Common reasons for hospitalization in urban diabetes patients. *Ethn Dis*. 2006;16:391-397.
95. Patil CG, Lad EM, Lad SP, et al. Visual loss after spine surgery: a population-based study. *Spine*. 2008;33:1491-1496.
96. HCUP Procedure Classes 2013. Healthcare Cost and Utilization Project (HCUP). November 2009. Rockville, MD: Agency for Healthcare Research and Quality. Available at: www.hcup-us.ahrq.gov/toolssoftware/procedure/procedure.jsp. Accessed October 25, 2012.
97. Inpatient Quality Indicators Overview. AHRQ Quality Indicators. March 2012. Rockville, MD: Agency for Healthcare Research and Quality. Available at: www.qualityindicators.ahrq.gov/modules/iqi_overview.aspx. Accessed October 12, 2012.
98. Prevention Quality Indicators Overview. AHRQ Quality Indicators. March 2012. Rockville, MD: Agency for Healthcare Research and Quality. Available at: www.qualityindicators.ahrq.gov/modules/pqi_overview.aspx. Accessed October 25, 2012.
99. Pediatric Quality Indicators Overview. AHRQ Quality Indicators. March 2012. Rockville, MD: Agency for Healthcare Research and Quality. Available at: www.qualityindicators.ahrq.gov/modules/pdi_overview.aspx. Accessed October 25, 2012.
100. Patient Safety Indicators Overview. AHRQ Quality Indicators. March 2012. Rockville, MD: Agency for Healthcare Research and Quality. Available at: www.qualityindicators.ahrq.gov/modules/psi_overview.aspx. Accessed October 25, 2012.
101. HCUP Chronic Condition Indicator (CCI). Healthcare Cost and Utilization Project (HCUP). Rockville, MD Agency for Healthcare Research and Quality. Available at: www.hcup-us.ahrq.gov/toolssoftware/chronic/chronic.jsp. Accessed October 25, 2012.
102. Radley DC, Gottlieb DJ, Fisher ES, Tosteson AN. Comorbidity risk-adjustment strategies are comparable among persons with hip fracture. *J Clin Epidemiol*. 2008;61:580-587.
103. Friedman B, Jiang HJ, Elixhauser A, Segal A. Hospital costs for adults with multiple chronic conditions. *Med Care Res Rev*. 2006;63:327-346.
104. HCUP Reports. Healthcare Cost and Utilization Project (HCUP). November 2012. Rockville, MD: Agency for Healthcare Research and Quality. Available at: www.hcup-us.ahrq.gov/reports.jsp. Accessed October 31, 2012.
105. HCUP Facts and Figures. Healthcare Cost and Utilization Project (HCUP). October 2011. Rockville, MD: Agency for Healthcare Research and Quality. Available at: www.hcup-us.ahrq.gov/reports/factsandfigures.jsp. Accessed October 31, 2012.
106. Owens P, Myers M, Elixhauser A, Brach C. Care of Adults With Mental Health and Substance Abuse Disorders in U.S. Community Hospitals, 2004—HCUP Fact Book No. 10. AHRQ Publication No. 07-0008, January 2007. Rockville, MD Agency for Healthcare Research and Quality. Available at: http://www.ahrq.gov/data/hcup/factbk10/. Accessed October 31, 2012.
107. HCUP Statistical Briefs By Topic. Healthcare Cost and Utilization Project (HCUP). September 2012. Rockville, MD: Agency for Healthcare Research and Quality. Available at: www.hcup-us.ahrq.gov/reports/sbtopic.jsp. Accessed October 31, 2012.
108. Agency for Healthcare Research and Quality. *2007 National Healthcare Quality Report*. Rockville, MD: U.S. Department of Health and Human Services, Agency for Healthcare Research

## Part 4: Alternative, Population-Based Data Sources

and Quality; February 2008. AHRQ Pub. No. 08-0040.
109. Agency for Healthcare Research and Quality. *2007 National Healthcare Disparities Report*. Rockville, MD: U.S. Department of Health and Human Services, Agency for Healthcare Research and Quality; February 2008. AHRQ Pub. No. 08-0041.
110. Cost-to-Charge Ratio Files. Healthcare Cost and Utilization Project (HCUP). September 2012. Rockville, MD: Agency for Healthcare Research and Quality. Available at: www.hcup-us.ahrq.gov/db/state/costtocharge.jsp. Accessed October 31, 2012.
111. HCUP Supplemental Files. Healthcare Cost and Utilization Project (HCUP). January 2010. Rockville, MD: Agency for Healthcare Research and Quality. Available at: www.hcup-us.ahrq.gov/toolssoftware/supplemental.jsp. Accessed October 31, 2012.
112. American Hospital Association Linkage Files. Healthcare Cost and Utilization Project (HCUP). October 2008. Rockville, MD: Agency for Healthcare Research and Quality. Available at: www.hcup-us.ahrq.gov/db/state/ahalinkage/aha_linkage.jsp. Accessed October 12, 2012.
113. HCUP NIS Trends Supplemental Files Healthcare Cost and Utilization Project (HCUP). May 2008. Rockville, MD Agency for Healthcare Research and Quality. Available at: www.hcup-us.ahrq.gov/db/nation/nis/nistrends.jsp. Accessed October 31, 2012.
114. HCUP KID Trends Supplemental Files. Healthcare Cost and Utilization Project (HCUP). May 2008. Rockville, MD: Agency for Healthcare Research and Quality. Available at: www.hcup-us.ahrq.gov/db/nation/kid/kidtrends.jsp. Accessed October 31, 2012.
115. HCUP Partners. Healthcare Cost and Utilization Project (HCUP). July 2010. Rockville, MD: Agency for Healthcare Research and Quality. Available at: www.hcup-us.ahrq.gov/partners.jsp. Accessed October 31, 2012.

**FIGURE 1.** HCUP Database Relationships

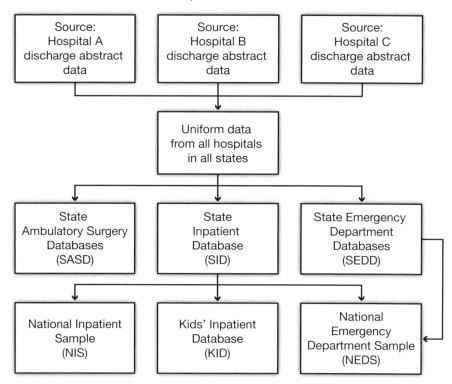

**TABLE 1.** Primary features of the HCUP databases

| | NIS | KID | NEDS | SID | SASD | SEDD |
|---|---|---|---|---|---|---|
| Target population | All discharges from community, nonrehabilitation hospitals in the US | Pediatric discharges from community, nonrehabilitation hospitals in the US | All emergency department visits from hospital-based emergency department units in community, nonrehabilitation hospitals in the US | All discharges from community, nonrehabilitation hospitals in the US | All ambulatory surgery visits from hospital-based ambulatory centers in community, nonrehabilitation hospitals in the US | All nonadmitted emergency department visits from hospital-based emergency department units in community, nonrehabilitation hospitals in the US |
| Sample frame | All discharges from community, nonrehabilitation hospitals in the participating HCUP Partner States * | Pediatric discharges from community, nonrehabilitation hospitals in the participating HCUP Partner States * | All emergency department visits from hospital-based emergency department units in community, nonrehabilitation hospitals in the participating HCUP Partner States * | All discharges from community, nonrehabilitation hospitals in the participating HCUP Partner States * | All ambulatory surgery visits from hospital-based ambulatory centers in community, nonrehabilitation hospitals in the participating HCUP Partner States * | All nonadmitted emergency department visits from hospital-based emergency department units in community, nonrehabilitation hospitals in the participating HCUP Partner States * |
| Sample strata | US region, urban or rural location, teaching status, ownership, bed size | State, uncomplicated births, complicated births, all other pediatric hospital stays | US region, urban or rural location, teaching status, ownership, trauma level | State, US region, urban or rural location, teaching status, ownership, bed size | State, US region, urban or rural location, teaching status, ownership, bed size | State, US region, urban or rural location, teaching status, ownership, trauma level |
| Sample unit | Hospital level (20% stratified sample) | Pediatric discharges (20% stratified sample) | Hospital emergency department level (20% stratified sample) | Contain the universe of encounters for HCUP Partner States, including encounters from hospital-affiliated and freestanding surgery centers | Some contain the universe of ambulatory surgery encounters for HCUP Partner States, including those from hospital-affiliated and freestanding surgery centers | Some contain the universe of emergency department visits for HCUP Partner states |
| Years covered | 1988-2010 | 1997, 2000, 2003, 2006, 2009 | 2006-2010 | 1990-2011 | 1997-2011 | 1999-2011 |

continued >

## Part 4: Alternative, Population-Based Data Sources

< continued from previous page

**TABLE 1.** Primary features of the HCUP databases

| | NIS | KID | NEDS | SID | SASD | SEDD |
|---|---|---|---|---|---|---|
| Number of participating states | Up to 40 | Up to 44 | Up to 29 | Up to 46 | Up to 30 | Up to 27 |
| Introductory reference | http://www.hcup-us.ahrq.gov/db/nation/nis/NIS_Introduction_2010.jsp | http://www.hcup-us.ahrq.gov/db/nation/kid/kid_2006_introduction.jsp | http://www.hcup-us.ahrq.gov/db/nation/neds/nedsdbdocumentation.jsp | http://www.hcup-us.ahrq.gov/db/state/siddist/SID_Introduction.jsp | www.hcup-us.ahrq.gov/db/state/sasddist/Introduction_to_SASD.pdf | www.hcup-us.ahrq.gov/db/state/sedddist/Introduction_to_SEDD.pdf |

* HCUP Partners.[115]

CHAPTER 22

# Medicare Databases

Renée J.G. Arnold, PharmD, RPh; and
Tammy G. Curtice, PharmD, MS, MBA

## 1. Introduction
This chapter provides an overview of Medicare data sources. First, there is a brief description of the Medicare program and its beneficiaries. Second, there is a description of the 3 types of Medicare data available: research identifiable files (RIFs), limited data set (LDS) files, and nonidentifiable data files. Third, we describe ways the data could be used in health and disease management programs. Finally, selected examples of published studies using Medicare data are reviewed, along with issues and limitations of using this data for research.

### The Medicare Program
Medicare became law July 30, 1965, under Title XVIII of the Social Security Act and is a compulsory health insurance program for the elderly financed by US federal payroll taxes and a voluntary insurance program for physician services subsidized with general tax revenues. The Centers for Medicare & Medicaid Services (CMS) is the federal agency that administers the program. As of 2008, Medicare provides coverage to approximately 45 million Americans. In 2006, Medicare spending accounted for 22% ($381 billion) of the total $1.76 trillion spent on personal health care in the United States (US).[1]

Public programs account for almost half (46%) of health care spending in the US and Medicare is the largest single purchaser. Medicare benefits are divided into 4 parts and are labeled "A" through "D." Part A pays for care provided to patients in hospitals, skilled nursing facilities, hospices, and some home health care programs. Part B provides coverage for physicians' and other practitioners' services, hospital outpatient and other outpatient facility services, home health (not covered under Part A), and other services such as diagnostic testing, durable medical equipment, ambulance services, limited preventative services, and some outpatient prescription drugs. Part C consists of Medicare Advantage and private health plans which cover all health care services. Part D is the voluntary outpatient prescription drug benefit that first became available in 2006. In 2007, Medicare program spending per enrollee was approximately $10,500.[1] Medicare is available for any individual who receives Social Security benefits, including those who are age 65 or older, are less than 65 years old with certain specified disabilities, or have end-stage renal disease (ESRD).

When individuals become eligible for Medicare, they are automatically enrolled in and receive Part A benefits. Although enrollment in Medicare Part B is voluntary, the majority of beneficiaries enrolled in the program choose to enroll in Part B. Medicare Part D covers most outpatient prescription drugs with a few exceptions that are covered by Part B or excluded from the benefit. Medicare patient cost-sharing consists of deductibles, copayments, coinsurance and premiums, which vary by coverage type. For example, Medicare Part A premiums vary according to the length of Medicare-covered employment. Part B premiums are based on a sliding scale according to beneficiary income. Part D premiums depend on the health plan in which the beneficiary chooses to enroll. Part D premiums are influenced by both the choice of medications available on the health plan's formulary and patient out-of-pocket costs. Medicare Advantage plans (Part C) cover the same services as Parts A, B, and D, but the cost-sharing (including premiums) may be structured differently.

The proportion of the US population that becomes eligible for Medicare each year is increasing. Simultaneously, those who have already qualified are living longer with chronic illnesses, creating a need for more effective methods of health and disease management to control potential health care costs. Therefore, research on the comparative effectiveness of different programs and tools to help contain costs, while maintaining or improving quality, has become increasingly important for the Medicare program. The Medicare population itself is an important one for researchers to understand, particularly those interested in evaluating health and disease management programs that target prevalent chronic conditions in the elderly—including diabetes, heart and lung diseases, and cancer—that represent some of the leading causes of illness, disability, and death, and account for a disproportionate share of United States health care expenditures.[2]

## Types of Medicare Data Available

Three types of Medicare data are available to researchers not working under a government contract for research purposes: RIFs, LDS files, and nonidentifiable data files. They are distinguished by the level of privacy review required before the release of data. Both the RIFs and LDS data are considered identifiable datasets. RIFs contain person-specific data on Medicare providers, beneficiaries and recipients, with submission of extensive documentation required to obtain access. Nonidentifiable data files contain aggregated data on beneficiaries and providers without personal information that could identify an individual.

Initially, researchers must submit applications materials to the Research Data Assistance Center (ResDAC), which then forwards data use applications to CMS for approval. Approval to use either the RIFs or LDS data sets is contingent on demonstrating to CMS that the research will directly benefit the beneficiaries or enhance administration of the Medicare program.

## Research Identifiable Files

RIF data are available from 1991 onward unless stated otherwise and include standard analytical files (SAFs), Medicare Provider and Analysis Review (MEDPAR) file, Medicare enrollment and vital statistics files, Beneficiary Annual Summary File (BASF), prescription drug event (PDE) data, chronic condition data warehouse (CCW) data, Hospital Outpatient Prospective Payment System (HOPPS), HOPPS – Partial Hospitalization Program (HOPPS PHP), and Medicare Physician Identification and Eligibility Registry (MPIER) files.[3] Table 1 describes these data.

**TABLE 1.** RIF Data Available from CMS

| | |
|---|---|
| **Standard Analytical Files (SAFs)** | Claims FOR institutional (inpatient, outpatient, skilled nursing facility (SNF), hospice or home health agency) and noninstitutional (physician and durable medical equipment) providers. |
| **Medicare Provider and Analysis Review (MEDPAR) Data** | Claims for inpatient hospital and SNF stays. |
| **Medicare Enrollment and Vital Statistics Files** | Demographic data on every beneficiary who was ever enrolled in the Medicare program. |
| **Beneficiary Annual Summary File (BASF)** | Enrollment, eligibility, vital statistics and summary information on service utilization. |
| **Prescription Drug Event (PDE) Data** | Information on demographics and utilization for the Medicare Part D prescription drug benefit |

## Limited Datasets

The difference between the RIF and the LDS data is the level of precision provided for certain identifying variables. In the LDS files, service dates are replaced by quarter and year, beneficiary's age is aggregated to 5-year intervals, and the geographic precision is the county rather than ZIP code in the RIF. LDS data are available in standard and searchable versions. The standard LDS files are 100% or 5% sample copies of the master data file. The searchable LDS files allow researchers to select 100% of records from up to 8 states. LDS files include SAFs, MEDPAR files, denominator data, HOPPS files, HOPPS PHP files, ESRD composite rate payment system data, and ambulatory surgical center (ASC) payment system data. Table 2 describes these data.

**TABLE 2.** LDS Data Available from CMS

| | |
|---|---|
| **Standard Analytical Files (SAFs)** | Claims for institutional (inpatient, outpatient, skilled nursing facility (SNF), hospice or home health agency) and noninstitutional (physician and durable medical equipment) providers. |
| **Medicare Provider and Analysis Review (MedPAR) Data** | Claims for inpatient hospital and SNF stays. |
| **Denominator File** | Demographic and enrollment information about each beneficiary and is available for fiscal years 1999 forward. |

*continued >*

Part 4: Alternative, Population-Based Data Sources

< continued from previous page

**TABLE 2.** LDS Data Available from CMS

| Hospital Outpatient Prospective Payment System (HOPPS) Data | Select claim-level data derived from hospital outpatient PPS claims, including fields such as bill type, principal and other diagnoses, outlier payments, and ambulatory payment classification (APC) rates. |
|---|---|
| HOPPS Partial Hospitalization Program (HOPPS PHP) Data | Select claim-level data derived from partial hospitalization program services. It includes mental illness and substance abuse disorders treatment furnished by hospitals and community mental health centers. |
| End-stage Renal Disease Composit Rate Payment System Files | Facility outpatient claims for individuals with end-stage renal disease. |
| Ambulatory Surgical Center (ASC) Payment System Data | Service utilization summary data by ASC suppliers. |

## Nonidentifiable Data

The aggregate-level information found in the nonidentifiable datasets includes: Medicare cost reports, health care information system (HCIS) data, Part B carrier summary data files, Part B national summary data files, provider of services files, hospital service area files, physician/supplier procedure summary master files, unique physician identification number (UPIN) directory and group file, Medicaid drug claim statistics, and prescription drug plan formulary and pharmacy network files. These are detailed in Table 3.

**TABLE 3.** Nonidentifiable Data Available from CMS

| Medicare Cost Reports | Provider information such as facility characteristics, utilization data, cost and charges by cost center (in total and for Medicare), Medicare settlement data and financial statement data in the Healthcare Provider Cost Reporting Information System (HCRIS). |
|---|---|
| Health Care Information System (HCIS) Data | Summary Medicare Part A (inpatient, SNF, Home Health Agency Parts A and B, and Hospice) and Medicare Part B (outpatient) data based on the type and state of the institutional provider. |
| Part B Carrier Summary Data File | These data are at the carrier level and show allowed services, charges, and payment amounts by Healthcare Common Procedure Coding/Current Procedural Terminology (HCPC/CPT). |
| Part B National Summary Data File | The data sets are summarized by meaningful Healthcare Common Procedure Coding/Current Procedural Terminology, (HCPC/CPT), code ranges. |
| Provider of Services File | This data file includes the provider name, number, and address. |
| Hospital Service Area File | This file is based on inpatient claims data by calendar year and includes discharge information, length of stay, total charges. |

continued >

< continued from previous page
**TABLE 3.** Nonidentifiable Data Available from CMS

| Physician/Supplier Procedure Summary Master File | All Part B carrier claims stored in the National Claims History Repository. |
|---|---|
| Unique Physician Identification Number Directory and Group File | Select information on practitioners enrolled in the Medicare program. The directory file has data from 2003 through 2007 and the group file has annual data from 2004 through 2007. The UPIN was discontinued as of June 2007 and replaced with the National Provider Identifier (NPI), which is not available for public use. |
| Medicaid Drug Claims Statistics | This file summarizes the number of claims paid for by Medicaid within the 60 groups from Medi-Span's Therapeutic Classification System with data available for 2003. |
| Prescription Drug Plan Formulary and Pharmacy Network Files | This file contains formulary and pharmacy network data for Medicare prescription drug plans and Medicare Advantage prescription drug plans. |

## 2. Requesting Centers for Medicare & Medicaid Services Data

### Research Identifiable Files

CMS requires that ResDAC review all requests for RIFs for completeness and accuracy prior to submission to CMS. There are 3 types of information packets that must be assembled to allow purchase/download and use of Medicare files: (1) New Use Request for new data, (2) Reuse (Re-release) Request to reuse data originally released for another purpose and (3) Amendment/Update to existing Data Use Agreement (DUA) Request to make a request for additional years of data for the same project. Requests to reuse data requires 2 additional documents—Certification of Reuse Form (to whom the data was originally released) and a Sample Letter of Support for Original Requester form if someone other than the original requestor will be using the data.

### Limited Dataset Files

Researchers requesting LDS files may send these requests directly to CMS, bypassing ResDAC review. Documentation includes: a written request letter, 2- to 3-page research application, LDS DUA, LDS Order Form and check or money order for payment in full. Similar to those for RIFs, requests are for New Use Request and Reuse/Re-release Request.

## 3. Use of Medicare Databases in Health and Disease Management

Real-world examples using Medicare data to inform health and disease management decisions and programs are important for understanding the potential value of these data. The Medicare Health Support program provides one example. In addition, select published studies using Medicare data for health management and outcomes assessment are summarized. Lastly, the Surveillance Epidemiology and End Results (SEER) and Medicare database project are described.

## Medicare Health Support Program: Traditional Fee-for-Service Medicare

The Medicare Health Support (MHS) program was designed to offer self-care guidance and support to chronically ill beneficiaries to help them manage their health, adhere to their physician's plan of care, and, overall, to reduce their health risks.[4] Care coordination between the health plan and providers was a key component of this program. In addition, resources and education were available to patients for appropriate and successful self-care.

The MHS initiative[4] was initially referred to as the Voluntary Chronic Care Improvement Pilot Program under Traditional Fee-for-Service Medicare. This program was supported by Section 721 of the Medicare Modernization Act of 2003 and was changed to the name Medicare Health Support (MHS) prior to implementation. CMS designed this program with the goal of reducing health risks, improving quality of life for patients, and providing financial savings. The MHS program was designed in 2 phases, with Phase I lasting 3 years, starting in 2005, and Phase II following, based on the evaluation of Phase I results. The program is operated by Medicare Health Support Organizations (MHSOs) who were awarded participation by CMS.

There were approximately 100,000 chronically ill beneficiaries who participated in the MHS programs. These beneficiaries represented both urban and rural areas and the programs were run by the 5 Active Phase I MHSOs in Central Florida (Green Ribbon Health), Tennessee (XL Health Corporation), Chicago, Illinois (Aetna Health Management LLC), Maryland and the District of Columbia (Healthways Inc.), and Western Pennsylvania (Health Dialog Services Corporation). All of the programs were active for 2 to 3 years and ended in August 2008.

The benefits of the MHS programs included the potential to reduce Medicare program spending, highlighting the value of care coordination and disease management interventions for older and sicker patients, determining the most effective programs and identifying barriers to success for future Medicare disease management interventions. Unfortunately, Phase I results demonstrated that the program did not meet its target for financial savings. Furthermore, the programwide fees paid to the MHSOs were 5 to 11% higher than typical Medicare management fees.[4,5]

## Examples of Retrospective Use of Medicare Databases

Medicare databases can be used to answer questions and inform decisions about health care programs. These data, although not collected specifically to answer health research questions, are rich with information. For example, using the Medicare datasets, disease prevalence can easily be estimated, including the capability to compare disease incidence over several years. In addition, disease costs and outcomes (for example, hospitalizations or physician visits) can be estimated.

The types of questions that can be posed and answered will depend on the specific dataset being used and the type of information contained in the database. For example, some datasets include cost information and can be useful for health care decision makers when trying to identify which types of health interventions provide the most value. Unfortunately, while there are no published studies using the Medicare databases with a primary focus on disease management, there are studies published that focused more broadly on health outcomes. Included in this discussion are examples of published studies that help to provide an understanding of the types of research that have been done with these data and the type of information that can be produced.

Dillavou and colleagues[6] used a 5% inpatient Medicare (MEDPAR) sample to evaluate changes in health outcomes over time in patients who had undergone abdominal aortic aneurysm (AAA) repair. The methodology stated that beneficiary encrypted files were used, so it is assumed they were RIFs. Data were obtained for the years 1994 through 2001. The authors also obtained a similar sampling for 2002 and 2003 with increased encryption as a 5% LDS. Information contained in the database included patient demographic data, diagnostic and procedure codes, discharge status, payment information, and location of treatment. Raw numbers of patients obtained from the 5% files were multiplied by 20 to estimate yearly nationwide totals. Ultimately, data from 16,124 records were analyzed, representing 322,480 patients with an AAA diagnosis.

Similarly, Kleindorfer and colleagues[7] compared use of recombinant tissue plasminogen activator (rt-PA) as noted in Medicare and a nationwide hospital database, the Premier Hospital database. The Premier Hospital database allowed cross-referencing to a pharmacy coding database in acute ischemic stroke. Both articles specified that the populations did not include Medicare beneficiaries in managed care plans (accounting for roughly 5% of Medicare enrollment in 2005) in the MEDPAR data and, by definition, patients under 65 years old. Kleindorfer found that using only MEDPAR data, rt-PA use is underestimated, due primarily to diagnosis and/or medication miscoding.

## SEER-Medicare Database

The Surveillance Epidemiology and End Results (SEER)-Medicare database is an initiative that links 2 large population-based data sources to provide information on Medicare-aged people with cancer.[8] This database can be used for a variety of research studies, including health and disease management research. The SEER data come from cancer registries and include clinical, demographic and cause of death information for individuals with cancer. The Medicare data come from Medicare claims collected from eligibility until death. By linking these 2 datasets, there is a unique opportunity for research in an older population suffering from cancer. There have already been numerous outcomes research studies published using this population, with the data available for additional studies.[9]

## 4. Data Quality and Availability Issues with Medicare Data

There are a number of data quality and availability issues that researchers must consider before using Medicare data. For example, MEDPAR files only contain data on inpatient hospital stays. Therefore, following a patient through outpatient visits upon hospital discharge will require linking of these data to outpatient SAFs. Also, in contrast to a Medicare MEDPAR file or inpatient SAF case, in which a single hospitalization corresponds to a single record, outpatient visits and claim records in the outpatient SAF do not have a 1-to-1 correlation. Consequently, an office visit may cover multiple services, for example, medical care, diagnostic radiology, and laboratory, with separate charges generating one or several claim records.

Conversely, a Medicare claim record can contain charges stemming from one or more office visits. Therefore, to estimate outpatient numbers and costs accurately, one must first scan claims records for each patient and assign all services and charges incurred on the same date to a unique visit record. The result will be a new file derived from the outpatient SAF that has one record per visit consolidating all costs associated with that visit. The researcher who is unfamiliar with Medicare data may choose to use MEDPAR data rather than the inpatient SAF because MEDPAR contains data consolidated per hospital visit (94% of all inpatient visits are consolidated into single claims for each visit) rather than as multiple claims for the same visit. In addition, it is important to account for the potential for reversals of claims data. These often appear months after the encounter and tend to be for the exact same amount—only negative.

Since there are multiple databases that often must be accessed to determine how a patient's disease has been managed, that is, an episode of care, the researcher must create a relational database containing data on individual patients. It is often necessary to link data from multiple fields (for example, age, sex, race) to obtain a unique patient identifier to carry across all datasets. Moreover, if data are sought across multiple years, codes that identify medical conditions or procedures may have changed or may be nonspecific or otherwise invalid.

These databases are primarily constituted by an elderly sector of the population (approximately 40 million patients), thereby, not generalizable to younger populations. Furthermore, because the databases are very large, Medicare typically suggests using a large database server running Microsoft Structured Query Language (SQL) in full SQL Server, Oracle or Sybase, thus limiting the ability of the lone researcher/program manager to perform the required functions on a personal computer. Moreover, these datasets were not developed for clinical analysis—requiring certain assumptions, for example, if a kidney rejection is antibody-treated vs. corticosteroid-treated. Finally, only charges are indicated, meaning that adjustments such as cost-to-charge ratios may be necessary to ascertain true costs of an HDM program.

## References

1. Medicare Payment Advisory Commission (MedPAC). A data book, healthcare spending and the Medicare Program. June 2008. Available at: http://www.medpac.gov/documents/Jun-08DataBook_Entire_report.pdf. Accessed February 28, 2010.
2. Linden A, Adler-Milstein J. Medicare disease management in policy context. *Health Care Financ Rev.* 2008;29:1-11.
3. ResDAC. Medicare data file descriptions, RIF data. February 24, 2010. Available at: http://www.resdac/umn.edu/Medicare/data_file_descriptions.asp. Accessed March 8, 2010.
4. Centers for Medicare & Medicaid Services. Fact sheet: completion of phase I of Medicare Health Support Program. Available at: http://www.cms.hhs.gov/CCIP/downloads/EOP_Fact_Sheet_FINAL_012808.pdf. Accessed February 28, 2010.
5. Disease Management Association of America. Benefits of Medicare health support. January 2007. Available at: http://www.dmaa.org/advocacy_mhs.asp. Accessed February 28, 2010.
6. Dillavou E, Muluk S, Makaroun M. A decade of change in abdominal aortic aneurysm repair in the United States: have we improved outcomes equally between men and women? *J Vasc Surg.* 2006;43:230-238.
7. Kleindorfer D, Lindsell C, Brass L, et al. National US estimates of recombinant tissue plasminogen activator use: ICD-9 codes substantially underestimate. *Stroke.* 2008;39:924-928.
8. National Cancer Institute, Health Services and Economics, SEER-Medicare Linked Database. March 2010. Available at: http://healthservices.cancer.gov/seermedicare/. Accessed March 8, 2010.
9. National Cancer Institute. Surveillance epidemiology and end results. March 2010. Available at: http://healthservices.cancer.gov/seermedicare/overview/publications.html. Accessed March 8, 2010.

CHAPTER 23

# Veterans Health Administration

Mariam K. Hassan, BPharm, PhD; and Dennis W. Raisch, RPh, PhD

This chapter provides an overview of Veterans Health Administration (VHA) data sources and the Department of Veterans Affairs (VA) Health Care system and population, followed by a description of the VHA data resources available on national and local levels. The focus of the chapter is the National Patient Care Databases (NPCD), which is sufficient for most health care and cost-effectiveness research studies of VA patients. We describe the utility and validity of the VA databases and discuss the strengths and limitations of VHA data sources. We note that the VA data are constantly evolving, so we recommend readers supplement their understanding by accessing the VA websites at www.va.gov and the VA Information Resource Center (VIReC) at http://www.virec.research.va.gov/.

## 1. The Veterans Administration Health Care System

The Veterans Health Administration is one of 3 divisions of the United States (US) VA. The VHA manages and implements a single health care system for US veterans and is a comprehensive health care system with facilities that provide inpatient and outpatient medical, dental, pharmacy, and prosthetic services. Additionally, the VHA provides domiciliary, nursing home, community-based residential care, and health and rehabilitation programs for homeless veterans, as well as sexual trauma counseling and alcohol and drug dependency treatment. Thus, the VHA is the largest centrally directed health care system in the US.[1]

VHA is an insurer as well as provider of care for veterans and operates more than 1,400 health care sites throughout the country, including affiliations with 107 academic health systems. The VHA health care system, as of 2008, operated through 21 Veteran Integrated Service Networks (VISNs) that regionally manage 153 medical centers, 731 community-based outpatient clinics, 135 nursing homes, 209 readjustment counseling centers (Vet Centers) and 47 domiciliaries. There is at least one VHA medical center in each state, Puerto Rico, and the District of Columbia. VHA offers a standard medical benefits package, which covers various outpatient and inpatient services.

Most veterans must be enrolled into the VHA system, a process that is initiated by the veteran, to receive benefits. Exceptions are veterans with a service-connected disability of 50% or more, those seeking care for a service-connected disability, and veterans who were discharged from the military within 1 year but have not yet been rated for a VA disability benefit. The VA has a priority enrollment system based on degree of service-connected disability, degree of disability, prisoner of war classification, income, wealth (assets), and date and place of military service. Veterans with service-connected disability or in low-income groups have priority access to VHA benefits.

In 2007, the US veteran population was about 23.8 million and predominantly male (~92.5%) with a median age of 61 years for men and 47 years for women. Due to the priority-based enrollment system, veterans who receive VHA benefits are a special population who are likely to be in low-income groups, less educated, older, unemployed or underemployed, African Americans and/or have a greater number of chronic health conditions.[2] In 2007, about 5.5 million veterans received health care treatments at the VHA. The patients who receive care in the VHA tend to remain in the system over long periods so longitudinal data on their care are usually available.

## 2. Veterans Administration Data Resources

Throughout all facilities, the VHA maintains identical electronic clinical information on all health care provided to veterans. Access to any VA data requires approval by an institutional review board (IRB), the researcher's local VA research review committee, and the VA's information resources management (IRM) department. In addition, researchers must maintain current VA training certification including, but not limited to, applicable VA information privacy and security, the Health Insurance Portability and Accountability Act of 1996 (HIPAA), and good clinical research practices. The integrated system of software applications that supports all patient care delivery in the VA is called the Veterans Health Information Systems and Technologies Architecture (VISTA). The Computerized Patient Record System (CPRS) is the graphical interface for VISTA through which health care providers record and access health care data.

Therefore VISTA, through CPRS, is the backbone of all health care utilization data, clinician notes, test results, and laboratory data. The National Patient Care Database (NPCD) is created through monthly extracts of data from VISTA at all VA facilities. NPCD is maintained by the VHA Office of Information at the Austin Information Technology Center (AITC) in Austin, Texas. The data are made available quarterly, and at the end of the fiscal year the quarterly data are combined into annual datasets.

The following sections provide brief descriptions of NPCD datasets that are important to researchers who use the large national VA databases as well as local VA data. Additionally, more comprehensive descriptions of all aspects of VA databases are found on the VA Information Resource Center (VIReC) website at http://www.virec.research.va.gov/. VIReC, established in 1998, provides a wealth of information to support researchers who wish to learn about or use the VA datasets, including educational seminars, newsletters, concerns with VA data, VA patient Medicare utilization data, and information regarding the approval process required to access the data. The 4 national VA data sources primarily used by researchers are: VA Medical SAS Datasets, VA Vital Status File, VA Decision Support System (DSS), and the VA/Centers for Medicare & Medicaid Services (CMS) Data.

## Veterans Administration Medical SAS® Datasets

The VA Medical SAS datasets are also referred to as the NPCD Hospital Data, often referred to as the Patient Treatment File (PTF), contain hospitalization information on all veterans who received care within VHA system or were reimbursed by the VA. Four datasets for inpatient care include main (demographics, diagnoses, length of stay), bed section (diagnoses and length of stay for specialty portion of a stay), [International Classification of Disease, Version 9 (ICD-9)] coded procedures, and surgery (ICD-9 coded surgeries).

In addition, the PTF also provides up to 13 ICD-9 discharge diagnosis codes (6 digits) and 5 ICD-9 procedure codes for each hospital episode. The discharge information includes information on date and time of discharge, transfer to another hospital, death, regular discharge, and length of stay in hospital. This file also contains information on health care received at VA nursing homes and on outpatient surgery. PTF data extend from 1976 to the present, although not all fields are present in earlier versions. More comprehensive data are available since the 1990s.

The Outpatient Care File (OPC) contains data on all outpatient care received by veterans at VA clinics. The OPC contains records on each outpatient visit per day. The information includes patient demographics, date, time of visit, clinic identifier, and diagnosis and procedures for the visit. Up to 10 ICD-9-CM diagnosis codes and 20 Current Procedural Terminology (CPT)—4 procedure codes are recorded. Visits to different clinics, laboratories or other outpatient facilities for each day are also recorded.

## Vital Status File

The Vital Status File provides death information on veterans who receive VA benefits. This file collects information on date of death from the PTF (VA inpatient), Beneficiary Identification and Records Locator Subsystem (BIRLS)—Death File, Medicare Vital Status, and Social Security Administration (SSA) death file.

## Veterans Administration Decision Support System

The VA decision support system (DSS) was developed and implemented in the 1990s to integrate data from clinical and financial systems in support of VA resource allocation decisions. DSS data can be used by researchers at 3 levels of aggregation: production, summary reports, and national data extracts (NDEs). Production databases include cost data, clinical data regarding resource utilization and patient outcomes, laboratory and pharmacy data, and workload.

The DSS summary reports are standardized reports but have the option to customize to obtain station-centric and patient-centric reports, financial user reports, and clinical reports. NDEs for clinical data include radiology, occurrence of lab test, lab results, and pharmacy including both inpatient and outpatient. Financial NDEs include the discharge, inpatient treating specialty, and outpatient files. Additionally, cost datasets have been developed from DSS data by the Health Economics Research Center (HERC). HERC utilized regression analyses to estimate regionally adjusted costs of typical health care encounters.[3] Estimates from HERC are applied to patient encounters, resulting in cost values for patient encounters.

## VA/CMS Data (Medicare and Medicaid)

Because a number of VA patients are also eligible for Medicare and/or Medicaid, it is important for researchers to consider adding patient-specific CMS data to their research analyses. Information on diagnosis and treatment received by veterans outside the VA is available through VIReC if the patient is also Medicare or Medicaid eligible. VIReC maintains such data using unique patient identifiers that can be linked across the systems. Special approval from the VHA is necessary to access such data and there are specific forms required by VIReC. The Medicare claims files are usually available to VIReC 9 months after the end of calendar year. Access to Medicaid claims data is typically delayed longer after the calendar year. VIReC performs quality checks prior to making the data available.

## Additional National and Regional VA Databases

Other data warehouses include the national Pharmacy Benefits Management (PBM) data and VISN data warehouses. The VA PBM administers the formulary for the VA system. The PBM database contains records of all prescriptions dispensed at any VA outpatient pharmacy or Consolidated Mail Outpatient Pharmacy (CMOP) since 1999. The database contains related information regarding the prescription such as generic drug name, dose, quantity, costs (cost of the drug product from the supplier), formulary status, and prescribing physician. The database includes information about controlled substance use and utilization of medications stored and administered in a clinic or on a ward.

The PBM also captures laboratory test and result data. The laboratory data are controlled and made available after approval by the PBM. For use of PBM data, researchers must provide IRB approval, a copy of the study protocol, and a completed data request to VA PBM. The VA PBM then provides a custom extract of the data file created based on researcher's needs.

The VISN data warehouses encompass regional data that may be more comprehensive than NPCD data. These data are controlled regionally and often use specific formatting and software that improves the search and screening of information. Existence and availability of these warehouses vary by VISN. A research proposal approved by the appropriate VA research committee and IRB is necessary, in addition to meeting other requirements specific to the VISN and/or individual medical centers.

## Local Veteran Administration Data

The VISTA database is maintained at the local level and contains the most detailed clinical information through electronic health records for each patient. It is the primary source for national VA datasets. All information on patients treated at VA medical centers are recorded including information on patients' medical and health care utilization histories, demographic information, medication use, practitioner information, diagnoses, laboratory data, and procedures.

The VISTA database is produced and maintained at the local VA medical center level so there may be slight site-to-site differences in level of information detail. Some information in VISTA is available in text or other forms resulting in increased complexity of retrieval and analysis. Data may need to be manipulated in order to use standard statistical software to analyze them. VISTA contains identifiable patient information making access for researchers more restricted and complicated than data from the national data extracts.

## 3. Utility of Veteran Administration Databases for Health and Disease Management Research and Evaluation

Veteran Health Administration data are ideal for various health and disease management research because researchers can use them to identify various clinical or operational problems and areas of unmet need within the VA system and provide input into the development of preventive services and disease management programs. The data are extensive and complete regarding medical and pharmaceutical care received by veterans, as well as VA costs of care. Since most veterans who enroll use the VA as their primary provider for many years, data are longitudinal. The information in the national database is consistent across all facilities and is well documented, making the data attractive for retrospective cost-effectiveness analyses (CEA).

A concern, however, is the potential for selection bias, because factors that influence prescribing decisions may not be evident in the databases. Further, limitations related to the generalizability of the VA population outside of the VHA system must be borne in mind when using these data for any analyses.

The linkages in VA databases enable researchers to perform longitudinal studies on various outcomes such as hospitalizations and readmissions, length of stay, outpatient visits, inpatient and outpatient procedure utilizations and costs. Depending on the disease area of interest, patients can be identified using ICD-9-CM codes from PTF and OPC files. Outcomes data can be analyzed at the patient, provider, regional, and national levels.

Inpatient and outpatient data can be linked to PBM or DSS datasets to study patterns of medication use, medication adherence, physician prescribing behavior, and medication costs. The link between pharmacy and medical files allows evaluation of VA formulary decisions or changes in terms of impact on patient outcomes rather than just drug acquisition costs.[4] By linking medical or PBM files to the Vital Status File researchers can perform studies of survival following diagnosis or treatment.[5] However, the Vital Status File does not provide information on cause of death.

Surveys using patient-reported outcomes questionnaire have been conducted among the VHA population to assess quality of life and functioning outcomes.[6] Administrative data can be merged with such survey data to study patient-reported outcomes along with service utilization by different disease conditions and by geographic regions represented by the VHA population.[7,8]

Due to its comprehensive nature and extensive detail, VISTA and the local electronic medical charts can be used to identify early development of conditions before they appear on claims records. This information can be used to identify patients with risk factors, initiate screening programs, and develop other targeted interventions. Other outcomes including glycosylated hemoglobin levels among diabetes patients, blood pressure levels, cholesterol levels and electrocardiograms can be monitored over time for veterans using VISTA data. Disease complications that develop over time such as those related to diabetes can also be studied.[9]

For each VA medical facility, VISTA files provide information on inpatient and outpatient utilization in addition to clinical information. One of the features of VISTA is an electronic clinical reminder system that has been used to provide prescribing or monitoring recommendations for health providers concurrently with patient visits while using the electronic medical record.

Studies of VA databases have also demonstrated methods for adequately estimating costs.[3,10-12] For instance, the VA national database can be augmented with DSS data to assure all discharges are captured.[12] The estimates can be incorporated into the cost analyses. HERC's encounter-level estimate of VA costs is an example.[3]

## 4. Strengths and Limitations of VHA Data

VHA has the largest integrated health care database in the US.[1] VHA data provide comprehensive information on inpatient, outpatient and pharmacy services at the national level, and detailed clinical information at the local level. Inpatient, outpatient, and pharmacy data are validated and available to researchers annually. Data allow for longitudinal assessment of outcomes over several years due to the consistent use of unique patient identifiers.

In addition to the restricted generalizability mentioned above, VA databases contain information specifically on veterans who receive health care within the system.[2] Researchers should note that the veterans who seek care in the VA are a unique population who are generally older, more commonly male, and have a lower-socioeconomic status than average for the US population in general. They also typically have more comorbidities and/or greater disease severity than found in the general population.

As with all large datasets, VA data are vulnerable to different coding errors[13] especially for admitting diagnosis for hospitalizations.[14] The validity of the VA national datasets has been established and reported in several studies.[3,15-17] Researchers have also described the methods for addressing potential limitations.[13,18-21] For example, a study was conducted to compare outpatient clinic stop data from NPCD and the electronic medical record identified 1% of nonmatching dates and 1% of nonmatching procedures.[21] These appeared to be due to limitations of data entry of the clinic stop information in which clinic stops by a patient exceeded number of fields allowed.

DSS has also been assessed with researchers concluding that inpatient data in NPCD were "almost perfectly matched."[10] Methods for costing of VA national data from DSS have been established and validated.[3] It has been shown that, for mortality data, there is a need to combine 4 datasets to achieve sufficient quality for research: BIRLS Death File, Medical SAS Inpatient Datasets, Medicare Vital Status, and Social Security Administration Death Master File.[21,22]

# References

1. Kizer KW, Demakis JG, Feussner JR. Reinventing VA health care: systematizing quality improvement and quality innovation. *Medical Care.* 2000;38:7-16.
2. Morgan RO, Teal CR, Reddy SG, et al. Measurement in Veterans Affairs health services research: veterans as a special population. *Health Serv Res.* 2005;40:1573-1583.
3. Barnett PG. Determination of VA health care costs. *Med Care Res Rev.* 2003;60:124S-141S.
4. Sales MM, Cunningham FE, Glassman PA, et al. Pharmacy benefits management in the Veterans Health Administration: 1995 to 2003. *Am J Manag Care.* 2005;11:104-112.
5. Ho PM, Fihn SD, Wang L, et al. Clopidogrel and long-term outcomes after stent implantation for acute coronary syndrome. *Am Heart J.* 2007;154:846-851.
6. Kazis LE, Miller DR, Skinner KM, et al. Patient-reported measures of health: the Veterans Health Study. *J Ambul Care Manage.* 2004;27:70-83.
7. Gage H, Hendricks A, Zhang S, et al. The relative health related quality of life of veterans with Parkinson's disease. *J Neurol Neurosurg Psychiatry.* 2003;74:163-169.
8. Weeks WB, Kazis LE, Shen Y, et al. Differences in health-related quality of life in rural and urban veterans. *Am J Public Health.* 2004;94:1762-1767.
9. Kupersmith J, Francis J, Kerr E, et al. Advancing evidence-based care for diabetes: lessons from the Veterans Health Administration. *Health Aff.* 2007;26:w156-w168.
10. Yu W, Barnett PG. *Reconciliation of DSS Encounter-Level National Data Extracts and the VA National Patient Care Database: FY2001-FY2002 Technical Report 9.* Menlo Park, CA: Health Economics Resource Center; 2003.
11. Barnett PG. Review of methods to determine VA health care costs. *Med Care.* 1999;37: AS9-AS17.
12. Barnett PG, Rodgers JH. Use of the decision support system for VA cost-effectiveness research. *Med Care.* 1999;37:AS63-AS70.
13. Kashner TM. Agreement between administrative files and written medical records: a case of the Department of Veterans Affairs. *Med Care.* 1998;36:1324-1336.
14. Halpern J. The measurement of quality of care in the Veterans Health Administration. *Med Care.* 1996;34:MS55-MS68.
15. Phibbs CS, Bhandari A, Yu W, et al. Estimating the costs of VA ambulatory care. *Med Care Res Rev.* 2003;60:54S-73S.

16. Yu W, Wagner TH, Chen S, et al. Average cost of VA rehabilitation, mental health, and long-term hospital stays. *Med Care Res Rev.* 2003;60:40S-53S.
17. Wagner TH, Chen S, Barnett PG. Using average cost methods to estimate encounter-level costs for medical-surgical stays in the VA. *Med Care Res Rev.* 2003;60:15S-36S.
18. Borzecki AM, Wong AT, Hickey EC, et al. Can we use automated data to assess quality of hypertension care? *Am J Manag Care.* 2004;10:473-479.
19. Kaboli PJ, McClimon BJ, Hoth AB, et al. Assessing the accuracy of computerized medication histories. *Am J Manag Care.* 2004;10:872-877.
20. Maynard C, Chapko MK. Data resources in the Department of Veterans Affairs. *Diabetes Care.* 2004;27(suppl 2):B22-B26.
21. Sohn MW, Arnold N, Maynard C, et al. Accuracy and completeness of mortality data in the Department of Veterans Affairs. *Popul Health Metr.* 2006;4:2.
22. Fisher SG, Weber L, Goldberg J, et al. Mortality ascertainment in the veteran population: alternatives to the National Death Index. *Am J Epidemiol.* 1995;141:242-250.

CHAPTER 24

# The Role of Patient Registries

Jayashri Sankaranarayanan, MPharm, PhD; Teresa Hartman, MLS; and William Crown, PhD

This chapter provides an overview of the potential roles that patient registries have for health and disease management especially in the monitoring of safety and in measuring health outcomes. The chapter begins with an introduction to patient registries including definitions and their relationship to comparative effectiveness research (CER). This is followed by sections on guidance for registry development and conceptual applications of registries. The next section classifies registries as product-specific or disease-specific with selected examples and discusses combining primary and electronic data into registries with a case study. Finally, the chapter ends with a section discussing the advantages and limitations of patient registries in studying health and disease management.

Patient registries are commonly defined as prospective, observational cohort studies of patients with, or at risk for, a particular disease and/or receiving a specific treatment or intervention. The National Committee on Vital and Health Statistics (NCVHS) serves as an advisory body to the Department of Health and Human Services (HHS) on the nation's health data, statistics and national health information systems policy.[1] The NCVHS defines a medical or public health registry as "an organized system for collection, storage, retrieval, analysis, and distribution of information on individuals who have either a particular disease, a condition (for example, a risk factor) that predisposes a health-related event to occur, or prior exposure to substances (or circumstances) known or suspected to cause adverse health effects."[2] The FDA in its guidance to the industry has supported this definition.[3] The International Society of Pharmacoeconomics and Outcomes Research (ISPOR) special interest group on patient registries defines a *patient registry* as a "prospective observational study of patients with certain shared characteristics (eg, particular disease, risk factor or exposure) that mainly collects continuing and supporting data over time on well-defined outcomes of interest for analysis and reporting to fulfill the direct purpose of the registry."[4]

Patient registries have gained importance as a mechanism for answering questions on real-world outcomes posed by practitioners, payers, policy makers, and consumers to inform health and disease management practices. Among others, these include the impact of medications and other treatments on the natural history of disease, clinical effectiveness, resource use, overall cost, quality and access to care in health and disease management.[5] Registries can provide real-world evidence of clinical practice, patient outcomes, safety, comparative effectiveness and cost-effectiveness of interventions to inform these questions.[6]

In response to widespread geographic variation in treatment patterns for patients with similar medical conditions, the United States government launched a major policy initiative on CER in 2009 to inform the health care reform debate.[7] With the growing emphasis on CER,[6,8] the current and potential role of registries in CER is included in this chapter to the extent that it informs the design and evaluation of health and disease management programs. The potential role of registries for CER is much broader as it has been defined as:

> ... the conduct and synthesis of research comparing the benefits and harms of different interventions and strategies to prevent, diagnose, treat and watch health conditions in "real-world" settings. The purpose of this research is to improve health outcomes by developing and spreading evidence-based information to patients, clinicians, and other decision makers, responding to their expressed needs, about which interventions are most effective for which patients under specific circumstances.[7]

CER involves head-to-head comparisons of medical and pharmacological treatments, as well as treatment processes such as health and disease management programs.

Two important components of any observational analysis are a robust research design and accurate measurement of appropriate outcomes and control variables. With a focus on longitudinal, primary data collection, well-designed and well-performed patient registries[9] offer a promising vehicle for monitoring product safety and for testing the comparative effectiveness of interventions in health and disease management programs. When developing registries it is important to balance the accuracy and comprehensiveness of evidence versus the urgency of a public health problem, the types of available interventions, and the risks to public health that could come from a wrong conclusion drawn from observational data.[10]

This is particularly true when health care policy makers, payers, and other stakeholders will use results from analyses of registry data related to the comparative effectiveness and safety of alternative strategies in health and disease management. Therefore, care must be taken to differentiate registries (that is, the means of data collection, storage and all operational aspects of registry set-up and maintenance) and the various epidemiological study designs that can be carried out using registry data. This chapter deals primarily with the former.

# 1. Guidance on Registry Development for Health and Disease Management

To guide the design, implementation, analysis, interpretation, and evaluation of the quality of a registry, the Effective Health Care Program of the Agency for

Healthcare Research and Quality (AHRQ) published 2 editions of a handbook.[6,8] Study outcomes and the desired impact of a given program will guide how investigators match the registry objectives to suitable design and operational elements.[6,8,10] Pragmatic considerations such as potential challenges and solutions are also factors. High-quality data can be obtained from registries by following good practice in planning, design, data elements, and data sources, as well as ethics, privacy, and governance.[6,8] The quality of evidence obtained from registries can be increased by planning ways to assure the quality and the reporting of the data.

Once a registry is identified as the most appropriate approach for addressing the research question, investigators and advisors should be selected based on expertise and experience. Investigators explain the purpose of the registry, define the scope and target population, assess whether or not developing the registry is feasible, and secure funding. A plan for governing and overseeing a registry is important and should clearly address the overall direction. When setting up a registry it is important to specify data elements in advance, establish procedures for institutional review board (IRB) approval processes to protect patient privacy, identify quality metrics for measuring outcomes, and set an analytic and publication plan.[8]

Using suitable procedures to protect the confidentiality of patient information (such as IRB approval and obtaining patient consent for participating in the study), it is often possible to link electronic medical records (EMR) data from treatment centers (for example, hospitals with cardiovascular units, diabetes clinics, oncology centers) with medical claims and enrollment information for patients. Other linkages, such as vital statistics data, can provide key end points, such as mortality information, that are typically missing in administrative claims databases.

Beyond collecting quality data in a registry, the appropriate analysis of these data requires an understanding of specific analytic challenges confronting any observational study, including controlling for the impact of confounders, selection bias, measurement error and other issues.[6,8,10] Statistical methodologies for the analysis of observational data have advanced considerably in recent years. Propensity score methods for creating balanced comparison cohorts, structural equation modeling to understand better the process of care and determinants of outcomes for different treatment cohorts, and instrumental variables to control for confounding are just a few of the advanced statistical methodologies that can help researchers to draw reliable inferences from observational data such as that collected in registries.[10]

Principles of accessing registry data and managing change need to be established in advance as it is particularly important to plan for the entire lifespan of a registry; including how and when the registry will end and plans for transitioning the registry. A registry may be stopped because it has satisfied its original purpose, is unable to satisfy its purpose, is no longer relevant, or is unable to obtain funding, staffing, or other support.[6] Thus, a registry's design and operation are driven by its classification (for example, a disease or product registry), and founded by early and comprehensive planning.

## 2. Application of Registry Data

Regulatory agencies such as the Food and Drug Administration (FDA) in the US and the European Medicines Agency (EMA) in Europe are placing growing emphasis on postlaunch safety surveillance for newly approved products[5] in health and disease management. There is a long history of government payers outside of the US wanting and considering information on the comparative benefits and costs of new treatments when making coverage and reimbursement decisions.[11] Public and private payers in the US are beginning to ask that manufacturers provide effectiveness data on treatments in actual clinical practice in addition to the efficacy reported in controlled settings of clinical trials.

For health and disease management, reasons for developing registries may include: a) estimating the size of a suspected problem; b) determining the incidence of disease uncovering and/or exploring suspected disease clusters; c) examining trends of a disease over time; d) examining trends in health care delivery, e) assessing delivery of services and identifying high-risk groups; and f) documenting patient types served by a health provider. In addition, registries may be used to address research questions such as the impact of specific exposures on long-term health outcomes in the general population, and etiologic hypothesis generation by identifying cases for case-control studies (for example, as a source of potential transplant donors and potential clinical trial participants).[5]

The application of registry data for generating clinical effectiveness and health care use information is increasingly critical. These data help agencies to review technologies and to assess a product's effectiveness (including costs) periodically in the years following its introduction. Registries offer the ability to address, in one comprehensive program, various study objectives across disciplines, and to provide important disease- and product-specific data. To comply with postapproval regulatory requirements, safety information and clinical effectiveness data increasingly are collected using registries.

Registries also represent an opportunity to prospectively collect and report on other outcomes, such as health care resource utilization, patient-reported outcomes of HRQOL, and patient satisfaction following implementation of a program or approval of a new product. A national survey of oncologists suggests there is physician support for federally funded comparative effectiveness data to assist their central role in deciding how and when to use expensive cancer treatments for their patients.[12] Thus, registries could also be used to produce comparative effectiveness data to design and deliver cost-effective health and disease management programs.

## 3. Classification of Registries

Registries are classified according to how their populations are defined. Disease-specific registries focus on populations with a particular disease or groups of similar diseases while product-specific registries consider populations with specific product exposures. Disease or condition registries include patients having the same diagnosis (for example, a rare disease such as cystic fibrosis, or a chronic illness, such as obesity, heart failure, diabetes, or end-stage renal disease) or having the disease for a more limited period of time (for example, infectious diseases).[6]

Potential patients for inclusion in a registry are actively identified by referral sources often associated with the registry (for example, hospital discharge records). Data tend to be collected longitudinally on people enrolled in the registry. Product registries include patients who have been exposed to particular biopharmaceutical products or medical devices and systematically collect adverse event information on the thousands of patients receiving the product. The use of registries in health and disease management is most similar to product registries as they may be used to evaluate the outcomes of patients exposed to a particular program or management strategy.

A literature review from 1998 to 2008 showed that there are numerous registries available worldwide and some of these are described below including the potential impact for health and disease management; a few representative product-specific and disease-specific registries are also summarized in Table 1. There is a growing role for registries that combine primary and electronic data and these are discussed in detail in the subsequent subsections.

## Product-Specific Registries

Product registries are set up by many manufacturers of medications in fulfillment of pharmacovigilance activities as well as by states and countries. Such registries have become increasingly common in recent years. Although a review published in 2007 showed an average of 1.5 drugs withdrawn from the US market in each year since 1993, some withdrawals have an impact on large numbers of people.[13]

From selected registries,[14-20] one example of a product-specific registry is the Clozaril National Registry (CNR) that was initiated to monitor patients at risk for developing potentially fatal agranulocytosis secondary to antipsychotic treatment with clozapine. It is an epidemiologic database created and maintained by Novartis with mandated white blood cell counts and demographic data on every patient receiving clozapine in the United States.[14] Data collected in another product-specific registry, the Outpatient Parenteral Antimicrobial Therapy (OPAT) Outcomes Registry demonstrated that osteomyelitis can be safely and effectively treated with outpatient parenteral antibiotics such as vancomycin and ceftriaxone.[15]

These registries and others demonstrate how data may be shared effectively with the medical community to help physicians in weighing potential risks and benefits of treatment for individual patients.[16] Product registries typically lack a comparator thus they play a limited role in CER; though these data can inform the risk-benefit ratio of the treatment(s) or intervention(s) under routine conditions as one important aspect of CER. Nevertheless, product registries are useful for understanding the real-world safety and effectiveness of specific treatments and may provide input to analyses of the relative effectiveness of a given treatment among alternative patient subgroups.

## Disease-Specific Registries

Disease registries are, by their nature, well suited to support health and disease management and CER. These are registries set up by specialists or expert investigators. Patients are enrolled during a routine health care service or when experiencing an acute event or exacerbation of an underlying disease such as hospitalization for a myocardial infarction or ischemic stroke.[6] They may also enroll voluntarily through the volunteer recruiting sites on the Internet.

One of the best-known disease registries is the Surveillance, Epidemiology, and End Results (SEER) cancer registry, which is supported by federal funds and the National Cancer Institute. It routinely compiles data from specific population-based cancer registries from different areas of the United States.[2,21-23] There are several important findings from SEER registry. One study found elderly patients with lung cancer were less likely to see a cancer specialist and consequently did not receive chemotherapy.[21] Another finding is that mortality rates were lower when complex surgical oncologic procedures were performed by specialized surgical teams in hospitals.[22] A third finding suggests that local health organizations can improve the care of Hispanic women by providing culturally suitable public health interventions to encourage them to undergo cervical cancer screenings.[23]

A final example of an important disease registry is a myelodysplastic syndrome/myelodysplasia (MDS) conducted by the Slone Epidemiology Center at Boston University.[24] This registry collects real-world data from across all US states on the effect of treatment on patient's physical, emotional, social and economic outcomes. While not many physicians in small practices have implemented electronic health record (EHR) systems, at least one organization set up simple registries for chronic disease tracking that helped their practice deliver high rates of preventive services.[25]

Disease registries provide the advantage of longitudinal data collection on considerable number of patients. Though the advantages have not been fully capitalized upon, the registry framework has been used to collect health-related quality of life (HRQOL), treatment patterns, health care use, and pharmacoeconomic data.[26] This information is increasingly requested by countries to support drug coverage and reimbursement decisions.

Government entities have also sponsored disease registries that inform health and disease management. One example is the Congenital Defects registry funded by the federal government and managed by the Centers for Disease Control. In this registry, the protective effect of increased periconceptional folate and fortification of selected foods on the risk of neural tube defects is studied.[2,5] State governments also operate many registries ranging from registries of people diagnosed with a particular disease (for example, sexually transmitted diseases) to state cancer registries which are useful for identifying issues of access to early diagnosis[27] and treatment.[28] These data help providers and policy makers target interventions that can improve health and disease management.

Disease registries collecting a broad range of data on treatments, confounders, clinical outcomes, and health care utilization are promising vehicles for collecting data on patient outcomes to support health and disease management and CER. For example, disease registries capturing clinical outcomes and all treatments received by patients with a given condition such as major depression could enable comparisons of outcomes for specific patient subgroups treated with various pharmacological, behavioral, and combination therapies.

Because the number of potential interventions is extraordinarily large, it is important to focus on areas in which more evidence is needed in health and disease management and has the potential to improve patient care. Several examples of disease registries and their objectives are summarized in Table 1.[29-44] Disease registries present immense opportunities to realize improvements in health and disease management, significantly improving the practice of medicine and quality of care in the community.

## Combining Primary and Electronic Data in Registries—A Growing Role?

Given the significant investment needed to execute clinical trials and prospective registry studies, it is instructive to consider how secondary use of administrative claims or electronic medical record data can contribute to the planning, design and implementation to increase the likelihood of success of using a combination registry. Large medical claims and EHR databases have a number of desirable properties including significant sample size, ability to observe use of treatments in real-world settings—for example, in patients with multiple comorbidities and being treated with concomitant drugs—as well as the observation of treatment patterns in actual clinical practice. In isolation, medical claims and EHR databases have substantial limitations (discussed below) that can often be reduced through database linkage and the addition of primary data collection.

In addition to clinical measures of effectiveness and safety, the growing interest in CER is motivated by a desire to understand better patterns of health care use among various patient subgroups receiving different treatments for the same condition. Combination registries with linked medical claims and/or EHR data facilitate the ability to construct large numbers of subgroup comparisons without the need for conducting multiple clinical trials or several more narrowly focused registries.

The American Recovery and Reinvestment Act (ARRA) allocated more than $20 million to the adoption of EHR in clinical practice to support the delivery of care to patients, as well as to create the research infrastructure to support CER.[45] This should substantially enhance the technical capability to link clinical and administrative claims data, although mechanisms for doing so will need to ensure that patient privacy is maintained in accord with legislation related to protected health information (PHI) to achieve this purpose.

Combining administrative claims data and/or EHR data with prospectively collected patient registry data may offer the opportunity to improve the comprehensiveness of economic data collected in registries while simultaneously reducing the cost of primary data collection—allowing primary data collection to focus upon data elements that cannot be extracted from the electronic data. Limitations of retrospective patient recall include difficulty remembering the drugs that they take, dosages, refill dates, visits to the doctor, procedures performed, diagnoses, and even hospitalizations. These types of information are captured by administrative claims data and, to a lesser extent, EHR systems, thus providing a way to leverage these data and focus on other elements collected in a registry.

Claims databases have well-known limitations in terms of the quality of clinical information they contain but they often provide detailed information on health care utilization across multiple treatment settings for large numbers of patients. Conversely, EHR data can be rich clinically but often lack information on patient treatments and outcomes outside specific treatment settings. Combining claims and EHR data also promotes such activities as checking the reliability of diagnostic coding in the claims data against the medical record.

Neither medical claims nor EHR data provide information on patient-reported outcomes such as HRQOL, or much insight into the motivations behind the patient and provider health care patterns reflected in the data. Therefore, an ideal combination registry of prospective data on HRQOL collected from patients receiving different treatments for a particular condition in clinical practice could be combined with administrative data on their patterns of health care utilization from claims data, as well as laboratory results, body mass index, and blood pressure data from an EHR. Similarly, combination registry studies can obtain information from patients about their reasons for medication refill decisions, as well from doctors about reasons influencing their prescribing decisions. It is expected that, at least in the United States, the growing availability of electronic claims and EHR data, coupled with advances in data linkage technologies, will lead to increased opportunities to carry out combination registry designs in place of traditional prospective studies.

## Using Administrative Claims and EHR Data for Registry Design and Preparation

The design of future registries can be improved using administrative claims data and EHR databases, even with the limitations inherent to these resources. Data contained in the claims and EHR records could spotlight geographical areas of disease prevalence, patterns of physician treatment methods and medical procedures, or drug dispensing habits, which could lead to more efficient patient recruitment efforts by the registry through improved identification of target sites and practices. Using the real-world data housed in claims databases could also help determine the sample size needed to identify statistical significance of outcomes.[10]

For planning studies conducted within large national health plans or other payer organizations the medical claims offer another important advantage—the claims capture details on patterns of health care utilization that do not need to be collected from patients who may have poor recall.[46] This enables the survey to focus more selectively on data not captured such as health care not reimbursed by insurance (for example, over-the-counter pharmacy utilization, HRQOL, and other patient-reported outcomes). In turn, data collection becomes more cost-efficient, thereby enabling a given registry to include a greater number of patients—improving the power of the study to detect statistically significant differences in health economic or patient-reported outcomes across treatment cohorts.

## Case Study: Evaluating a Registry Protocol for Nonsmall Cell Lung Cancer

Suppose we wish to evaluate the feasibility of a registry for nonsmall cell lung cancer, NSCLC.[47] Deidentified medical claims can be used to investigate the geographic location of potential sites for the study. Using a database of deidentified administrative claims and enrollment data from a national managed care organization covering approximately 15 million lives annually was used, the geographically diverse population data were accessed using Health Insurance Portability and Accountability Act (HIPAA) compliant techniques, and no identifiable protected health information (PHI) was extracted.

First all patients in the database, age 18 or older, with evidence of the following 2009 International Classification of Diseases, Ninth Revision, Clinical Modification (ICD-9-CM) Diagnoses Codes for NSCLC were identified:

- 162.3: Malignant neoplasm of upper lobe, bronchus, or lung
- 162.4: Malignant neoplasm of middle lobe, bronchus, or lung
- 162.5: Malignant neoplasm of lower lobe, bronchus, or lung
- 162.8: Malignant neoplasm of other parts of bronchus or lung

Searching through the database, we identified the geographic distribution of 1,732 patients, along with their 1,069 treating physicians. This sampling frame of 1,069 physicians could be the initial potential site list for a registry. If experienced investigators are desired, the list of physicians can be cross-referenced with the subset of physicians who are experienced clinical investigators from the FDA's Bioresearch Monitoring Information System (BMIS). Moreover, by linking information from ClinicalTrials.gov, other nonsmall cell lung cancer studies being conducted in various geographic areas can be identified to further assess the feasibility of recruiting particular sites for the registry. This information can be viewed all the way down to the local level. One can even take account of the distance between the ZIP codes of the potential patients and the investigators.

## 4. Advantages of Using Registry Data

Interpretations from registry data could result in changes in the standard of care or highlight problems that must be further investigated to inform health and disease management of certain conditions.[48] The advantages of using registry data can be realized by understanding the rationale for patient registries in health and disease management. By design, randomized trials address many of the challenges faced in observational data analysis.[11] So why not conduct randomized trials instead of collecting registry data? One issue is cost.

Randomized trials can be more expensive than observational studies. With CER, the number of comparisons needed may be very large and running the necessary number of trials might be prohibitively expensive and time-consuming. Similar issues apply to assessments of patient outcomes for alternative patient subpopulations. In addition, there may be ethical issues in randomizing patients to treatment when there is no evidence the treatment will be efficacious or safe.

Finally, there are various design issues typical of clinical trials that limit their generalizability to real-world patient populations—restrictive inclusion and exclusion criteria, limited length of follow-up and sample size, and carefully controlled treatment protocols to name just a few.[10] Also, clinical trials may produce estimates of average treatment effects that mask variation in treatment response among subpopulations not prospectively considered in clinical trials. Intent-to-treat analyses may distort inferences about treatment effectiveness since they do not account for tolerability and other factors that may affect adherence.

Like individual clinical trials, it is common for systematic reviews of alternative treatments also to find no evidence of differences in outcomes. In such cases, one response is to conduct subanalyses to understand better the characteristics of responders and nonresponders. Further, though clinical trials are designed to detect statistically significant differences in the primary clinical end points, they rarely are powered to detect statistically significant differences in health economic outcomes or patient-reported outcomes (unless they are prespecified outcomes of the trial). Therefore, substantially larger sample sizes are needed to test hypotheses at comparable levels of statistical significance and clinical relevance.[10]

In the hierarchy of evidence, most observers would agree that pragmatic trials specifically designed to measure health economics and outcomes research end points would probably do the best job of producing evidence on the comparative effectiveness of alternative medical and drug treatments in health and disease management. The analysis of real-world data is fraught with a host of potential challenges. Problems of measurement error, missing variables, confounding (eg, confounding by indication), 2-way causation and other issues can undermine the ability to draw reliable statistical inferences about comparative treatment effectiveness or safety.

Randomized pragmatic trials with few inclusion and exclusion criteria and real-world follow-up offer a methodological design for dealing with such issues. Yet because such trials are expensive to undertake, nonrandomized study designs are commonly used to fill the evidence gap. Nevertheless, registries using nonrandomized design may provide reliable evidence if they are properly designed and analyzed using suitable multivariate statistical methods. Registries often tend to be large and will play a role in capturing critical health economic or patient-reported outcomes and powering hypothesis generation for future studies. Further, because of the expense of conducting clinical trials, registries will likely play an important role in providing real-world evidence about the comparative effectiveness of treatments in several patient subpopulations in health and disease management programs.

## 5. Limitations and Challenges in Registry-Based Data Collection

Data abstraction by untrained individuals without proper guidance can cause errors compromising the quality of the data in a registry. Therefore, designing clear case record forms is needed to ease burden of data abstraction and frequent auditing of abstracted data.[49] Another source of error can be from patient-reported data. Collecting detailed health care use data from patients is difficult as recall can be inaccurate or incomplete. Much of this information resides in large medical claims databases, which is the reason these databases are often used for health care utilization studies of medical or pharmacological technologies.

On the other hand, medical claims databases typically lack clinical detail and reliability of diagnostic coding has been shown to vary widely by condition. Also, they lack information on patient-reported outcomes such as HRQOL or reasons for medication adherence behaviors. Although some administrative claims databases include prescription data as well as medical data, they do not include all relevant information such as use of over-the-counter medications and herbals, or potentially important behavioral health variables such as exercise, diet, and other behaviors. There are instances, however, when it is possible to link administrative claims data with detailed clinical information such as that available from an EHR.

Generally, these situations involve large health care provider organizations or payers such as commercial health plans or government agencies that have access to the PHI of the patients. At present, we are a long way from systematically being able to link EHR data for all patients to administrative claims. One significant challenge is that a high percentage of medical records are still paper in the US.[50]

Another challenge is the lack of standards and uniformity in electronic medical record systems. Nevertheless, for conditions in which patients are treated in specialty centers such as diabetes, cardiology, or cancer, EHR data are much more commonly available and linkage with administrative data may be possible. The result would be a large improvement in availability of health care services use data across treatment settings, as well as reduced data collection costs. Overall, because of the costs of actively seeking and linking data from multiple sources overtime, registries are expensive.

There is no guarantee the design or analysis technique can fully protect against bias, such as channeling new treatments to sicker patients in registry data. In general, the more robust the up-front planning on data collection, the better the job that such methods can do in controlling for confounding factors, such as unobserved disease severity, that may be the real reason behind variation in patient outcomes. Adhering to established checklists when reporting registry results can improve the quality of future studies, which is a major concern.[49,51-57] Such checklists include those of ISPOR,[49] Transparent Reporting of Evaluations with Nonrandomized Designs (TREND),[51] and Consolidated Standards Of Reporting Trials (CONSORT) guidelines[52] developed for randomized controlled trials. Numerous guidelines address the challenges of drawing appropriate statistical inferences from analyses of observational data [for example, Good Epidemiological Practice (GEP)[53] and Strengthening the Reporting of Observational Studies in Epidemiology (STROBE)[54]].

There is continuing debate in the hierarchies of the evidence community about traditional methods of grading levels of evidence, their underlying assumptions, their shortcomings in assessing certain types of evidence (for example, benefit vs. harm), and their interscale consistency in evaluating the same evidence.[6,49,51-57] The Grading of Recommendations Assessment, Development, and Evaluation (GRADE) Working Group proposed a robust approach that addresses some of these decision-making issues.[56,57]

To encourage collaboration, reduce duplicative efforts, and improve transparency for patient registries, AHRQ awarded a contract to design and develop a Registry of Patient Registries (RoPR) database. The database will be developed with input from the potential users of the database in order to remain responsive to users' needs. The RoPR will be designed as a searchable central catalog to locate patient registries in the US.[58]

## 6. Conclusion

In summary, this chapter provides a brief overview of the potential utility of registries for health and disease management to familiarize the readers; and is not a comprehensive literature review on this topic. Regulatory authorities, commercial and government payers, and other health care stakeholders around the world are requiring evidence of effectiveness, safety, and economic value of interventions including health and disease management programs to support evidence-based medicine, as well as coverage and reimbursement decisions. Product registries inform the safety of biopharmaceutical products and medical devices. Disease or combination registries offer the opportunity to collect the information on compara-

Part 4: Alternative, Population-Based Data Sources

tive effectiveness research of multiple interventions.

**TABLE 1.** Selected Registries from 1998 to 2008

| Name | Nation | Objective/Goal | Ref. # |
|---|---|---|---|
| **Product** | | | |
| Clozaril National Registry | USA | Reviews registry data on clozapine-related morbidity and mortality | 14 |
| Acyclovir in Pregnancy Registry | International | Assess outcomes of acyclovir-exposed pregnancies, effects of drug | 16 |
| International Lamotrigine Pregnancy Registry | International | Frequency of/maternal drug dose of birth defects in lamotrigine-exposed pregnancies | 16 |
| WHO Vaccine Trial Registry | International | Registry collects vaccine studies | 18 |
| Lousiana Immunization Network for Kids Statewide | USA | Was accessed successfully for records after the hurricane disaster | 19 |
| Swedish Prescribed Drug Registry | Sweden | Estimate prevalence of inappropriate drug use among elderly, with associated patient characteristics | 20 |
| **Disease** | | | |
| Active Liver Transplant Recipient Registry | USA | Analyze donor availability and selection criteria | 29 |
| FACT: French National Registry of Acute Coronary Syndromes (ACS) | France | Identify delays for medical admission, epidemiology, and modalities | 30 |
| National Registry of Acute Coronary Syndromes | Portugal | Assess current situation and compliance with ACS guidelines | 31 |
| Cystic Fibrosis (CF) Foundation National Patient Registry | USA | Identify risks for women with CF-related pregnancy | 32 |
| Global Registry of Acute Coronary Events (GRACE) | International | Analyze outcomes of ACS patients; improve quality of care | 33 |
| OSCAR Registry - Registry of Acute Coronary Syndromes | France | Describe medical management of ACS patients | 34 |
| National Registry of Acute Ischemic Coronary Syndromes (RENASICA) | Mexico | Assess current treatment practices | 35 |
| Canadian Registry of Atrial Fibrillation (CARAF) | Canada | Identify atrial fibrillation patient population and symptoms | 36 |
| Association of the French Cancer Registries (FRANCIM) | France | How treatment of colorectal cancer can be assessed using registries | 37 |
| National Registry of Myocardial Infarction 4 (MRMI-4); CRUSADE registry (Can rapid risk stratification of unstable angina patients suppress adverse outcomes?) | USA | Impact on guidelines, updates on patient treatment; explore outcomes | 38 |

**TABLE 1.** Selected Registries from 1998 to 2008

| Name | Nation | Objective/Goal | Ref. # |
|---|---|---|---|
| Canadian Inherited Marrow Failure Registry (CIMFR) | Canada | Identify disease progression and significant outcome development | 39 |
| Acute Decompensated Heart Failure National Registry (ADHERE) | USA | Showed delays/underuse of guideline recommended therapies at discharge | 40 |
| Chronic Back and Neck Pain Registry | Finland | Determine rehabilitation effects on sick absences and analgesic purchase | 41 |
| Swedish Registry of Congenital Malformations | Sweden | Identify maternal age and parity, sex rate, and birth weight distribution | 42 |
| Statewide Acute Stroke Registry | USA | Compare in-hospital with out-of-hospital stroke outcomes | 43 |
| General Practice Research Database (GPRD) | United Kingdom | Investigate as data source for primary care health and disease management | 44 |

# References

1. National Committee on Vital and Health Statistics (NCVHS). Introduction to the NCVHS. http://www.ncvhs.hhs.gov/intro.htm. Accessed March 5, 2010.
2. National Committee on Vital and Health Statistics. Frequently asked questions about medical and public health registries. http://www.ncvhs.hhs.gov/9701138b.htm. Accessed March 5, 2010.
3. US Food and Drug Administration (FDA). Guidance for industry: good pharmacovigilance practices and pharmacoepidemiologic assessment. 2005. http://www.fda.gov/downloads/RegulatoryInformation/Guidances/UCM126834.pdf. Accessed September 20, 2012.
4. Gemmen E, Faria C. Patient registries: a taxonomy for the design, development and implementation. International Society for Pharmacoeconomics and Outcomes Research (ISPOR) Annual Meeting. 2009. Available at: http://www.quintiles.com/elements/media/presentations/patient-registries-taxonomy-design-development-and-implementation.pdf. Accessed March 3, 2010.
5. Sankaranarayanan J, Mason HL. Medical or public health registries: evidence of impact on standards for health care in the United States. *ISPOR Connections*. 2003;9:3-4. http://www.ispor.org/news/index_new.asp. Accessed March 3, 2010.
6. Gliklich RE, Dreyer NA, eds. Registries for Evaluating Patient Outcomes: A User's Guide. 2nd ed.(Prepared by Outcome DEcIDE Center [Outcome Sciences, Inc. d/b/a Outcome] under Contract No.HHSA29020050035I TO3.) AHRQ Publication No.10-EHC049. Rockville, MD: Agency for Healthcare Research and Quality. September 2010. Available at: http://www.effectivehealthcare.ahrq.gov/ehc/products/74/531/Registries%202nd%20ed%20final%20to%20Eisenberg%209-15-10.pdf. Accessed March 12, 2010.
7. Federal Coordinating Council for Comparative Effectiveness Research. Report to the President and Congress. US Health & Human Services: June 30, 2009 http://www.hhs.gov/recovery/programs/cer/cerannualrpt.pdf. Accessed September 26, 2012.
8. US Agency for Healthcare Research and Quality. Registries for Evaluating Patient Outcomes: A User's Guide (Full report: AHRQ Publication No. 07-EHC001-1. Summary report: AHRQ Publication Number 07-EHC001-2 ed.). Rockville, MD: US Department of Health and Human Services, Public Health Service, Agency for Healthcare Research and Quality; April 2007. Available at: http://effectivehealthcare.ahrq.gov/repFiles/PatOutcomes.pdf. Accessed November 23, 2008.

**Part 4: Alternative, Population-Based Data Sources**

9. Hartz S, Huse D. The role of patient registries in disease management and outcomes research. *Value Health*. 1998;1(1):87. Abstract DA2.
10. Crown WH, Marshall D, Barr CE. Health economics & analysis in clinical development. *Appl Clin Trials*. 2007;16:44-57.
11. Johnson ML, Crown W, Martin BC, et al. Good research practices for comparative effectiveness research: analytic methods to improve causal inference from nonrandomized studies of treatment effects using secondary data sources: The ISPOR good research practices for retrospective database analysis task force report—Part III. *Value Health*. 2009;12:1062-73.
12. Neumann PJ, Palmer JA, Nadler E, et al. Cancer therapy costs influence treatment: a national survey of oncologists. *Health Aff*. 2010;29:196-202.
13. Issa AM, Phillips KA, Van Bebber S, et al. Drug withdrawals in the United States: a systematic review of the evidence and analysis of trends. *Curr Drug Saf*. 2007;2:177-85.
14. Honigfeld G, Arellano F, Sethi J, et al. Reducing clozapine-related morbidity and mortality: 5 years of experience with the Clozaril National Registry. *J Clin Psychiatry*. 1998;59 (suppl 3):3-7.
15. Tice A. The use of outpatient parenteral antimicrobial therapy in the management of osteomyelitis: data from the Outpatient Parenteral Antimicrobial Therapy Outcomes Registries. *Chemotherapy*. 2001;47(suppl 1):5-16.
16. Reiff-Eldridge R, Heffner CR, Ephross SA, et al. Monitoring pregnancy outcomes after prenatal drug exposure through prospective pregnancy registries: a pharmaceutical company commitment. *Obstet Gynecol*. 2000;182:159-163.
17. Gaudino JA, deHart MP, Cheadle A, et al. Childhood immunization registries: gaps between knowledge and action among family practice physicians and pediatricians in Washington state, 1998. *Arch Pediatr Adolesc Med*. 2002;156:978-985.
18. Robertson SE, Mayans MV, El-Husseiny A, et al. The WHO Vaccine Trial Registry. *Vaccine*. 2001;20:31-41.
19. Boom JA, Dragsbaek AC, Nelson CS. The success of an immunization information system in the wake of Hurricane Katrina. *Pediatrics*. 2007;119:1213-1217.
20. Johnell K, Fastbom J, Rosen M, et al. Inappropriate drug use in the elderly: a nationwide register-based study. *Ann Pharmacother*. 2007;41:1243-1248.
21. Earle CC, Neumann PJ, Gelber RD, et al. Impact of referral patterns on the use of chemotherapy for lung cancer. *J Clin Oncol*. 2002;20:1786-1792.
22. Begg CB, Cramer LD, Hoskins WJ, et al. Impact of hospital volume on operative mortality for major cancer surgery. *JAMA*. 1998;280:1747-1751.
23. Centers for Disease Control and Prevention (CDC). Invasive cervical cancer among Hispanic and non-Hispanic women: United States, 1992-1999. *MMWR Morb Mortal Wkly Rep*. 2002;51:1067-1070.
24. Slone Epidemiology Center. Patient registries at Slone: MDS. http://www.bu.edu/prs/mds/ Accessed August 9, 2008.
25. Ortiz DD. Using a simple patient registry to improve your chronic disease care. *Fam Pract Manag*. 2006;13:47-48, 51-52.
26. Kennedy L, Craig AM. Global registries for measuring pharmacoeconomic and quality-of-life outcomes: focus on design and data collection, analysis and interpretation. *Pharmacoeconomics*. 2004;22:551-568.
27. Sankaranarayanan J, Watanabe-Galloway S, Sun J, et al. Rurality and other determinants of early colorectal cancer diagnosis in Nebraska: a 6-year cancer registry study, 1998-2003. *J Rural Health*. 2009;25:358-365.
28. Sankaranarayanan J, Watanabe-Galloway S, Sun J, et al. Age and rural residence effects on accessing colorectal cancer treatments: a registry study. *Am J Manag Care*. 2010;16:265-273.
29. Abougergi MS, Rai R, Cohen CK, et al. Trends in adult-to-adult living donor liver transplant organ donation: the Johns Hopkins experience. *Prog Transplant*. 2006;16:28-32.
30. Dujardin JJ, Steg PG, Puel J, et al. FACT: French national registry of acute coronary syndromes. Specific study of French general hospital centers. *Ann Cardiol Angeiol*. 2003;52:337-343.

31. Ferreira J, Monteiro P, Mimoso J. National Registry of Acute Coronary Syndromes: results of the hospital phase in 2002. *Rev Port Cardiol.* 2004;23:1251-1272.
32. Fiel SB. Pulmonary function during pregnancy in cystic fibrosis: implications for counseling. *Curr Opin Pulm Med.* 1996;2:462-465.
33. Philippe F, Larrazet F, Dibie A, et al. Management of acute coronary syndromes in a new French coronary intensive care unit: the first four years of activity in the GRACE registry (Global Registry of Acute Coronary Events). *Ann Cardiol Angeiol.* 2005;54:68-73.
34. Lablanche JM, Amouyel P, Hoden S. The OSCAR registry: registry of acute coronary syndromes. *Ann Cardiol Angeiol.* 2003;52:205-211.
35. Lupi Herrera E; The RENASICA Cooperative Group. National Registry of Acute Ischemic Coronary Syndromes (RENASICA). Mexican Cardiology Society. *Arch Cardiol Mex.* 2002;72 (suppl 2):S45-S64.
36. Kerr C, Boone J, Connolly S, et al. Follow-up of atrial fibrillation: the initial experience of the Canadian Registry of Atrial Fibrillation. *Eur Heart J.* 1996;17(suppl C):48-51.
37. Launoy G, Maurel J, Grosclaude P, et al. Value of cancer registries in the evaluation of colorectal cancer treatment. *Rev Epidemiol Sante Publique.* 1996;44(suppl 1):S22-S32.
38. Silva MA, Donovan JL, Gandhi PJ, et al. Platelet inhibitors in non-ST-segment elevation acute coronary syndromes and percutaneous coronary intervention: glycoprotein IIb/IIIa inhibitors, clopidogrel, or both? *Vasc Health Risk Manag.* 2006;2:39-48.
39. Steele JM, Sung L, Klaassen R, et al. Disease progression in recently diagnosed patients with inherited marrow failure syndromes: a Canadian Inherited Marrow Failure Registry (CIMFR) report. *Pediatr Blood Cancer.* 2006;47:918-925.
40. Fonarow GC; ADHERE Scientific Advisory Committee. The Acute Decompensated Heart Failure National Registry (ADHERE): opportunities to improve care of patients hospitalized with acute decompensated heart failure. *Rev Cardiovasc Med.* 2003;4(suppl 7):S21-S30.
41. Suoyrjo H, Hinkka K, Oksanen T, et al. Effects of multidisciplinary inpatient rehabilitation for chronic back or neck pain: a register-linkage study of sickness absences and analgesic purchases in an occupational cohort. *Occup Environ Med.* 2008;65:179-184.
42. Carlgren LE, Ericson A, Kallen B. Monitoring of congenital cardiac defects. *Pediatr Cardio.* 1987;8:247-256.
43. Gargano JW, Wehner S, Reeves M. Sex differences in acute stroke care in a statewide stroke registry. *Stroke.* 2008;39:24-29.
44. Charlton RA, Cunnington MC, de Vries CS, et al. Data resources for investigating drug exposure during pregnancy and associated outcomes: the General Practice Research Database (GPRD) as an alternative to pregnancy registries. *Drug Saf.* 2008;31:39-51.
45. US Department of Health and Human Services. Secretary Sebelius releases $27.8 million in Recovery Act funds to expand the use of health information technology. http://www.recovery.gov/News/press/Pages/20090929_HHS_PR_HealthIT.aspx. Accessed March 3, 2010.
46. Bhandari A, Wagner T. Self-reported utilization of health care services: improving measurement and accuracy. *Med Care Res Rev.* 2006;63:217-235.
47. De-Identified Normative Health Information (dNHI) Database of Insurance Claims. http://www.optuminsight.com/life-sciences/solutions/value-strategy/marketing-analytics/clin-formatics-data-mart/overview. Accessed October 18, 2012.
48. Pass HI. Medical registries: continued attempts for robust quality data. *J Thorac Oncol.* 2010;5(6 suppl 2):S198-S199.
49. Motheral B, Brooks J, Clark MA, et al. A checklist for retrospective database studies—report of the ISPOR Task Force on Retrospective Databases. *Value Health.* 2003;6:90-97.
50. Blumenthal D. Launching HITECH. *N Engl J Med.* 2010;362:382-385.
51. Des Jarlais DC, Lyles C, Crepaz N, et al. Improving the reporting quality of nonrandomized evaluations of behavioral and public health interventions: the TREND statement. *Am J Public Health.* 2004;94:361-366.
52. CONSORT (Consolidated Standards of Reporting Trials) Statement (online). Available at: http://www.consort-statement.org/. Accessed October 18, 2012.

Part 4: Alternative, Population-Based Data Sources

53. Good Epidemiological Practice (GEP) – International Epidemiological Association (IEA) Guidelines for proper conduct of epidemiological research. http://webcast.hrsa.gov/conferences/mchb/mchepi_2009/communicating_research/Ethical_guidelines/IEA_guidelines.pdf. Accessed October 18, 2012.
54. von Elm E, Altman DG, Egger M, et al. The Strengthening the Reporting of Observational Studies in Epidemiology (STROBE) statement: guidelines for reporting observational studies. *Ann Intern Med.* 2007;147:573-577.
55. Concato J, Shah N, Horwitz RI. Randomized, controlled trials, observational studies, and the hierarchy of research designs. *N Engl J Med.* 2000;342:1887-1892.
56. Atkins D, Eccles M, Flottorp S, et al. Systems for grading the quality of evidence and the strength of recommendations I: critical appraisal of existing approaches The GRADE Working Group. *BMC Health Serv Res.* 2004;4:38.
57. Atkins D, Best D, Briss PA, et al. Grading quality of evidence and strength of recommendations. *BMJ.* 2004;328:1490.
58. Registry of Patient Registries (RoPR): Project Overview. http://effectivehealthcare.ahrq.gov/ehc/products/311/1114/DEcIDE40_Registry-of-patient-registries_FinalReport_20120531.pdf. Accessed October 18, 2012.

CHAPTER 25

# Randomized Controlled Trial Data

Mariam K. Hassan, BPharm, PhD; and
Jayashri Sankaranarayanan, MPharm, PhD

This chapter describes the use of data from randomized controlled trials (RCTs) to evaluate the effectiveness of health and disease management programs. In this section, we provide an overview of the need for data from RCTs and the measurement of different outcomes, followed by a discussion on strengths and limitations of RCT data.

Health and disease management programs offer various strategies for promoting targeted improvements in health or better managing and controlling disease. These interventions include programs aimed at prevention, diagnostic testing and screening, medication adherence, and patient and provider education. However, development and implementation of a health and disease management program in any health care setting can be challenging and expensive. To make evidence-based decisions about which health and disease management programs to implement, policy makers need reliable and valid estimates to measure the impact of a proposed intervention.

Appropriate experimental and observational studies are needed to demonstrate the likelihood for improved patient outcomes and cost-savings as a result of the health and disease management program. RCTs are the gold standard among clinical study designs and their application for evaluating health and disease management programs can play a key role in determining the outcomes as a result of program implementation.[1] Appropriate randomization could potentially reduce threats related to validity such as selection bias and confounding, thereby increasing the value of the assessment to inform decision making of practitioners, health care system leaders and policy makers.

## 1. Need for Randomized Controlled Trial Data

The aim of evaluation of a health and disease management program is to provide sound evidence to demonstrate that an intervention leads to improvement in health outcomes. This evidence is critical to support decision making if a program is to be implemented on a wider scale across a broader range of health care settings. In the face of questions about the effectiveness of health and disease management programs, vendors who provide services need accurate and conclusive data from methodologically strong studies to demonstrate improvement in outcomes and cost-neutrality or -savings resulting from their program's intervention.[2-4]

Program outcomes can be difficult to quantify and assess as they are susceptible to various biases and confounding factors that remain unaccounted for in most program evaluations.[5] Factors such as age, gender, comorbidities, and time-related effects can impact outcomes above and beyond the intervention and confound the results. The RCT design can provide reliable and valid data regarding the impact of interventions on outcomes as the randomization eliminates selection bias and potential confounding factors on the outcomes.[1]

In nonrandomized comparisons, it is difficult to attribute differences in outcomes to the interventions with certainty. Furthermore, providers may selectively assign patients who may benefit from one intervention over another. This also introduces bias as changes in outcomes may be due to the assignment process rather than the intervention itself. In RCTs, randomization distributes measurable and unmeasurable variables similarly between the control and intervention groups so that observed changes in outcomes can be attributed to the intervention.[6]

## 2. Measuring Health and Disease Management Outcomes in Randomized Control Trials

### Data Needs

The goals of a health and disease management program will determine which data are required and collected in a trial. In order to evaluate the impact of a program, it is important to determine the data needs in advance and to integrate an effective data collection strategy in the trial. The first consideration in developing a data collection strategy is to assess how the intervention may impact different outcomes in the short- and long-term. For example, consider the effectiveness and cost-effectiveness evaluation of a health and disease management program designed to manage type 2 diabetes among patients in an outpatient setting.[7] If the program intervention is effective, it will result in improvements in clinical outcomes, such as blood pressure, cholesterol levels or glucose control. The program could prevent worsening of diabetes symptoms that lead to emergency room visits or hospitalizations. Consequently, outcomes such as patient satisfaction and health status may be affected. Some of the changes due to the intervention may occur immediately while others will be affected directly or indirectly over time. Therefore, data needed to evaluate this diabetes program include clinical data such as HbA1c, LDL, HDL and total cholesterol, and blood pressure measurements at each assessment time point and economic data on relevant health care utilization such as hospitalizations, emergency room visits, drug therapy, glucose monitor and strips, surgical procedures, and health care personnel time, and associated costs for the cost-effectiveness analysis.[7]

If the patient-reported outcomes (PRO) are important to the decision maker, the data collection strategy should include selecting appropriate questionnaires and allocating time for patients to respond to the PRO questionnaire at each assessment point. If the goal of the evaluation is to determine the long-term impact of the program then the trial duration will have to be of adequate length to obtain long-term data. This would involve deciding the appropriate trial duration to capture long-term effects, planning to retain patients during the course of the trial and to have continuous access to all utilization data incurred during the trial period.

## Data Source

For each outcome measured in an RCT, a valid and reliable source of data has to be ascertained. Different data sources available to researchers include patient interviews, medical chart reviews, laboratory reports, and administrative claims databases.[8] While considering a data source for a study, it is important to consider the reliability and validity of the data source as well as convenience of using this data. Medical chart review may be expensive, cumbersome, or incomplete if the patient goes to multiple providers.

Alternatively, data could be collected from administrative claims, hospital and laboratory reports, patient assessments and patient interviews if the information on the outcome of interest is available in these data sources. There may not be a single data source available for different types of data requirements. Claims data may not contain information on health care services that are not covered by the health plan or information on clinical outcomes. Researchers may have to arrange access to multiple data sources depending on the needs of the evaluation.

## Data Collection

In RCTs, researchers randomly assign patients to the control and treatment groups and collect data at baseline (or the point of randomization) and at follow-up time points. At the end of the trial, outcomes from all groups are compared and differences in outcomes are attributed to the intervention.[6,9]

In most cases, data collection procedures can be set up as a part of the health and disease management program. At each patient visit, data collection on clinical end points, patient-reported outcomes and health services used can be carried out along with other procedures in the program. If needed, additional data from medical charts, patient interviews and diaries, and administrative claims can be extracted for patients participating in the program to supplement the RCT data. The duration of the trial may need to be extended to fulfill the need for long-term data. Institutional Review Board (IRB) approval needs to be obtained, as well as appropriate informed consent from the patient to participate in the trial and allow data collection.

## Outcome Measurement

### Clinical Outcomes

Many health and disease management program evaluations, especially those based on clinical outcomes, integrate clinical data collection into the program. Clinical assessments are usually carried out during patient visits. For example, impact of a work-site cholesterol control management program was assessed based on serum cholesterol levels. Venipuncture specimens were obtained at the trial sites at baseline and at follow-up visits from patients to evaluate the effectiveness of the program.[10] In an another program evaluating nurse case management, tests on HbA1c, the primary study outcome, fasting glucose levels, fasting lipid levels and serum creatinine levels were ordered for the participating patients as a part of an HMO-sponsored health and disease management program.[11]

Medical charts also offer comprehensive information on clinical outcomes for patients. Information on patient medical history, diagnostic information, laboratory test results, and prescribed medications can be ascertained from medical charts. Some clinical information, such as diagnosis and procedures performed that were covered by a health plan could also be obtained from administrative databases. However, there is usually a lag before these claims are processed and available in datasets.

## Utilization and Cost Outcomes

Trial data on resource utilization is usually collected from medical charts, patient self-report, or administrative claims data. Medical charts can be abstracted to review resource utilizations including hospitalizations or emergency room visits, laboratory tests, outpatient visits, or consultations by specialists.

Patient interviews can be useful when patients have multiple providers and their complete resource use cannot be obtained from any one source. This involves using patient diaries, mail or telephone surveys, or face-to-face interviews to ask patients about various health care services they received. A patient daily diary or log book could be used to reduce recall bias. If detailed information on resource utilization, such as specific medical procedures or laboratory tests performed is needed, patient interview may not be reliable. Standardized questionnaires or forms can be developed to collect information on resource use. These forms could be divided into hospital resource use, outpatient resource use, pharmacy use for both prescription and nonprescription drugs. Patient self-report is also a good source to collect indirect costs due to missed work days, lost wages and caregiver time.

Information on health care utilization and costs can also be obtained from administrative databases, such as hospital or outpatient billing records or managed care claims databases. These databases capture inpatient, outpatient, and pharmacy claims of services provided to the patient and can be comprehensive sources of health care utilization and costs. The diagnosis associated with each service claim can be identified using specific International Classification of Diseases, Ninth Revision, Clinical Modification (ICD-9-CM) codes. Different outcome measures, such as hospitalization rates and costs, various types of outpatient visits such as psychotherapy or physical therapy, medical procedures, use of prescription drugs and their refill pattern can be collected using administrative databases. Unique patient identifiers are available, usually in the form of encrypted social security number, to track patients within these databases. Appropriate IRB approval is needed to access patient identifier information from the databases.

## Patient-Reported Outcomes

Patient-reported outcomes (PROs) can be reports provided by the patient on patient functioning, symptom control, satisfaction with treatment, adherence, or quality of life. Patient interviews or patient diaries are commonly used to obtain data on PROs. To collect PROs, validated questionnaires are available for different disease states and for specific outcomes such as depression symptoms, disability, and quality of life.[12]

Patient interviews or diaries can also be used to collect data on process of care and patient satisfaction. For example, Quality Enhancement by Strategic Teaming (QuEST) intervention, a multifaceted intervention involving a team of health care providers to improve care for major depressive disorder (MDD) patients, was evaluated based on its impact on process of care and outcomes of care. The assessment was done using patient telephone interview data for both process of care and outcomes of care. Process of care was measured based on changes in the quantity of guideline-concordant pharmacotherapy and psychotherapy. Patients were asked if they received a recommendation from a medical provider to visit another physician or therapist for depression treatment. Pharmacotherapy was assessed based on patient self-report if they received an antidepressant at or above minimum dose for at least 3 months. Outcomes were measured based on improvement in depressive symptoms, physical functioning and patient satisfaction.[13]

Some program evaluations may be based on different types of outcomes and require multiple sources of data. As an example, a health and disease management program implemented in a Health Maintenance Organization (HMO) population was evaluated based on clinical outcomes such depression severity, patient-reported outcomes, such as functional status, and economic outcomes, such as health care utilizations. The program targeted patients with depression who were not adequately treated and were high utilizers of nonpsychiatric health services. Depression severity was measured using the Hamilton Depression Rating Scale (HDRS) and functional status using the Medical Outcomes Study 20-item short form (SF-20) subscales. These were assessed via telephone interviews with the patients. Health care utilization during hospitalization and outpatient visits were determined from HMO administrative claims data for 1 year before and 1 year after study randomization.[14]

## 3. Strengths and Limitations

Before a new HDM program is deemed effective and can be broadly implemented, decision makers need robust evidence that subsequent changes in outcomes are associated with the intervention. Though observational study data are an important source of evidence to evaluate HDM programs, they do not control for potential confounding, especially that induced by unmeasured variables.[15,16] Thus it becomes difficult to establish a cause-effect relationship between the HDM program and outcomes. Because of the nature of properly designed RCTs, postintervention changes in outcomes can be reasonably attributed to the program itself. The strong internal validity of RCT data is its main strength, increasing the usefulness of the evaluation and providing stronger evidence than observational data regarding the effectiveness of HDM programs to support decision making. These data can be used to evaluate the effectiveness of programs in terms of different outcomes and to support decisions on selection between different interventions and implementation on a wider scale.

Certain limitations of RCTs should be considered before using RCT data or this approach to evaluate program implementation. One of the major limitations of RCT data is the limited external validity or lack of generalizability. The health care providers involved in the intervention may not be representative of real-world practices and providers where the HDM program may be implemented.[17] Patients recruited and consented into RCTs may be different from the target population with regard to several factors such as demographics, socioeconomic status and medical comorbidities.[18] Of note, patients participating in preventive interventions have been shown to have higher socioeconomic status and education and to be more receptive to healthy lifestyle interventions.[19] Thus, the most important strength of the data from the RCTs is the high-internal validity and a critical caveat is the potential for low-external validity.

A pragmatic limitation is that RCTs may not be feasible due to funding restrictions or high-dropout rates among participants.[20,21] Data collection in RCTs can be expensive, especially follow-up data in trials with longer duration.[21] Patient recruitment and dropout issues create challenges in obtaining adequate sample size for such evaluations. In addition, if the trial is unblinded, patients' or providers' preference for the intervention may bias the outcomes.[18] Lastly, RCTs are not an option when it may be unethical to assign patients to certain interventions. For example, the control group cannot be denied access to necessary health education or important medical intervention if there is certainty that it will benefit the patient.[17,22] Observational studies may be more appropriate alternatives where RCTs are not feasible or relevant to the program evaluation.

Different data sources used in RCTs may have some limitations associated with them. With administrative databases, there is usually a lag time before claims are processed and when they are available in administrative datasets. If an RCT is using data from different sources, clinical outcomes may be measured immediately at the site, but it may take time to collect related economic outcomes. RCTs collecting PRO data should be aware of recall bias and use short patient recall periods.

## 4. Conclusion

RCT data can provide valid and reliable estimates to evaluate the effects of HDM programs. Because of concerns regarding generalizability of RCT data, researchers should exercise caution in extrapolating findings of a particular study population for implementation of the HDM program. Despite the challenges of conducting RCTs and the associated costs, RCT data may be essential when evidence of causality is needed to support decision making regarding HDM programs.

## References

1. Evans D. Hierarchy of evidence: a framework for ranking evidence evaluating healthcare interventions. *J Clin Nurs*. 2003;12(1):77-84.
2. Carroll J. Health plans demand proof that DM saves them money. *Manag Care*. 2000;9(11):25-30.
3. Fireman B, Bartlett J, Selby J. Can disease management reduce health care costs by improving quality? *Health Aff* (Millwood). 2004;23(6):63-75.
4. Sidorov J, Shull R, Tomcavage J, et al. Does diabetes disease management save money and improve outcomes? A report of simultaneous short-term savings and quality improvement associated with a health maintenance organization-sponsored disease management program among patients fulfilling health employer data and information set criteria. *Diabetes Care*. 2002;25(4):684-689.
5. Johnson A. Measuring DM's net effect is harder than you might think. *Manag Care*. 2003;12(6):28-32.
6. Akobeng AK. Understanding randomised controlled trials. *Arch Dis Child*. 2005;90(8): 840-844.
7. Gary TL, Batts-Turner M, Bone LR, et al. A randomized controlled trial of the effects of nurse case manager and community health worker team interventions in urban African-Americans with type 2 diabetes. *Control Clin Trials*. 2004;25(1):53-66.
8. Abarca J, Armstrong E. Improving the use of data sources in disease management programs. *Dis Manage Health Outcomes*. 2001;9(9):459-471.
9. Roberts C, Torgerson D. Randomisation methods in controlled trials. *BMJ*. 1998;317(7168):1301.
10. Fielding JE, Mason T, Kinght K, et al. A randomized trial of the IMPACT worksite cholesterol reduction program. *Am J Prev Med*. 1995;11(2):120-123.
11. Aubert RE, Herman WH, Waters J, et al. Nurse case management to improve glycemic control in diabetic patients in a health maintenance organization: a randomized, controlled trial. *Ann Intern Med*. 1998;129(8):605-612.
12. Emery MP, Perrier LL, Acquadro C. Patient-reported outcome and quality of life instruments database (PROQOLID): frequently asked questions. *Health Qual Life Outcomes*. 2005;3:12.
13. Rost K, Nutting P, Smith J, et al. Improving depression outcomes in community primary care practice: a randomized trial of the quEST intervention: quality enhancement by strategic teaming. *J Gen Intern Med*. 2001;16(3):143-149.
14. Katzelnick DJ, Simon GE, Pearson SD, et al. Randomized trial of a depression management program in high utilizers of medical care. *Arch Fam Med*. 2000;9(4):345-351.
15. Byar DP. Problems with using observational databases to compare treatments. *Stat Med*. 1991;10(4):663-666.
16. Byar DP. Why data bases should not replace randomized clinical trials. *Biometrics*. 1980;36(2): 337-342.
17. Hannan E. Randomized clinical trials and observational studies guidelines for assessing respective strengths and limitations. *J Am Coll Cardiol Intv*. 2008;1:211-217.
18. McKee M, Britton A, Black N, et al. Methods in health services research: interpreting the evidence: choosing between randomised and non-randomised studies. *BMJ*. 1999;319(7205): 312-315.
19. Davies G, Pyke S, Kinmonth AL. Effect of non-attenders on the potential of a primary care programme to reduce cardiovascular risk in the population: family heart study group. *BMJ*. 1994;309(6968):1553-1556.

**Part 4: Alternative, Population-Based Data Sources**

20. Moher D, Dulberg CS, Wells GA. Statistical power, sample size, and their reporting in randomized controlled trials. *JAMA*. 1994;272(2):122-124.
21. Stables RH. Observational research in the evidence based environment: eclipsed by the randomised controlled trial? *Heart*. 2002;87(2):101-102.
22. Hellman S, Hellman DS. Of mice but not men: problems of the randomized clinical trial. *N Engl J Med*. 1991;324(22):1585-1589.

For more information on randomized controlled trials, please see Part 5 of this book.

CHAPTER 26

# Genetics Databases

Christopher R. Frei, PharmD, MSc; Russell T. Attridge, PharmD, MSc; and Bradi L. Frei, PharmD, MSc

This chapter illustrates how existing databases with genetic information can be used for health and disease management. This chapter highlights databases from NIH's SNP Health Association Resource (SHARe), an epidemiological genetics initiative that provides genetic and clinical datasets to researchers worldwide. Databases are characterized by organ system, including cardiovascular disease, stroke, cancer, diabetes, and mental health. Access policies, associated costs, advantages, and limitations of each database are described. This chapter concludes with a discussion regarding current perspectives and future challenges for genetics databases that are to be used for health and disease management.

The United States Agency for Healthcare Research and Quality (AHRQ) has previously sought to identify databases capable of value-based assessments for emerging gene-based diagnostic and therapeutic technologies.[1] AHRQ hoped that such databases would enable them to monitor test utilization and quantify health and fiscal benefits, but unfortunately concluded that no existing databases met this need. The agency maintained that "health care policy makers, providers, and payers need data on how specific genetic tests and related interventions impact short- and long-term health outcomes, including information on cost-effectiveness." Finally, the agency further concluded that "information is currently lacking on the use of gene-based tests and the outcomes of clinical interventions based on these tests."[1]

## 1. Genetic Concepts

Early human genetics research focused on identifying genetic variants responsible for human disease (fundamental discovery). The completion of comprehensive genetics programs, such as the Human Genome Project or the International HapMap Project, coupled with advances in molecular biology and bioinformatics, has led to an explosion in the development and widespread availability of gene-based approaches to diagnosis and treatment. Therefore, genetics research has since refocused on translating knowledge of fundamental genetic discoveries into therapeutic interventions (knowledge translation). The core concept of knowledge translation is simple, but its application is elusive. Conceptually, the idea is to utilize genetic information to assist treatment decisions and improve patient health. Gene-based diagnostic tests and therapies have emerged for cancer, HIV/AIDS, and many other common human diseases.

Oncology provides one of the best examples of the clinical utility of gene-based tests. Cytogenetic testing for chronic myelogenous leukemia (CML) determines the type of cancer and predicts response to a selected treatment.[2] Initially, the testing is used to determine the presence of a specific genetic abnormality, the Philadelphia chromosome. The Philadelphia chromosome is a result of a translocation of parts of chromosome 9 and chromosome 22, which forms the *bcr-abl* gene. The goal of treatment is to deactivate the *bcr-abl* protein. One of the first targeted medications developed to combat CML was imatinib (Gleevec®). Second-generation targeted medications include nilotinib (Tasigna®) and dasatinib (Sprycel®). Genetic tests continue to be used during treatment and after remission to monitor response to therapy. In this way, the genetic tests play an integral part in the diagnosis, treatment, and management of CML.

Genetic testing is a key factor in the treatment decision process for human immunodeficiency virus/acquired immune deficiency syndrome (HIV/AIDS). In the past, health care providers have cautiously used abacavir for the treatment of HIV because its use is associated with about a 5% risk of a severe hypersensitivity reaction. However, the ability to test for a specific allele (the HLA-B*5701 allele) helps clinicians to identify patients who might suffer a hypersensitivity reaction.[3] These advances have led to clinical practice changes that include a recommendation to conduct genetic screening for this allele prior to initiating abacavir therapy and a strong recommendation against the use of abacavir in patients identified as having this allele.

## 2. Application of Genetics Databases for Health and Disease Management

As gene-based diagnostic and treatment strategies become part of routine patient care, a third research approach is necessary to transform health care systems. Such an approach is needed to explore issues including: mechanisms to facilitate timely utilization, barriers to equitable distribution, real-world effectiveness, and economic value. Large genetics databases may be the best way to study these issues. In order to make genetic databases useful for the evaluation of health and disease management programs, such databases must contain patient-level genetic, clinical, health, and economic outcomes data, undergo rigorous validation and be representative of the target population. Unfortunately, no existing databases currently meet all of these criteria.

## 3. Existing Databases with Genetic Information

This section describes some of the available databases (Table 1), highlights their strengths and weaknesses, and outlines the general steps needed to access these databases. In 2007, the NIH made a major commitment to the science of epidemiological genetics by establishing SHARe.[4] The goal of the SHARe project is to conduct genomewide association studies (GWAS) from multiple, large National Heart, Lung, and Blood Institute (NHLBI) cohorts to generate knowledge on cardiovascular disease, lung disease, diabetes, and other disorders.[5] This project and others are available online, many through the National Center for Biotechnology Information's (NCBI) database of Genotypes and Phenotypes (dbGaP). Robust collections of data from existing large-scale clinical studies are centrally located and accessible at no charge.[6]

## Cardiovascular Disease

### Framingham SHARe

The NIH SHARe, one of the pioneering programs in the world of integrated genetics databases, performs and maintains genomewide association studies over large NHLBI patient cohorts. The first SHARe database, made publicly available in 2008, focuses on data from over 9,000 subjects involved in the landmark Framingham Heart Study (FHS). The FHS encompasses 3 generations of individuals since it was first started in 1948; it now includes over 15,000 subjects and has provided an enormous wealth of knowledge about cardiovascular disease.

The SHARe includes an extensive amount of genetic information about these patients, including analysis of over 550,000 SNPs and a variety of microsatellite markers. All of the clinical data are from the original and follow-up studies of the FHS and include variables such as blood pressure, body mass index (BMI), lab values (for example, fasting blood glucose, total and HDL cholesterol), lifestyle factors (for example, smoking history), biomarkers (for example, fibrinogen, C-reactive protein), and electrocardiographic information (for example, QT intervals).

Since the original study, investigators have amplified the study scope to include genetic information obtained from patient blood samples, with the latest phase resulting in this SHARe database. Additionally, almost 90 substudies of these patients are available and adding to the impressive amount of genetic information documented on these patients. Patient-level, deidentified data from the SHARe program are available at dbGaP. There is no fee for accessing the databases at dbGaP; however, for the protection of the participants, interested researchers must submit a request for authorization to ensure that the research plans are consistent with the informed consent agreements of the patients. The SHARe data are now being utilized across multiple disciplines and are a source of great future interest.[7-9]

### Study of the Effectiveness of Additional Reductions in Cholesterol and Homocysteine Genome Wide Association Study of Statin-Induced Myopathy

The Study of the Effectiveness of Additional Reductions in Cholesterol and Homocysteine (SEARCH) database contains clinical and genetic data from 175 patients involved in the ongoing research.[10] SEARCH was a randomized trial of over 12,000 patients with a previous myocardial infarction that sought to determine if

80 mg of simvastatin daily conferred any additional benefit over 20 mg of simvastatin daily. After 6 years of follow-up, 98 patients in the 80-mg group were said to have either definite or incipient myopathy and a follow-up study was performed to search for genetic causes.[11]

Genetic information was obtained from 90 of those 98 individuals and matched with 85 patients in the 80-mg group that did not show signs of myopathy. No individual-level data are currently available.[12] Clinical information forthcoming will include data regarding basic demographics, comorbidities (for example, diabetes), kidney function (for example, estimated glomerular filtration rate, serum creatinine), medications (for example, amiodarone, calcium channel antagonists), and myopathy status. Data may be accessed through NCBI's dbGaP.

## Stroke

### Ischemic Stroke Genetics Study

The Ischemic Stroke Genetics Study (ISGS) is a 5-center, case-controlled study that aims to find associations between ischemic strokes and polymorphisms of genes that are involved in coagulation and platelet function.[13] The raw data are available on NCBI's dbGaP and are available for qualified researchers to use in independent studies. In addition to SNP data, this resource includes clinical information, which comprises vital signs, laboratory tests, imaging results, and patient treatments. Stroke subtype, time of stroke onset, and post-stroke evaluations including the NIH Stroke Scale, the Barthel Index, the Oxford Handicap Scale, and the Glasgow Outcome Scale are also available.[13]

## Cancer

### Genome-Wide Association Study of Neuroblastoma

The Genome-Wide Association Study of Neuroblastoma is a database containing the genetic variants associated with clinically aggressive neuroblastomas in children. Data published in June 2008 demonstrated that children homozygous for certain alleles at chromosome *6p22* are more likely to have metastatic disease, oncogene amplicification, and relapse.[14] As a substudy, a GWAS was performed on a total of 1,032 case subjects using SNP genotypes and copy number variants. Study participants were of European ancestry with a median age of 10 years. Case subjects were defined as having a diagnosis of either neuroblastoma or ganglioneuroblastoma; all were registered in the Children's Oncology Group. Available data include pathological information such as the site of tumor origin, disease stage using the International Neuroblastoma Staging System, the International Neuroblastoma Pathology Classification, and genetic data such as the MYCN oncogene copy number and DNA index.[14]

# Diabetes

## Genetics of Kidneys in Diabetes

GoKinD, the Genetics of Kidneys in Diabetes study, is a collection of data from case-control singletons and trios (1 singleton and 2 parents) aiming to identify genes that increase susceptibility to diabetic nephropathy in type 1 diabetics.[15] The study analyzed 3,043 patients and collected information on patient demographics, diabetic history, renal function, and other characteristics of diabetes (for example, hypertension, hyperlipidemia, retinopathy, and neuropathy). Of the case patients, approximately two-thirds were classified as having end-stage renal disease (ESRD); one-third demonstrated persistent proteinuria.[15] Genetic information, including allele and genotype frequencies, was also collected on 1,825 type 1 diabetics through the Genetic Association Information Network (GAIN).

GAIN is a publicly and privately funded organization dedicated to assisting in GWAS for common diseases.[16] The database is restricted to those conducting research on type 1 diabetes and its related disorders. Information regarding additional patients in the study (not included in the GAIN database) is available by a separate process through the National Institute of Diabetes and Digestive and Kidney Diseases (NIDDK).

# Mental Health

## Linking Genome-Wide Association Study of Schizophrenia

Interested individuals may gain access to information on 5,066 phenotyped case-control subjects in a GAIN database available through dbGaP.[17] The sample population includes people of European and African ancestry with a full set of genetic information to include genotype intensity data for all participants. Cases are people greater than 18 years of age who have been formally diagnosed (using DSM-IV criteria from the *Diagnostic and Statistical Manual of Mental Disorders*) with either schizophrenia or schizoaffective disorder. The database includes mental health information such as age of onset, the presence/absence of disease characteristics [for example, positive symptoms (hallucinations, delusions) and negative symptoms (alogia, avolition, flat affect)], consensus ratings from the DSM-IV schizophrenia criteria, and other diagnoses (for example, bipolar disorder), as well as genetic information.

It also includes demographics such as income, education, race/ethnicity, and housing, marital, and employment status. Database information may be used for any genetic studies, except for a subset of patients who have consents only allowing genetic studies of schizophrenia and related disorders. Researchers also have the presence of the Psychiatric GWAS Consortium (PGC) to aid in interpretation of the increasing number of GWAS. The PGC is an international group that performs *mega-analyses* across the field of psychiatry to find the strongest associations between genetics and disease.[18]

## International Multi-Center ADHD Genetics Project

Attention Deficit Hyperactivity Disorder (ADHD) is a disorder estimated to affect 3 to 10% of children and 2 to 4% of adults in the United States.[19,20] There is great interest in learning more about the role genetics plays in ADHD.[21] The International Multi-Center ADHD Genetics (IMAGE) project, a European multicenter project, has used a methodical approach to screen for novel genes and gene systems involved in ADHD in a population of over 1,400 families.[22]

Derived from the IMAGE project patients, the GAIN database analyzes 958 parent-child trios (2,835 total subjects) with the goal of creating a 600,000 tag-SNP association study. Accompanying the genetic data, dbGaP has phenotypic and clinical information available that includes age, sex, DSM-IV ADHD diagnosis subtypes, IQ, medication status, parental information, personality traits, and parent and teacher results from the Strengths and Difficulties Questionnaire (SDQ). Researchers must also be approved by the National Institute of Mental Health (NIMH), and use of this database is restricted to ADHD genetic studies and may not be used by those seeking financial gain. A published review of GWAS in ADHD may be useful to interested researchers.[23]

## Center for Inherited Disease Research: Genome-Wide Association Study in Familial Parkinson's Disease

An ever-present concern of older age, Parkinson's disease (PD) is associated with great morbidity and has piqued the interest of many researchers hoping to improve care for these patients. This study resulted from the combined efforts of 2 major NIH-funded PD genetics studies, PROGENI and GenePD. When combined, over 1,000 PD families (1,991 total subjects) are included, with all cases having a positive family history of the disease. Controls were obtained from the NINDS repository and are non-Hispanic subjects with no history of neurological disease.

Combining genetic information obtained in both studies regarding novel genes related to PD, the Center for Inherited Disease Research (CIDR) study provides an opportunity to better relate these genes to disease, ultimately leading to a better understanding and better care for these patients. Phenotypic data are also available and include variables such as age of onset, family history of disease, medication history (for example, prior response to levodopa), ethnicity, and smoking history. Also included are results of the Unified Parkinson's Disease Rating Scale (UPDRS), the presence/absence of PD signs and symptoms (for example, bradykinesia, cerebellar signs, gait, resting tremor, rigidity, etc.), and Mini Mental Status Exam (MMSE) results.

## Mayo-Perlegen Linked Efforts to Accelerate Parkinson's Solutions Collaboration

Additional means to improve knowledge about PD have been advanced through the efforts of groups like the Linked Efforts to Accelerate Parkinson's Solutions (LEAPS) Collaboration. In March 2008, the LEAPS group made the genetic and clinical data associated with a 2005 PD study by Maraganore et al. publicly available for further analysis.[24] The study, a multitiered high-resolution genome scan, was able to identify genes that may increase a person's susceptibility to PD. In the beginning, almost 200,000 SNPs were genotyped in sibling pairs discordant for PD. After identifying possible associations, these SNPs were matched with unrelated controls, and the list of association genes continued to narrow. After combining analyses with additional statistical tests, the most significant SNPs tagged the same genetic locus, PARK10, as most associated with PD. Available genetic data include SNP analysis of all the study individuals (1,550 patients). Diagnosis and demographic characteristics are also available. Perlegen Sciences ceased operations in 2009; however, interested researchers may still gain access to these data through dbGaP.

## Other Databases

### The Wellcome Trust Case Control Consortium

The Wellcome Trust Case Control Consortium (WTCCC) was formed to take advantage of technological advances in genetics and apply those to common diseases. Genotypic data collected by the WTCCC span over multiple disease states (eg, type 1 and type 2 diabetes, coronary heart disease, hypertension, bipolar disorder, rheumatoid arthritis, and inflammatory bowel disease), with over 2,000 case subjects from each of the disorders. An additional 1,000 samples are available from patients with multiple sclerosis, autoimmune thyroid disease, ankylosing spondylitis, and breast cancer.

Phenotypic data are limited, as the only individual-level data available to include chromosomal information, age at onset or collection, geographical region, and sex.[25] More detailed phenotypic information is available; however, this requires an agreement with the principal investigator of the original case collection. As with most other genome-based studies, the population is almost entirely Caucasian. Because this database is more genetic in nature, integrating clinical and phenotypic data would require more effort on the part of the researcher, but is still feasible through collaboration. Interested researchers can gain access after approval of the Consortium Data Access Committee.

### National Eye Institute Age-Related Eye Disease Study

Age-related macular degeneration (AMD) is a principal cause of registered blindness in the US. Cataracts, defined as lens opacities in the eye, often lead to significant vision loss and are the leading cause of visual impairment in the US.[26,27] With no effective preventative treatments available, researchers undertook the Age-Related Eye Disease Study (AREDS) in 1992. Completed in 2005, the AREDS includes nearly 5,000 patients with varying degrees of disease severity for both AMD and age-related cataracts.

The purpose of the AREDS was to gather information regarding the progression and the associated risk factors of these disorders. The AREDS also evaluated the use of an assortment of available vitamins and minerals. The clinical trial was carried out for 6.5 years with 5 additional years of follow-up, and blood samples obtained from 600 patients have been used in a genomewide association scan available through dbGaP. Basic demographic information (for example, age, sex, BMI, smoking history) and relevant medical information (for example, AMD status, type of cataract, history of diabetes, cancer, angina, blood pressure, and multivitamin use) are available.

## 4. Conclusion

As scientific interest in genetic databases continues to escalate, the need for high-quality, accessible databases is becoming increasingly important. There is also great need to improve these databases so that they are appropriate for the evaluation of health and disease management programs. Unfortunately, the existing databases are mostly focused on *fundamental discovery* and there is very little attention given to *knowledge translation* or *health care transformation*. In September 2008, the United States President's Council of Advisors on Science and Technology called for near-term investments in genetics resources like these to enable "tools and resources essential to move beyond genomic discoveries to personalized medicine products and services of patient and public benefit."[28]

One practical approach for improving the capabilities of the existing and emerging databases is to utilize and report better measures of effectiveness, include information on costs of genetic tests and resulting treatments, and make better use of validated utility instruments. There remain significant scientific, economic, regulatory, and social hurdles that must be overcome to translate genetic knowledge into clinically meaningful benefits. These include patient concerns that their genetic information will be used against them by insurers, employers, and researchers.

## References

1. DeStefano F, Whitehead N, Lux LJ, Lohr KN. Infrastructure to monitor utilization and outcomes of gene-based applications: an assessment. (Prepared by RTI International DEcIDE Center under Contract N. HSA2902200500361.) AHRQ Publication No. 08-EHC012. Rockville, MD: Agency for Healthcare Research and Quality; May 2008.
2. Hughes T, Deininger M, Hochhaus A, et al. Monitoring CML patients responding to treatment with tyrosine kinase inhibitors: review and recommendations for harmonizing current methodology for detecting BCR-ABL transcripts and kinase domain mutations and for expressing results. *Blood*. 2006;108(1):28-37.
3. Mallal S, Phillips E, Carosi G, et al. HLA-B*5701 screening for hypersensitivity to abacavir. *N Engl J Med*. 2008;358(6):568-579.
4. NIH launches extensive open-access dataset of genetic and clinical data. http://www.nih.gov/news/pr/oct2007/nhlbi-01.htm. Accessed October 23, 2012.

5. Framingham SNP health association resource (SHARe). http://www.ncbi.nlm.nih.gov/projects/gap/cgi-bin/study.cgi?study_id=phs000007.v4.p2. Accessed October 23, 2012.
6. Mailman MD, Feolo M, Jin Y, et al. The NCBI dbGaP database of genotypes and phenotypes. *Nat Genet*. 2007;39(10):1181-1186.
7. Piccolo SR, Abo RP, Allen-Brady K, et al. Evaluation of genetic risk scores for lipid levels using genome-wide markers in the Framingham Heart Study. *BMC Proc*. 2009;3(suppl 7):S46.
8. Karasik D, Dupuis J, Cho K, et al. Refined QTLs of osteoporosis-related traits by linkage analysis with genome-wide SNPs: Framingham SHARe. *Bone*. 2010;46(4):1114-1121.
9. Cupples LA, Heard-Costa N, Lee M, Atwood LD. Genetics Analysis Workshop 16 Problem 2: the Framingham Heart Study data. *BMC Proc*. 2009;3(suppl 7):S3.
10. Bowman L, Armitage J, Bulbulia R, et al. Study of the effectiveness of additional reductions in cholesterol and homocysteine (SEARCH): characteristics of a randomized trial among 12064 myocardial infarction survivors. *Am Heart J*. 2007;154(5):815-823.
11. Link E, Parish S, Armitage J, et al. SLCO1B1 variants and statin-induced myopathy—a genome-wide study. *N Engl J Med*. 2008;359(8):789-799.
12. National Center for Biotechnology Information, National Institutes of Health, U.S. Department of Health and Human Services. The study of the effectiveness of additional reductions in cholesterol and homocysteine (SEARCH) genome wide association study (GWAS) of statin-induced myopathy. http://www.ncbi.nlm.nih.gov/projects/gap/cgi-bin/study.cgi?study_id=phs000141.v1.p1. Accessed October 23, 2012.
13. Meschia JF, Brott TG, Brown RD Jr, et al. The Ischemic Stroke Genetics Study (ISGS) Protocol. *BMC Neurol*. 2003;3:4.
14. Maris JM, Mosse YP, Bradfield JP, et al. Chromosome 6p22 locus associated with clinically aggressive neuroblastoma. *N Engl J Med*. 2008;358(24):2585-2593.
15. Mueller PW, Rogus JJ, Cleary PA, et al. Genetics of Kidneys in Diabetes (GoKinD) study: a genetics collection available for identifying genetic susceptibility factors for diabetic nephropathy in type 1 diabetes. *J Am Soc Nephrol*. 2006;17(7):1782-1790.
16. National Human Genome Research Institute, National Institutes of Health, U.S. Department of Health and Human Services. Genetic association information network (GAIN). http://www.genome.gov/pfv.cfm?pageID=19518664. Accessed October 23, 2012.
17. National Center for Biotechnology Information, National Institutes of Health, U.S. Department of Health and Human Services. Genome-wide association study of schizophrenia. http://www.ncbi.nlm.nih.gov/projects/gap/cgi-bin/study.cgi?study_id=phs000021.v2.p1. Accessed October 23, 2012.
18. Sullivan PF, de Geus EJ, Willemsen G, et al. Genome-wide association for major depressive disorder: a possible role for the presynaptic protein piccolo. *Mol Psychiatry*. 2009;14(4):359-375.
19. Burd L, Klug MG, Coumbe MJ, Kerbeshian J. Children and adolescents with attention deficit-hyperactivity disorder: 1. Prevalence and cost of care. *J Child Neurol*. 2003;18:555-561.
20. Kessler RC, Adler L, Ames M, et al. The prevalence and effects of adult attention deficit/hyperactivity disorder on work performance in a nationally representative sample of workers. *J Occup Environ Med*. 2005;47:565-572.
21. Brookes K, Xu X, Chen W, et al. The analysis of 51 genes in DSM-IV combined type attention deficit hyperactivity disorder: association signals in DRD4, DAT1 and 16 other genes. *Mol Psychiatry*. 2006;11(10):934-953.
22. Kuntsi J, Stevenson J. Hyperactivity in children: a focus on genetic research and psychological theories. *Clin Child Fam Psychol Rev*. 2000;3(1):1-23.
23. Franke B, Neale BM, Faraone SV. Genome-wide association studies in ADHD. *Hum Genet*. 2009;126(1):13-50.
24. Maraganore DM, de Andrade M, Lesnick TG, et al. High-resolution whole-genome association study of Parkinson disease. *Am J Hum Genet*. 2005;77(5):685-693.
25. The Wellcome Trust Case Control Consortium (WTCCC). http://www.wtccc.org.uk/. Accessed October 23, 2012.

**Part 4: Alternative, Population-Based Data Sources**

26. The Age-Related Eye Disease Study (AREDS): design implications. AREDS report no. 1. *Control Clin Trials*. 1999;20(6):573-600.
27. Thorisson GA, Muilu J, Brookes AJ. Genotype-phenotype databases: challenges and solutions for the post-genomic era. *Nat Rev Genet*. 2009;10(1):9-18.
28. Priorities for Personalized Medicine, Report of the President's Council of Advisors on Science and Technology, September 2008. http://www.whitehouse.gov/files/documents/ostp/PCAST/pcast_report_v2.pdf. Accessed October 23, 2012.

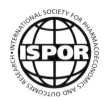

# PART 5

# Statistical Approaches and Methods

CHAPTER 27  Introduction ................................................................. 335

CHAPTER 28  Primary Data Types and How They Are Analyzed Statistically:
             *Demonstration Projects* ................................................. 340

CHAPTER 29  Primary Data Types and How They Are Analyzed Statistically:
             *Randomized Controlled Trials* ........................................ 343

CHAPTER 30  Primary Data Types and How They Are Analyzed Statistically:
             *Natural Experiments* .................................................. 347

CHAPTER 31  Primary Data Types and How They Are Analyzed Statistically:
             *Prospective Designs* ................................................... 350

CHAPTER 32  Primary Data Types and How They Are Analyzed Statistically:
             *Retrospective Designs* ................................................ 355

CHAPTER 33  Statistical Methods for Randomized Controlled Trials:
             *Hypothesis Testing* .................................................... 360

| CHAPTER 34 | Statistical Methods for Randomized Controlled Trials: Discrete Outcomes | 365 |
|---|---|---|
| CHAPTER 35 | Statistical Methods for Randomized Controlled Trials: Continuous Outcomes | 374 |
| CHAPTER 36 | Statistical Methods for Randomized Controlled Trials: Survival Analysis | 381 |
| CHAPTER 37 | Statistical Methods for Randomized Controlled Trials: Confounders | 388 |
| CHAPTER 38 | Statistical Methods for Randomized Controlled Trials: Missing Data in Outcomes Research Studies | 393 |
| CHAPTER 39 | Statistical Methods for Randomized Controlled Trials: Sample Selection Bias Issues | 398 |
| CHAPTER 40 | Statistical Methods for Randomized Controlled Trials: Propensity Scores | 405 |
| CHAPTER 41 | Statistical Methods for Randomized Controlled Trials: Instrumental Variables Methods | 409 |
| CHAPTER 42 | Statistical Methods for Randomized Controlled Trials: Heckman Selection Models | 415 |
| CHAPTER 43 | Statistical Methods for Randomized Controlled Trials: Bootstrap Method | 419 |
| CHAPTER 44 | Statistical Methods for Randomized Controlled Trials: Model Validation | 423 |
| CHAPTER 45 | Statistical Methods for Randomized Controlled Trials: Nonparametric Statistical Methods | 427 |

CHAPTER 27

# Introduction

Joel Hay, PhD

This chapter introduces statistical methods and approaches used to evaluate health and disease management (HDM) programs. While there are many approaches to study design and data collection for HDM evaluation, each strategy implies a set of statistical analysis approaches that is feasible and/or optimal. Appropriate statistical evaluation is crucial to informed HDM policy. Use of the wrong statistical approach is a primary cause of biased or otherwise inappropriate assessment of relative benefits and clinical outcomes.

The first section of this chapter discusses study design and data collection approaches, indicating the strengths and weaknesses of each approach. The second section deals with randomized controlled trials (RCTs) since these are the gold standard for generating unbiased treatment effects. The final section describes a variety of statistical issues that relate to non-RCT study designs. Such study designs are subject to a wide variety of threats to internal validity, and thus require more complex statistical analysis than RCTs. The primary advantages of non-RCT study designs are that they are generally less expensive and require less study time than RCT study designs. While this chapter is not intended to cover any of the statistical methods in detail, it will provide an introduction to the concepts of statistical evaluation of HDM interventions.

## 1. Background

Much of health care is either unnecessary, wasteful, or harmful.[1, 2] Dr. David Eddy has estimated that only 15% of medical care is evidence based.[3] One study has found that only 11% of cardiovascular treatment guidelines are based on multiple randomized controlled trials or meta-analyses of randomized controlled trials while 48% of these guidelines are based only on expert opinion, anecdotal evidence, or existing standard of care.[4]

Rather than using subjective opinion or other qualitative assessments, researchers evaluate empirical data on HDM interventions statistically to determine which therapeutic approach is preferable and whether or not the study findings are robust. These quantitative empirical analyses allow the researcher to draw valid and reliable inferences as to which medical treatments are appropriate. Evidence-based medicine (EBM) is the framework for establishing best medical and health care practices, and statistical methods and approaches are key to determining the evidentiary bases for all types of HDM interventions. There is a well-established hierarchy of clinical evidence, based on available treatment data:[3,5]

- **Level of Evidence A:** Recommendation based on evidence from multiple randomized trials or meta-analyses.

- **Level of Evidence B:** Recommendation based on evidence from a single randomized trial or nonrandomized studies.

- **Level of Evidence C:** Recommendation based on expert opinion, case studies, or standards of care.

This evidence hierarchy has been validated in the literature. Randomized controlled trials are the only way to guarantee that the observed HDM intervention effect is caused by the intervention and not due to some observable or unobservable confounder. Patsopoulos and colleagues evaluated peer-reviewed articles in the medical literature with high-citation counts (more than 10 in 2 years following publication), and found that RCTs and meta-analyses of RCTs accounted for 76% of all of these highly cited articles.[6] Ioannidis looked at all articles published in the 3 highest-impact factor journals (*New England Journal of Medicine*, *JAMA* and *Lancet*) between 1990 and 2003—they were cited more than 1,000 times in the medical literature. Of all of the original clinical research studies meeting these criteria, 5 of 6 highly cited nonrandomized studies had been contradicted by or had found stronger treatment effects than later studies on the same interventions, while only 9 of 39 randomized controlled trials (p=.008) were similarly challenged or contradicted by later studies. Ioannidis demonstrated that, due to the paucity of RCTs and meta-analyses of RCTs in the scientific literature, most published peer-reviewed research findings are false.[7]

Unfortunately, while there are numerous studies supporting the clinical and economic values of HDM interventions,[8] all of the Class A RCT studies on health and disease management interventions are not favorable to these interventions, either because there are no favorable demonstrated clinical effects, or there are no favorable clinical effects that can be justified on a cost basis.[9-13] For example, the most comprehensive of these RCT demonstration projects is a CMS-sponsored demonstration involving 15 separate randomized controlled trials of coordinated care interventions in 18,402 Medicare patients involving 1,018 physicians and a variety of health care institutions around the US with 18.4 to 37.0 average months of follow-up across the 15 sites.[14]

As Ayanian wrote in an accompanying *JAMA* editorial[15]:

> The financial and clinical results of this careful evaluation were sobering. Only 2 of the 12 largest programs had a statistically significant effect on the annual number of hospital admissions. ... When program fees were incorporated in the analysis, total expenditures were 8% to 41% higher (p < .10) in the

intervention groups than the control groups for 9 of the 12 largest programs, and no programs reduced expenditures. In the clinical domain, the interventions had only sporadic effects on process measures of quality of care, such as vaccinations, cancer screening, or diabetes services, and had minimal or no effects on patients' functional status and health-related quality of life.

It is hard to identify any other example in health care in which the quality and rigor of the medical evidentiary basis for such a negative finding on the clinical and economic values of an intervention is so strong and robust. If after reviewing these disease management RCT trials, one still takes the position that *more evidence is needed* regarding the lack of benefits for disease management interventions, one is in essence denying the value of evidence-based outcomes research itself in informing health care policy decisions. There are very few medical interventions that have generated so many thousands of patient-years of rigorous medical and economic outcomes follow-up in independent RCTs. As a society we cannot possibly devote such medical effectiveness research resources to evaluating even the most important medical interventions if the result of unpleasant but scientifically solid findings is to take the position that *more research is needed*. The only reasonable conclusion is that disease management programs are not clinically effective or cost-effective. It is time to design new interventions beyond the disease management paradigm that have a chance of demonstrating more positive outcomes.

The purpose of this section of the book is to introduce the various statistical techniques and study designs that are available for health and disease management program evaluation. As the various chapters demonstrate, there are varieties of techniques and designs each with its advantages and disadvantages. However, not all statistical techniques and study designs are equivalent. The gold standard for establishing that a specific intervention causes a specific clinical, economic or humanistic outcome will always be the RCT study design. A major reason why this is so is because the RCT, if conducted properly, requires only the simplest of statistical analyses (for example, independent group t-tests) to evaluate an intervention. When study subjects are randomly assigned to treatment or placebo, and yet there is found to be a statistically significant difference in prespecified outcome measures at the conclusion of the study period, this difference is highly unlikely to have occurred by random chance. It is difficult or impossible to argue that there is some observable or unobservable confounder that is actually causing the differences rather than the intervention itself.

RCTs are not easy or always feasible. Nevertheless, given that the US health care sector currently costs $2.7 trillion per year and about $900 billion of that spending may be useless or harmful, as a society we can afford to conduct more RCT evaluations of a wide variety of medical interventions. More importantly, we cannot afford not to do so. People are developing a variety of strategies to conduct RCTs more cheaply and quickly, including Bayesian adaptive trial study designs and pragmatic comparative effectiveness study designs.[16] Others are developing hybrid RCT study designs that overcome the problems associated with inability to blind treatment assignment or with outcomes reporting bias.[17]

There are many legitimate reasons for non-RCT study designs and statistical methods. In fact, given the infinite number of treatment comparisons and study populations that could be evaluated, most research will not be conducted feasibly through RCT study designs. There are some distinct advantages of non-RCT study designs, including cost, convenience and the fact that most non-RCT study subjects and treatment providers (particularly in retrospective study designs) are unaware that they are being studied and thus do not alter their behavior or refuse to participate because they are being evaluated.[18]

While advances have been made in statistical methods for detecting treatment selection bias and estimating unbiased treatment effects in non-RCT settings, these methods are complex and vulnerable to a variety of misspecification concerns.[18,19] Generally, they include propensity score methods, sample selection methods and instrumental variables. In particular, when analyzing treatment effects in non-RCT settings, the results are generally dependent on the choice or availability of observable statistical covariates, the assumed error distributions, model functional forms, sample sizes, selection bias correction method, treatment of missing values and untestable assumptions regarding (asymptotic) correlations between model stochastic error terms and observable variables. Since most of these statistical analysis specification issues can be resolved in a variety of plausible and mutually exclusive ways, depending on available data and choice of statistical methods, statistical analysis of non-RCT study data is much less likely to generate robust and objective results than statistical analysis of RCT study data.

Since most statistical analysis of HDM programs is likely to require methods that are more complex than those needed for RCT study evaluation, it is useful to provide an introductory review of many of the most commonly used statistical methods and study designs. Like any powerful tool, statistics should be used carefully and appropriately, and only by those possessing a full grasp of the methodological assumptions and limitations inherent in any statistical approach.

# References

1. Gawande A. The cost conundrum: what a Texas town can teach us about health care. The New Yorker Online. June 1, 2009. Available at: http://www.newyorker.com/reporting/2009/06/01/090601fa_fact_gawande. Accessed June 21, 2009.
2. Goldhill D. How American health care killed my father. The Atlantic Online. September 2009. Available at: http://www.theatlantic.com/magazine/archive/2009/09/how-american-health-care-killed-my-father/307617/6/. Accessed September 15, 2009.
3. Brownlee S. *Overtreated: Why Too Much Medicine Is Making Us Sicker and Poorer*. New York, NY: Bloomsbury; 2007: 237.
4. Tricoci P, Allen J, Kramer J, et al. Scientific evidence underlying the ACC/AHA clinical practice guidelines. *JAMA*. 2009;301(8):831-841.
5. Evans D. Hierarchy of evidence: a framework for ranking evidence: evaluating healthcare interventions. *J Clin Nurs*. 2003;12:77-84.
6. Patsopoulos N, Analatos A, Ioannidis J. Relative citation impact of various study designs in the health sciences. *JAMA*. 2005;293:2362-2366.
7. Ioannidis JPA. Why most published research findings are false. *PLoS Med*. 2005;2(8):e124.
8. Fitzner K, Fox K, Schmidt J, Roberts M, Rindress D, Hay J. Implementation and outcomes of commercial disease management programs in the United States: the disease management outcomes consolidation survey. *Dis Manag J*. 2005;8(4):253-264.
9. Esposito D, Brown R, Chen A, et al. Impacts of a disease management program for dually eligible beneficiaries. *Care Financ Rev*. 2008;30:27-45.
10. Martin DC, Berger ML, Anstatt DT, et al. A randomized controlled open trial of population-based disease and case management in a Medicare Plus Choice health maintenance organization. Prev Chronic Dis. [serial online] October 2004. Available at: http://www.cdc.gov/pcd/issues/2004/oct/04_0015.htm. Accessed June 21, 2009.
11. Brown R, Peikes D, Chen A, Ng J, Schore J, Soh C. *The Evaluation of the Medicare Coordinated Care Demonstration: Findings for the First Two Years*. Princeton, NJ: Mathematica Policy Research Inc.; 2007. Available at: http://www.mathematica-mpr.com/publications/PDFs/mccd-firsttwoyrs.pdf. Accessed January 14, 2009.
12. Chen A, Brown R, Esposito D, Schore J, Shapiro R. Report to Congress on the Evaluation of Medicare Disease Management Programs. February 14, 2008. Available at: http://www.mathematica-mpr.com. Accessed June 21, 2009.
13. Esposito D, Brown R, Chen A, Schore J, Shapiro R. Impacts of a disease management program for dually eligible beneficiaries. *HCFR*. 2008;30(1):27-45.
14. Peikes D, Chen A, Schore J, et al. Effects of care coordination on hospitalization, quality of care, and health care expenditures among Medicare beneficiaries: 15 randomized trials. *JAMA*. 2009;301(6):603-618.
15. Ayanian J. The elusive quest for quality and cost savings in the Medicare program. *JAMA*. 2009;301(6):668-670.
16. Luce BR, Kramer JM, Goodman SN, et al. Rethinking randomized clinical trials for comparative effectiveness research: the need for transformational change. *Ann Intern Med*. 2009;151:206-209.
17. Long Q, Little RJ, Lin X. Causal inference in hybrid intervention trials involving treatment choice. *J Am Stat Assoc*. 2008;103(482):474-484.
18. Hay J. Appropriate econometric methods for pharmacoeconometric studies of retrospective claims data: an introductory guide. *J Manag Care Pharm*. 2005;11(4):344-348.
19. Angrist JD, Pischke JS. *Mostly Harmless Econometrics: An Empiricist's Companion*. Princeton, NJ: University Press; 2009.

CHAPTER 28

# Primary Data Types and How They Are Analyzed Statistically: Demonstration Projects

Pedro Plans-Rubió, MD, PhD, MSc

A demonstration project is a prospective observational study conducted to assess the acceptability, effectiveness, and implementation of new curative or preventive interventions in a community setting. In a demonstration project, it is necessary to develop an evaluation plan that identifies the outcomes to be measured at the individual, organization, and community levels (Table 1). The objective of the evaluation plan is to ensure that structural, process, and outcome improvements can be identified. Outcomes that are often evaluated in a demonstration project include effectiveness, resource use, and cost parameters, as well as metrics of the structure and processes necessary to provide the health intervention.

Basic information is acquired using a specific minimum data elements (MDE) form. The data collected in the evaluation must be detailed enough to answer key questions concerning intervention benefits for the community, but not overly burdensome for the respondents or those implementing the intervention. Summary measures can be proposed to obtain a synthetic measure of effectiveness when the health intervention may have an effect on multiple related outcomes. A summary measure should be broad enough to allow for comparisons with similar interventions, but also specific enough to the intervention being evaluated that it will be relevant to the evaluation at hand.

If an outcome is considered relevant to the demonstration project, health care costs are estimated taking into account the activities and resources used, and the cost per individual is calculated dividing total costs by the number of individuals. The cost-effectiveness of the intervention is estimated by comparing costs and effects in a sample of individuals from the community.

Effectiveness is assessed by comparing outcomes in a sample of individuals of the community to outcomes in a convenience sample, serving as a comparison group, which could be obtained from a nondemonstration community. In the differences-in-differences approach, pre-intervention outcomes differences between the community and the nondemonstration comparison group are also taken into account to assess effectiveness. As individuals in the intervention and comparison groups might differ on observable covariates, outcomes must be adjusted for these covariates using multivariable techniques to estimate the effectiveness.

A demonstration project can be conducted to assess the impact of a curative or preventive intervention in a community before deciding on its implementation at the regional or national level. It can provide information to explain how and why the intended outcomes were or were not achieved. This information, in turn, can inform which changes may be necessary to improve outcomes. Generalizability presents one limitation of results obtained from a demonstration project as outcomes may reflect characteristics unique to a specific community or communities participating in a demonstration project. Consequently, the results cannot necessarily be assumed to generalize to other communities. Care must be taken to interpret the results cautiously when extending the demonstration project findings beyond the population(s) studied.

# 1. Examples of Demonstration Projects

Demonstration projects have been used to assess the potential benefits associated with large public health programs. The Well-Integrated Screening and Evaluation of Women Across the Nation (WISEWOMAN) disease management demonstration project was developed in the United States to assess the feasibility and outcomes associated with a public health intervention aimed at reducing the risk for cardiovascular disease among low-income, underinsured and uninsured women in 14 states through a combination of screening and lifestyle modification.[1] Screening included information on blood pressure, cholesterol concentration, and smoking status. Outcomes were measured in terms of changes in cardiovascular risk factor levels and change in the 10-year probability of coronary heart disease over the 12-month period following enrollment. The impact of the intervention was evaluated by comparing the prevalence of risk factors and coronary heart disease risk among WISEWOMAN participants with those reported in the CDC's Behavioral Risk Factor Surveillance System.[1] The WISEWOMAN intervention resulted in reduced blood pressure, reduction in cholesterol levels, a lower smoking rate, improved dietary habits and physical activity, and lower projected 10-year risk for coronary heart disease. Cost-effectiveness was estimated in 2 subpopulations (Massachusetts and North Carolina), resulting in a cost of $637 per 1 % decrease in the 10-year risk of coronary heart disease.[2]

A second example includes the Breast Cancer Detection Demonstration Project (BCDDP).[3] For this project, 280,000 women were screened between 1973 and 1981 with a combination of mammography and breast physical examination. The study was developed without a control group, making it difficult to estimate the reduction in mortality caused by screening. Nevertheless, a comparison with US national statistics from the Surveillance, Epidemiology and End-Result program (SEER) indicated that screening improved relative survival rates in women aged under and over 50 years. Specifically, among women with invasive breast cancer detected by screening before age 50, 5-year survival was 88% in BCDDP versus 76% observed in the SEER program. This implies a 50% reduction in mortality at 5 years for women in the screening program. For women with breast cancer detected by screening after age 50 years, 5-year survival was 89% in the BCDDP and 74 % in the SEER program, implying a 58% reduction in mortality at 5 years.

Part 1: Statistical Approaches and Methods

# References

1. Finkelstein EA, Wittenborn JS, Farris RP. Evaluation of public health demonstration programs: the effectiveness and cost-effectiveness of WISEWOMAN. *J Womens Health*. 2004;13:625-633.
2. Finkelstein EA, Troped PJ, Will JC, Plaombo R. Cost-effectiveness of cardiovascular disease risk reduction program aimed at financially vulnerable women: The Massachusetts WISEWOMAN projects. *J Womens Health Gend Based Med*. 2002;11:519-526.
3. Seidman H, Gelb SK, Silverberg E, LaVerda N, Lubera JA. Survival experience in the Breast Cancer Detection Demonstration Project. *Cancer*. 1987;367:258-290.

**TABLE 1.** Determinants of Outcomes and Outcomes Evaluated in Demonstration Projects

| Level | Determinants of Outcomes | | Outcomes | |
|---|---|---|---|---|
| | Characteristics/ Structure | Process | Short-Term | Long-Term |
| Individual | • Health status<br>• Medical history<br>• Sociodemographic characteristics | • Screening<br>• Medication<br>• Treatment<br>• Follow-up | • Health effects<br>• Awareness<br>• Lifestyle changes<br>• Change in health status<br>• Change in access to care<br>• Costs | • Health effects<br>• Morbidity<br>• Mortality<br>• Quality of life<br>• Costs |
| Organization | • Personnel<br>• Resources<br>• Planning and coordination<br>• Clinical guidelines<br>• Data management systems | • Activities developed<br>• Personnel involved<br>• Resources used<br>• Data management<br>• Recruitment<br>• Training | • Cost-effectiveness | |
| Community | • Community organizations and institutions | • Involvement of organizations and institutions | • Community health<br>• Efficiency and equity in the distribution of health resources and health gains | |

CHAPTER 29

# Primary Data Types and How They Are Analyzed Statistically: Randomized Controlled Trials (RCTs)

Ashish Parekh, MS

Randomized controlled trials (RCT) are one of the simplest, most powerful, and revolutionary research tools. The RCT is a study in which people are allocated at random to one of several interventions or a control group.[1] According to Lachin and colleagues, RCTs are the most reliable forms of scientific evidence in health care because they demonstrate causality and eliminate treatment selection bias.[2] The study population in RCTs are called *participants* or *subjects*. Those who design and carry out the study and analyze the results are the *investigators*. The interventions provided to participants are sometimes referred as *clinical maneuvers*. In most cases, RCTs seek to measure and compare different outcome events that are present or absent in participants who receive the intervention compared to participants who receive the control or placebo.

RCTs are used to compare 2 or more interventions and are also referred to as *comparative studies*, though it is of note that not all comparative studies are RCTs. Usually one of the interventions is regarded as a standard of care for comparison, and the group of participants that receives it is referred to as the control group. Thus, the nomenclature *randomized controlled trial*. Furthermore, RCTs are known as experiments because investigators design the study and define the number of subjects, type of intervention and the regimen (amount, route and frequency). In summary, RCTs can be viewed as quantitative comparative controlled experiments in which a group of investigators studies 2 or more interventions in a set of individuals that is randomly allocated to receive either an intervention or standard comparator.[1]

RCTs are the most rigorous ways of determining whether or not a cause-effect relationship exists between treatment and outcome. There are several key features of a RCT:[3]

- Random allocation to intervention groups

- Patients, providers, and investigators are unaware of which treatment was given (*blinded*) until the study is completed—although such double-blind studies are not always feasible or appropriate

Part 5: Statistical Approaches and Methods

- Subjects and providers in RCTs know they are being watched, so they do not behave like they do when they are not being watched (also known as the Hawthorne effect)

- All intervention groups are treated identically with the exception of only the experimental treatment

- Patients are typically analyzed within the group to which they were allocated, irrespective of whether or not they experienced the intended intervention (intention to treat analysis)

- Analysis is focused on estimating the size of the difference in predefined outcomes between intervention groups

## 1. Random Allocation

Random allocation means that participants are assigned to one of the study groups by chance. The decision as to which group they will be in is not determined or influenced by the investigators, clinicians or study participants. By allocating participants randomly, the characteristics of the participants are expected to be similar, or balanced, across groups at the start of the comparison (baseline).[1] By keeping the groups balanced at baseline the investigators will be better able to isolate and quantify the impact of the interventions being studied while minimizing effects from other factors that could influence the outcomes (confounding factors).[1]

Randomization can be achieved in many ways. There are 2 rules that investigators must follow—first, they must define the rules that govern allocation in advance, and second, they must adhere to those rules throughout the whole study. One of the simplest methods of randomization is known as *flipping a coin* or *rolling a die*. This technique is rarely used because it does not leave an audit trail. Investigators sometimes use random number tables to generate sequences of numbers to determine random assignment to one group or another. The use of a random number table forces investigators to decide the correspondence between the numbers and the groups.[1] Two other types of randomization techniques are *restricted* randomization and *stratified* randomization.

Restricted randomization is used to ensure the numbers of participants in all study groups are as equal as possible. It is achieved by creating blocks of sequences that will ensure that the same number of participants will be allocated to the study groups within each block. Stratified randomization is used to keep the characteristics of the participants as similar as possible across each study group. In order to do this, the investigators must first identify factors (strata) that are known to be related to the outcome of the study. Once these factors are identified, the next step is to produce a separate block randomization scheme for each factor to ensure that the groups are balanced within each stratum.[1]

## 2. Sample Inclusion and Exclusion

Inclusion and exclusion criteria are defined as the medical or social standards determining whether a person may or may not be allowed to enter a clinical trial. These criteria are based on such factors as age, gender, the type and stage of a disease, previous treatment history, and other medical conditions. It is important to note that inclusion and exclusion criteria are not used to reject people personally, but rather to identify appropriate participants and keep them safe.[4]

When designing a clinical research study, it is important for the investigator first to decide which types of participants are appropriate to participate in the study and who should be excluded. Diligent adherence to those inclusion/exclusion criteria is needed, lest the study be weakened. The researchers must therefore find a balance between identifying the most appropriate participants to test a new therapy and casting a wide enough net to ensure that they will have enough participants to power the analyses sufficiently.[5]

Inclusion or exclusion criteria might be such factors as the age of the participants—many studies will only include people over 18 years old, for example—the date of diagnosis of the illness, other therapies, and other illnesses that might be present in the participant. Other criteria might be the stage of the illness—studies often exclude patients with very advanced illnesses—how active the participants are in their day-to-day routines, and the ability to take oral medications. It is important to explain the inclusion and exclusion criteria to all potential participants before they are enrolled in a study.[5]

## 3. Types of Trials

Randomized controlled trials are the gold standard for determining the effects of a health care intervention in a group of patients.[1] The broad aim of the clinical research investigation is to show that the treatments concerned are safe and efficacious to the extent that the risk-benefit ratio between the active and control treatments is favorable and acceptable.[6] There are several different types of trials that can take place during an RCT—open blind, single blind, double blind, and triple blind.

In an open-blind trial, both the clinician and patient know the intervention given. In these types of trials, the perceptions about the advantages of one treatment over another can influence assessments of outcomes. These are appropriate in instances when, for example, the intervention itself does not permit blinding (for example, pharmacotherapy versus surgical intervention) or when the advantages of an open-blind trial outweigh concerns regarding the influence of knowing the intervention. In a single-blind trial the patient is unaware of the allocated treatment, so potential bias in reporting of symptoms or events is minimized.

In a double-blind trial, neither the clinician nor patient knows which treatment is given. This type of trial has the advantage of controlling both the reporting and assessment bias.[6] Double blinding ensures that any preconceived views held by subjects and clinicians cannot systematically bias the assessment of outcomes. Intention to treat analysis maintains the advantages of random allocation, which may be lost if subjects are excluded from analysis through withdrawal or failure to comply.[3] Triple-blind trials are double-blind trials in which the statistician interpreting the results also does not know which intervention has been given.[7]

## 4. Limitations of Randomized Controlled Trials

RCTs are powerful tools that can be limited by both ethical and practical concerns. Exposing patients to an intervention believed to be inferior to current treatment is viewed as unethical. In other circumstances an RCT may be ethical but infeasible, because of difficulties with randomization or recruitment for example. During a trial, once an intervention becomes widespread, it would be difficult to recruit clinicians who are willing to experiment with alternatives. A third limiting factor is that RCTs can be more costly and time-consuming than other types of studies. Careful consideration must be taken when discussing their use and timing. Such examples include:

- Is the intervention developed well enough to permit evaluation?

- Is there preliminary evidence that the intervention is likely to be beneficial including some appreciation of the size of the likely treatment effect?

Given the constraints of RCTs, they still remain an ideal by which all new health care interventions for health and disease management should be evaluated using the RCT design.

## References

1. Jadad A, Enkin MW. *Randomized Controlled Trials*. Malden, MA: Blackwell BMJ Books Publishing; 2007.
2. Lachin JM, Matts JP, Wei LJ. Randomization in clinical trials: conclusions and recommendations. *Control Clin Trials*. 1998;9:365-374.
3. Sibbald B, Roland M. Understanding controlled trials: why are randomized controlled trials important? *BMJ*. 1998;(316):201.
4. U.S. National Institutes of Health, Department of Health and Human Services. Glossary of clinical terms. Available at: http://clinicaltrials.gov/ct2/info/glossary. Accessed September 13, 2008.
5. Hudson, C, Rutigliano R. Emerging Med. About clinical trials. Available at: http://www.emergingmed.com/pub_aboutclinicaltrials.asp. Accessed September 13, 2008.
6. Chan YH. Randomized controlled trials (RCTs): essentials. *Singapore Med J*. 2003;44(2): 60-63.
7. Day SJ, Altman DG. Blinding in clinical trials and other studies. *BMJ*. 2000;(321):504.

CHAPTER 30

# Primary Data Types and How They Are Analyzed Statistically: Natural Experiments

Hans Petersen, MS

The essence of the natural experiment is encapsulated by the familiar aphorism "serendipity favors the prepared mind." A natural experiment represents a serendipitous alternative to a controlled experiment. Circumstances suggesting a natural experiment represent an opportunity to study phenomena that might otherwise never be considered for a controlled experiment, either for practical or ethical reasons. Sometimes called a quasi-experiment, these experiments involve observation and analysis of data resulting from naturally occurring phenomena over which the observer has no control, yet these data exist in a form mimicking traditional experimental methods. Natural experiments create conditions in which some participants are forced or encouraged to receive a treatment or intervention they may not have selected but for the external (natural) shift in their environment. For example, the impact of the 2006 Massachusetts Health Care Reform Act on choice of treatment provider by the uninsured may be viewed as a natural experiment. Passage of the act was implemented irrespective of how the uninsured selected their treatment providers before or after the legislation went into effect.

Certain natural or manmade disasters also offer opportunities for natural experiments.[1] If one wished to study, for example, the psychological and/or health effects of real versus perceived exposure to the harmful effects of a nuclear accident, a study of the population in the vicinity of an actual nuclear accident could be carried out in much the same way as if the accident had been part of some deliberate, heinous experiment. If true exposure to radioactive fallout could be measured accurately, using careful sample selection criteria one could obtain readings from Geiger counters and administer the appropriate questionnaires to carry out this quasi-experiment.

Natural experiments are exogenous events that force treatment selection, such as that implicit to a randomized controlled trial and, therefore, potentially allow more accurate estimation of the unbiased treatment effects given that there is no treatment selection bias. In this sense, natural experiments are perfect instrumental variables (refer to Chapter 41 on Instrumental Variables Methods.)

Developers of Health and Disease Management programs (HDM) will sometimes be presented with opportunities to perform natural experiments based on occurrences within their health systems if the effects can be measured in the resulting claims data. In fact, retrospective natural experiments often can be performed using health care claims data coupled with additional knowledge of specific occurrences within the health system. This will hold true since, presumably, the data were collected both prior to, during and after the occurrence of interest. It is the researcher's task to take notice of the opportunity, formulate the hypothesis, and organize the existing data in a way that will permit investigation of the question of interest using methods that mimic as closely as possible the rigors of a controlled experiment.

Notwithstanding their fortuitous nature, natural experiments are still subject to limitations. In particular, because the experimental control the researcher is able to exert over the system being studied is necessarily limited to the organization and analysis of preexisting data, there is a possibility that unobserved or uncontrolled factor(s) will influence the outcomes. Variables influenced can be the dependent variable (the outcome), the exposure (perhaps a drug or the propensity for its use in treatment) or both (ie, a true confounder; see the Chapter 37 on Confounders). Hence, without taking extra care to control for potential bias and confounding in the data analysis, the results of a natural experiment have the same potential to be erroneous or misleading as those from any other observational study.

Sometimes, a natural experiment can arise from a policy change like one that was performed in the Military Health System (MHS).[2] The study examined the effects on drug utilization and expenditures using pharmacy claims data from male military service members 45 years of age and older and their families (N = 266,380). The data were extracted for a period representing 28 months surrounding the military's decision to restrict a leading uroselective alpha-blocker to third tier (nonformulary). Segmented regression models were used to estimate the effects of the new policy within the MHS with respect to drug utilization and expenditures. Not surprisingly, it was determined that the decision led to rapid migration from the newly designated third-tier drug to less expensive alternative medications.

Natural experiments represent an opportunity to employ existing claims data within an HDM program. Advantages of this method are myriad if one is fortunate enough to identify the ideal conditions in a claims database for the conduct of a natural experiment to test a specific hypothesis of interest. One of the greatest limitations in the use of any data from claims, naturalistic study or other nonrandomized source is that one can only "know what is known" through the data. This leaves investigators unaware of what data they might be missing (for example, confounders, patient characteristics, or other mediating variables) by virtue of the means by which the data are collected.

Furthermore, natural experiments do not often lend themselves to longitudinal follow-up as patients may change plans or be lost to follow-up for other administrative reasons. For example, in the case of administrative databases, patients have little incentive to maintain participation in a study beyond its intrinsic personal value. A nontrivial, practical caveat is that though many such serendipitous situations almost certainly exist in claims data, one must have the focused resources and be observant and lucky to recognize and exploit them in a timely manner. Thus, as the assessment of HDM becomes increasingly important, researchers will need to identify the proper circumstances in which to implement natural experiments and carry out analyses appropriate to the data to control adequately for potential confounding.

## References

1. Gallacher J, Bronstering K, Palmer S, et al. Symptomatology attributable to psychological exposure to a chemical incident: a natural experiment. *J Epidemiol*. 2007;61:506-512.
2. Devine JW, Conrad RC, Tiller KW. The effect of three-tier formulary adoption for alpha-blockers on drug utilization in the department of defense. *Value Health*. 2008;11:A23-A23.

CHAPTER 31

# Primary Data Types and How They Are Analyzed Statistically: Prospective Designs

Pedro Plans-Rubió, MD, PhD, MSc

A prospective study is a comparative and quantitative study in which a cohort of individuals is followed over time with the objective to assess the association between one or more independent variables and one or more dependent variables, such as a risk factor and a disease. Prospective studies are also called cohort or longitudinal studies. The term cohort is used to describe a group of individuals with defined similarities (for example, born during a particular year, receiving a specific treatment, exposed to a risk factor, or living in a particular place).

## 1. Design of a Prospective Study

In a prospective study, a cohort of individuals is divided into 2 or more groups based on the presence of an individual characteristic. For instance, individuals without coronary heart disease may be divided into those with and without hypercholesterolemia. Individuals are then followed for a period of time after which the presence of the disease or other outcome is determined in both groups. The prospective design is used for both observational and experimental studies (clinical trials).

In the Framingham Heart Study, a cohort of persons born in Framingham, Massachusetts, was followed for 50 years to assess the relationship between individual characteristics and the incidence of coronary heart disease and related mortality.[1] This assessment was conducted by dividing the cohort of individuals without cardiovascular disease into risk strata according to the presence of cardiovascular risk factors such as hypercholesterolemia and hypertension, and comparing the incidence of coronary heart disease and related mortality in individuals with and without the risk factors. This chapter is dedicated to the former, observational studies. In these studies, the progression of individuals over time is observed to identify the cause-and-effect relationship between treatments and outcomes; however subjects are not assigned at random to the treatment.[2]

## 2. Results in a Prospective Cohort Study

The analysis for a prospective study is conducted by comparing the frequency of development of the disease in individuals with and without the risk factor, or other individual characteristics under study. A cohort study can estimate the incidence in the population (i), exposed ($i_1$) and unexposed ($i_2$) individuals, the relative risk (RR), and the attributable risk (AR) that the outcome is associated with the risk factor. If the cohort of exposed (a+b) and unexposed (c+d) individuals is divided into those with the disease (a,c) and those without the disease (b,d), the relative risk of developing the disease over the observed period is obtained by dividing incidence in exposed and unexposed individuals (Table 1):

$RR = i_1/i_2 = [a/(a+b)]/[c/(c+d)]$.

The RR measures the strength of association between a risk factor and disease. A value of 1 indicates no difference between the risk groups. The excess risk is obtained from the difference between incidence rates in exposed and unexposed individuals: $(i_1-i_2)$. The attributable risk (AR) of the population, showing the proportion of the population risk that can be attributed or associated with the risk factor, is obtained from:

$AR = (i_1-i_2)/i_1$.

## 3. Differences between Cohort and Case-Control Studies

The primary difference between cohort and case-control studies is that case-control studies, a type of retrospective study, begin with the identification of a group of individuals with a diagnosis or condition (cases), and a second group of similar individuals without the disease or condition (controls).[3] Prospective studies provide stronger evidence of causality than retrospective studies (Figure 1). Case-control studies do not estimate incidence or relative risk, rather, they can estimate the likelihood of an association, or the odds ratio (Table 1):

OR=(ad)/(bc).

The odds ratio is considered an accurate, or equivalent, estimate of the RR when the incidence of disease is low, given that

$(a+b) \approx b$ and $(c+d) \approx d$.

In case-control studies, recall bias is possible since individuals with the disease may be more likely to recall the exposure to the risk factor under study than individuals without the disease.[3] The longitudinal observation of an individual over time, and the collection of data at regular intervals, can reduce recall bias in cohort studies.

In a cohort study, it is not possible to ensure that individuals receiving a treatment are similar on all covariates to those not receiving treatment, since individuals included in the study are not randomly assigned to the treatment. Potential bias can be reduced, however, through different methods, including matching, stratification and analytical adjustments. Matching may take place before outcomes are measured, whereas stratification by covariates and analytical adjustments are developed after outcomes have been collected.[2]

## 4. Pros and Cons of Cohort Studies

Prospective studies can provide stronger evidence of causality than case-control studies, and weaker evidence of causality than randomized controlled trials. Cohort studies can be conducted when it is not practical or ethical to perform a RCT to answer a research question, whereas case-control studies are more adequate than cohort studies for diseases with low incidence or those that require extremely long follow-up. Recall bias is typically lower in prospective cohort studies than in case-control studies, while cohort studies are more costly and take a longer time to generate useful data than case-control studies. RCTs, in the hierarchy of evidence, are superior to cohort studies because randomization limits the potential for bias. For this reason, RCT clinical research studies are more adequate than cohort studies to assess the efficacy and effectiveness of new drugs.

## 5. Examples of Prospective Cohort Studies

Cohort studies can be developed to assess beneficial and adverse effects of established drugs. Hippisley-Cox et al[4] assessed the beneficial and adverse effects of statins by developing a prospective cohort study in which a cohort was followed of 2 million primary health care patients aged 34-84 years in England and Wales. The group of new users of statins (exposed) was formed by 225,922 (10.7 %) patients. The study started in January 2002 and ended 6 years later in December 2008. Crude rates per 10,000 patients were determined in new users and nonusers, and the RR comparing both rates were calculated. Statins were, however, found to be associated with an increased risk for moderate or serious liver dysfunction, acute renal failure, moderate to serious myopathy, and cataracts. Table 2 presents adjusted RR for simvastatin.

Cohort studies can also be conducted to estimate the effectiveness of vaccine on a population. Ortqvist and colleagues[5] evaluated the effectiveness of influenza vaccination to reduce mortality in persons aged 65 years or older in Sweden. To examine this, a prospective cohort study was developed in which the RR of mortality was determined by comparing mortality rates in vaccinated and unvaccinated individuals who were followed during 3 influenza seasons.

The population followed was formed by the 260,000 residents of 65 or more years who resided in Stockholm County. The treatment evaluated was the trivalent split-virion influenza vaccine. The cohort of individuals vaccinated was determined from vaccination records. By linking this information to the population register corresponding to Stockholm County, each resident aged 65 or more years could be classified as exposed or unexposed to the influenza vaccine each year. The study showed that influenza vaccination was associated with a crude effectiveness in terms of reduction in all-cause mortality of 50%, 46% and 40%, during the 3 influenza seasons, respectively (Table 3). The vaccine effectiveness adjusted for demographic variables and comorbid conditions using Cox's proportional hazards regression was 14%, 19% and 1%, respectively.

## 6. Conclusion

Prospective study designs, specifically observational studies, provide a suitable alternative to the more restrictive randomized controlled trial design under specific conditions such as comparisons in which it is unethical to randomize patients. Observational studies also present the opportunity to complement data collected in randomized controlled trials to supplement and further the knowledge base obtained through this more restrictive design.

**TABLE 1.** Relative Risk (RR) and Odds Ratio (OR)

|  |  | Disease | | |
|---|---|---|---|---|
|  |  | Yes | No |  |
| Risk Factor | Present | a | b | a+b |
|  | Absent | c | d | c+d |
|  |  | a+c | b+d | a+b+c+d |

RR=a/(a+b)c/(c+d)    OR= adbc

**TABLE 2.** Relative Risk of Disease in Men and Women Treated with Simvastatin[2]

| Disease | Adjusted Relative Risk[3] (95 %CI) | |
|---|---|---|
|  | Women | Men |
| Rheumatoid arthritis | 0.96 (0.84-1.09) | 1.12 (0.96-1.32) |
| Parkinson's disease | 0.84 (0.71-1.00) | 0.84 (0.71-1.00) |
| Venous thromboembolism | 0.91 (0.83-0.99) | 0.88 (0.80-0.97) |
| Gastric cancer | 0.79 (0.55-1.13) | 0.83 (0.65-1.04) |
| Colon cancer | 0.89 (0.76-1.05) | 1.02 (0.90-1.17) |
| Renal cancer | 1.07 (0.86-1.32) | 1.10 (0.97-1.26) |
| Lung cancer | 1.10 (0.96-1.25) | 1.11 (1.01-1.23) |
| Melanoma | 1.02 (0.79-1.32) | 1.11 (0.88-1.40) |
| Prostate cancer | – | 1.05 (0.98-1.13) |
| Breast cancer | 1.09 (1.00-1.18) | – |
| Esophageal cancer | 0.69 (0.50-0.94) | 0.82 (0.68-0.99) |
| Moderate myopathy | 3.03 (2.35-3.91) | 6.14 (5.09-7.40) |
| Acute renal failure | 1.50 (1.23-1.83) | 1.61 (1.37-1.90) |
| Cataract | 1.20 (1.25-1.36) | 1.31 (1.25-1.38) |
| Liver dysfunction | 1.52 (1.38-1.66) | 1.54 (1.41-1.60) |

CI: confidence interval
[a] Relative risk adjusted for individual characteristics

Part 5: Statistical Approaches and Methods

**TABLE 3.** Effectiveness of influenza vaccination to reduce mortality

|  | Disease | | |
| --- | --- | --- | --- |
|  | 1998/1999 | 1999/2000 | 2000/2001 |
| No. of excess deaths in unvaccinated | 547 | 1019 | 206 |
| Crude vaccine effectiveness (%) | 50 | 46 | 42 |
| Adjusted vaccine effectiveness (%)[a] | 14 | 19 | 1 |
| 95% CI of effectiveness (%) | 5-23 | 11-27 | 0-11 |

[a] Vaccine effectiveness adjusted for population characteristics

# References

1. Dawber TR. *The Framingham Study: The Epidemiology of Atherosclerotic Disease*. Cambridge, MA: Harvard University Press; 1980.
2. Rosenbaum PR. *Observational Studies*. New York, NY: Springer; 2002.
3. Schlesselman JJ. *Case-Control Studies*. New York, NY: Oxford University Press; 1982.
4. Hippisley-Cox J, Coupland C. Unintended effects of statins in men and women in England and Wales: population based cohort study using the QResearch database. *BMJ*. 2010;340;c2197. Available at: http://www.bmj.com/content/340/bmj.c2197.pdf%2Bhtml.
5. Ortqvist A, Granath F, Askling J, Hedlund J. Influenza vaccination and mortality: prospective cohort study of the elderly in a large geographical area. *Eur Respir J*. 2007;30:414-422.

CHAPTER 32

# Primary Data Types and How They Are Analyzed Statistically: Retrospective Designs

Ashish Parekh, MS

A retrospective study is one in which the data, typically as medical or administrative records, have already been collected and are used to answer a research question about an outcome that has already occurred. Retrospective study design enables an investigator to examine hypotheses about possible associations between management strategies or risk factors and outcomes.[1] The advantage of a retrospective study design is that it provides a relatively inexpensive way to access data efficiently, as the information is readily available. In comparison, prospective studies require more time, effort, and resources to collect enough observations and outcomes to power statistical analyses. For some studies of medical conditions such as cardiovascular disease and diabetes, many years of data collection are required to achieve the statistical power needed to address study research questions.

## 1. Prospective versus Retrospective Studies

In a prospective study, the condition or risk factors of the patients are determined at baseline, the intervention(s) applied, and the outcome is measured after the period of time specified by the study design. In contrast, the intervention, initial (baseline) condition(s), and outcome(s) are obtained using existing information in a retrospective study.[2] Eligible subjects are identified to define a cohort for study and the subsequent occurrence of events, disease progression, or death is evaluated over the historical observation period.[3]

An example of a prospective study is one conducted by Mutsert and colleagues to investigate the association between nutritional status as measured by the subjective global assessment (SGA) scale and mortality in patients requiring chronic dialysis.[4] Patients with end-stage renal disease, aged 18 years and older, who were starting with their first renal replacement therapy were eligible for inclusion in the Netherlands Cooperative Study on the Adequacy of Dialysis-2 (NECOSAD-II) Study. The long-term and time-dependent relationship between SGA and mortality was calculated at 3 and 6 months after dialysis initiation and subsequently every 6 months over 7 years. Using Cox regression analysis, the researchers calculated hazard ratios for the baseline and time-dependent SGA measurements, adjusting for age, sex, treatment modality, primary kidney disease, and comorbidity. Severe protein energy wasting at baseline was associated with a twofold increase in mortality over 7 years in patients with end-stage renal disease.[4] This provides a typical example of a prospective cohort study in which exposure is assessed at baseline and outcomes are assessed over time to evaluate the relationship of baseline characteristics with the disease progression or mortality.[3]

To determine the association of plasma phosphate with renal function loss and mortality in predialysis patients diagnosed with chronic kidney disease (CKD) in stages IV–V, Voormolen and colleagues employed a retrospective study design using data extraction from medical records.[5] They identified patients diagnosed with CKD stage IV–V at 1 of 8 hospital outpatient clinics during the period 1999-2001 at the point when a referral to predialysis care was made. The clinical course of patients was followed using medical charts until patients required dialysis, time of death, or January 2003—whichever was earliest. The study found that renal function declined faster with higher phosphate levels at baseline and that high plasma phosphate is an independent risk factor for a more rapid decline in renal function and a higher risk of mortality during the predialysis phase. Conclusions drawn from this retrospective study indicate that plasma phosphate within the normal range is likely of vital importance in achieving the best outcomes among predialysis patients.[5]

The major strength of a prospective cohort study is the ability to control key aspects of data collection thereby increasing confidence in the interrelationships between intervention exposure, confounders, and end points; however, this is realized at a cost, because this design is both expensive and more time-consuming because of a usually long follow-up period.[3] On the other hand, the retrospective design can be time efficient at answering new questions using existing data. Researchers and analysts are limited, however, by working with data that have already been captured, often for another purpose than the one under investigation.[3]

**Figure 1.** Prospective versus retrospective study design. In a prospective study, the baseline state of the subjects is determined, the controlled intervention is applied, and then the outcome is measured. In a retrospective study, the intervention, baseline state, and outcome are obtained from existing information that was recorded for reasons other than the study.

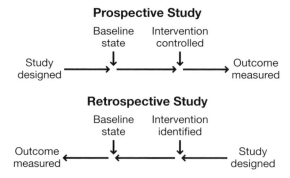

*Source:* Hess DR, Retrospective studies and chart reviews. *Respiratory Care.* 2004;49:1171-1174.

The design elements of retrospective and prospective studies are very similar as described by Hess.[6] These 10 steps outline the process from writing the study question, developing a hypothesis, and searching the literature to analyzing data, explaining the results and preparing a written report.

**TABLE 1.** Important Elements in a Retrospective Study Design*

1. Write the study question
2. Develop the hypothesis
3. Search the literature
4. Consider the statistical issues, such as sample size and how the results will be analyzed
5. Write the protocol: where the data will be found, what data will be needed, how data will be collected, how data will be analyzed
6. Obtain permission: institutional review board (patient?), data source (eg, medical records department)
7. Collect the data
8. Analyze the data
9. Explain the results
10. Write the report

\* Note that these are by and large the same as the elements of a prospective study design.
*Source:* 2. Hess DR

Most investigators view retrospective studies as "quick and dirty" because the data are quickly gleaned from existing records to answer a question.[6] When a prospective design is a viable option, then retrospective designs are discouraged. However, there are times when retrospective studies are beneficial and preferred such as with a pilot study to inform study design of a prospective study.[6] This approach allows investigators to focus the study question efficiently, clarify the hypothesis, determine an appropriate sample size, and identify feasibility issues for a prospective study.[6]

## 2. Retrospective Data Sources

Various sources of retrospective data are available and may be used alone or in combination with data from other sources depending on the requirements of the study. These sources include administrative databases, medical records, and interviews with individuals known to have exposure to an intervention, to possess a risk factor, and/or have been diagnosed with the condition being investigated. Researchers may conduct retrospective studies to study a rare outcome for which a prospective study is not feasible or to estimate efficiently the potential effect of an exposure on an outcome.[2] It is of note that retrospective study design precludes one from drawing causal inferences and conclusions from the results of the analyses. Examining a rare condition using retrospective study design can be much more efficient than using a prospective study approach because individuals who suffer from the condition can be identified through medical records or a database using knowledge from published literature to guide this process. In contrast, a prospective study requires sampling a large number of subjects to find the few cases of a rare condition.

## 3. Various Types of Retrospective Studies

Case reports, case series, case-control and cohort studies are general types of retrospective methods. A case report is a report of one unusual and/or instructive case (for example, symptoms not previously observed with a given medical condition, or an unexpected or new combination of medical conditions in one case).[6] A case series is a report of multiple similar unusual or instructive cases. Retrospective case series can be used to study a disease that occurs infrequently, or to generate a hypothesis that can be tested more rigorously in a prospective study.[6] An investigator can quickly estimate the effect of an exposure on outcomes by using a retrospective case-control study. Cases and controls are established based on the presence of the condition, and exposure is assessed by looking back over time. In this study, the case and control should be similar on all factors except the outcome of interest.[2]

If an investigator wishes to describe a population over time or obtain preliminary measures of association to develop future studies and interventions, a retrospective cohort study is the best option. By using administrative datasets, patient charts and conducting interviews, the researcher is able to identify the exposure and outcome information retrospectively.[2] Cohort studies are the best way to identify incidence and natural history of a disease. They are typically used to examine multiple outcomes after a single exposure.[7] Cohort studies should provide specific definitions of exposures and outcomes—it is important that these should be as objective as possible. The control group (unexposed) should be similar to the exposed in all important respects, with the exception of not having the exposure.[7] Retrospective cohort studies are also known as historic cohort studies, as indicated by the US National Cancer Institute. They define a historic cohort study as a research study in which the medical records of groups of individuals who are alike in many ways but differ by a certain characteristic (for example, female nurses who smoke and those who do not smoke) are compared for a particular outcome (such as lung cancer).[8]

## References

1. Shi L, Wu E, Hodges M, Yu A, Birnbaum H. Retrospective economic and outcomes analyses using non-US databases – a review. *Pharmacoeconomics*. 2007;25(7):563-576.
2. The National EMSC Data Analysis Resource Center. Retrospective Study. Available at: http://www.nedarc.org/nedarc/collectingData/chooseProjectDesign/retrospectiveStudy.html. Accessed March 27, 2009.
3. Euser AM, Zoccali C, Jager KJ, Dekker FW. Cohort studies: prospective versus retrospective. *Nephron Clin Pract*. 2009;113:c214-c217.
4. de Mutsert R, Grootendorst DC, Boeschoten EW, et al. Subjective global assessment of nutritional status is strongly associated with mortality in chronic dialysis patients. *Am J Clin Nutr*. 2009;89:787-793.
5. Voormolen N, Noordzij M, Grootendorst DC, et al. High plasma phosphate as a risk factor for decline in renal function and mortality in pre-dialysis patients. *Nephrol Dial Transplant*. 2007;22:2909-2916.
6. Hess DR. Retrospective studies and chart reviews. *Respir Care*. 2004;49(10):1171-1174.
7. Grimes DA, Schulz KF. Cohort studies: marching towards outcomes. *Lancet*. 2002;359:341-345.
8. US National Cancer Institute. NCI Dictionary of Cancer Terms. Available at: http://www.cancer.gov/dictionary?cdrid=286525. Accessed June 23, 2010.

CHAPTER 33

# Statistical Methods for Randomized Controlled Trials: Hypothesis Testing

Pedro Plans-Rubió, MD, PhD, MSc; and
Nalin Payakachat, BPharm, MSc, PhD

The principal theory (that is, hypothesis) tested in a research study is called the *null hypothesis*. Researchers state a hypothesis, or guess, about the outcome of the study at the beginning of the research process; typically after identifying the primary research question(s). The hypothesis presents the researcher's expectation of the outcomes of the study.[1,2] Hypotheses help researchers plan the design of their study and provide a framework for data analysis. A well-framed hypothesis will describe an expected relationship between the independent and dependent variables of a population, but often expresses it in terms of there being no relationship (null hypothesis) between the dependent and independent variables.

Hypothesis testing is a method for informing decisions using statistical criteria. It is used to answer questions such as: Is treatment A more effective than treatment B? Is the rate of survival related to one treatment rather than another? Is there a smooth dose-effect relationship for a specific treatment? The objective of hypothesis testing is to help draw conclusions about population parameters, comparison of means and proportions and the relationship between variables.

## 1. Context

In biomedical and related research, it is necessary to decide whether or not the empirical data are consistent with a prespecified null hypothesis. The null hypothesis is derived from one's prior understanding of the underlying mechanisms at play and is typically phrased in terms of no difference in effect between one or more treatments or interventions. For example, one might consider whether or not implementation of a nurse education health and disease management (HDM) program improves adherence to statin medication. In planning a prospective study (for example, a randomized controlled trial) to examine the impact of this program, the null hypothesis would be stated as "patients who receive the nurse education program have no difference in treatment adherence relative to control patients who do not receive the program." This sets up the condition to evaluate whether the observed differences in treatment adherence at the end of the trial are different enough to be attributed to the intervention rather than chance or random events.

## 2. Procedures for Hypothesis Testing

Hypothesis testing is done by asking and answering the null hypothesis. Every statistical measure is designed to test the null hypothesis, identified as H0, against one or more alternative hypotheses, H1...n. The goal of hypothesis testing is to reject or disprove the null hypothesis through statistical analysis of the data. When considering the therapeutic effect associated with a given intervention, the null hypothesis is that it is no better than the comparator, in other words, that the intervention has no additional therapeutic effect.

Traditionally, interventions have been compared to no intervention or placebo, testing the hypothesis that the new intervention has no effect. The alternative hypothesis is that the intervention has a therapeutic effect that can be either positive or negative relative to the comparator. A one-sided alternative hypothesis is that the drug can only have a positive effect, or only have a negative effect.

The approach is the same for testing most hypotheses:

1. Formulate the null hypothesis and the alternative hypothesis.

2. Chose the appropriate test statistic(s) to evaluate the null hypothesis.

3. Define the Type I error, alpha ($\alpha$), significance level for statistical testing. This is the probability of concluding there is a significant treatment effect by rejecting the null hypothesis when, in fact, there is no difference between the groups. The significance level ($\alpha$) must be prespecified; in many studies this p-value<0.05.

4. Collect data and calculate the test statistic for the sample.

5. Calculate the probability that the difference between the groups is at least as great as the one observed assuming the null hypothesis is true.

6. Determine whether or not the null hypothesis can be rejected. If the observed p-value is less than $\alpha$, the null hypothesis is rejected. If the observed p-value is greater than $\alpha$, the null hypothesis cannot be rejected.

## 3. Statistical Significance

Hypothesis testing results in a single decision: reject or do not reject the null hypothesis.[1] The null hypothesis is rejected when observed differences between the intervention groups meet the criteria described above indicating they are unlikely to have been produced by chance. In this situation, the difference is statistically significant and the estimated treatment effect is considered to be a statistically significant effect. Statistical significance is determined by the Type I error rate defined when designing a study to reject the null hypothesis. The null hypothesis cannot be rejected when observed differences are likely to be produced by chance. In this situation, differences are defined as not significant.

It is important to differentiate statistical significance from clinical significance and to recognize that the 2 are not one and the same, and indeed, may have different implications. The results of our previously described nurse education program may indicate that patients improve adherence to statin therapy by 1%, which is a statistically significant result (that is, not due to chance events). However, clinicians may not believe that a 1% improvement in adherence to statin therapy is sufficient to impact a patient's health meaningfully. Conversely, outcomes from the nurse education intervention may produce an estimated mean improvement in adherence of 50% relative to usual care, which clinicians may consider clinically important for achieving better health outcomes. However, such a result may not be statistically significant (usually because of small sample size) leading to the conclusion that the observed difference is due to chance and not statistically significant.

## 4. Statistical Error and Assumptions

A test statistic separates significant effects from random chance. Nevertheless, all hypothesis tests have risks of making the wrong conclusion (Table 1). The Type I ($\alpha$) error is the chance of concluding that a significant effect is present when in fact it is not. Conversely, the Type II error, or beta ($\beta$), is the likelihood of not detecting a significant effect when one exists. To perform a statistical test for any hypothesis, it is necessary to make assumptions about the data. Some tests require more strict assumptions than others to render the results valid. For example, with the t-test to compare means, it is necessary that the observations are drawn from independent and identically distributed random samples from a normal distribution with equal variance. To ensure appropriate use of a test statistic, analysis of the distributional assumptions should be incorporated as part of the hypothesis testing procedure.

## 5. Confidence Intervals

In analyzing the data, researchers can estimate a single value or point estimate of the parameter of interest (for example, sample mean) by direct calculation. Knowledge of the data distribution further permits researchers to calculate confidence intervals (CI) that reflect the range of values an estimated parameter might take within a specified level of confidence (for example, 95%). The CI establishes a range and specifies the probability of the true population value being within that range. For a symmetric CI, the point estimate calculated from the data will be halfway between the lower- and upper-confidence limits. The degree of confidence is expressed as a prespecified probability such as 90% or 95% CI. One can assert that should an experiment be repeated multiple times, the true value of the parameter will fall within the distribution of values 90% or 95% of the time, depending on which CI probability is chosen. The 95% CI around the mean obtained from one sample is often chosen to define the range of possible values as it is comparable to estimating the boundaries by taking plus or minus 2 standard errors from the parameter estimate.

## 6. A Health and Disease Management Example

Suppose one wants to test the impact of a new program to increase adherence to cholesterol-lowering drugs in patients with hypercholesterolemia (high LDL-cholesterol levels). This evaluation is carried out dividing a group of 80 patients into 2: those who participate in the new program and those who continue with usual care. The null hypothesis is that the new program is no better than usual care. One determines whether or not the no difference hypothesis can be rejected, based on the evidence from the sample of patients. The null hypothesis is specified as follows:

> H0: LDL-cholesterol reduction in the group participating in the new program is equivalent to LDL-cholesterol reduction in the group receiving usual care. This is equivalent to: (LDL-cholesterol reduction in the new intervention group) - (LDL-cholesterol reduction in the usual care group) = 0. The null hypothesis is tested against the alternative hypothesis, H1: the difference in LDL-cholesterol reduction between the 2 groups does not equal 0.

The efficacy of the new program to reduce LDL-cholesterol is assessed using the t-test[2] to compare mean LDL reduction in the new program group (n=40 patients) with the mean LDL reduction in the usual care group (n=40 patients). The study shows a mean LDL-cholesterol reduction of 72.3 mg/dl in the new program group and 48.2 mg/dl in the usual care group. The new program can therefore reduce LDL-cholesterol levels by 45%, while usual care can reduce LDL-cholesterol by 30%. The t-test indicates that these differences are statistically significant, with a p value <0.001 (Table 2). The t-test of programs such as SPSS[2] compares the variance of both groups, using the Levene test, and then compares the means assuming equal and unequal variances. In this example, the variances are not different, p>0.05 for F test indicates. The t-statistic calculated assuming equal variances has a value of 30.3 and is statistically significant with p<0.001. This indicates that the difference is sufficiently greater than 0 and the null hypothesis can be rejected; with the probability of a Type I error being lower than the prespecified significance level (p-value) of the statistical test. The conclusion of the study is that the new adherence program reduces LDL cholesterol more than usual care.

Part 5: Statistical Approaches and Methods

**TABLE 1.** Type I and Type II Errors in Hypothesis Testing

|  |  | Null Hypothesis (H0) | |
|---|---|---|---|
|  |  | True | False |
| **Risk Factor** | Reject $H_0$ | Type I error | Correct |
|  | Not reject $H_0$ | Correct | Type II error |

# References

1. Portney LG, Watkins MP. *Foundations of Clinical Research: Applications to Practice*. 3rd ed. Upper Saddle River, NJ: Prentice Hall; 2009.
2. Norusis JM. SPSS Statistics 17.0. *Statistical Procedures Companion*. Chicago, IL: Prentice Hall; 2008.

CHAPTER 34

# Statistical Methods for Randomized Controlled Trials: Discrete Outcomes

Rahul Jain, PhD; and Joel Hay, PhD

Discrete outcomes can be found in all types of study designs including randomized controlled trials, cohort studies, and cross-sectional studies. These outcomes or variables are not measured as a continuous string of values but rather as discrete units (for example, yes or no). Discrete measures, also known as *qualitative* or *categorical measures*, can be either independent or dependent variables defined as outcomes with 2 (binary) or more than 2 (categorical) categories—see Table 1 for examples. Outcomes may have obvious value ranking (for example, live or dead) and indicators for different categories may or may not be numerically quantifiable. For example, patients may be classified as having a diagnosis of heart failure, cancer, or diabetes, and while these might take a yes or no value, one cannot determine disease severity from a discrete measure.

In many evaluations of health and disease management programs the outcomes of interest are qualitative rather than quantitative. For example, one may be interested in whether or not a disease management program for asthma reduces the risk of hospitalization or emergency department (ED) visits. In this example, a majority of patients may never experience one of these outcomes, which occur infrequently. Thus, treating the dependent variable as continuous with so many zero entries for hospitalizations and ED visits would violate the assumption of a normal distribution and other statistical error distributional assumptions.

Discrete variables may also come from the transformation of continuous variables into groups or categories (both binary and categorical). This may be desirable when the variable measured has one or more threshold values with specific clinical meaning or policy relevance, or when the underlying numerical properties are unnecessary for the analysis. One example is the medication possession ratio (MPR), which is often used as proxy for adherence to medication. The MPR is a continuous variable that ranges from 0 to 1. When considering a health and disease management program aimed at improving medication compliance, a researcher might choose to classify patients as adherent using a prespecified MPR threshold (for example, greater than 0.80) and nonadherent otherwise. By classifying patients as *adherent* or nonadherent, the data are transformed from a continuous variable into a discrete variable.

The remainder of this chapter is broken down into 2 primary sections. First, it discusses regression analysis for binary outcomes and then regression analysis for categorical outcomes. Each section provides a brief introduction to appropriate regression techniques, followed by a discussion on the interpretation of the results and examples in the context of health and disease management.

## 1. Binary Outcomes

When a dependent variable is defined as binary and discrete, multivariate regression analysis proceeds with either least-square linear regression or with nonlinear regression models. This section introduces the use of these models with examples and a discussion on the interpretation of the estimates.

### The Linear Probability Model

In the linear probability model (LPM), the discrete outcome is expressed as a linear probability function of the explanatory (independent) variables. These models are called *linear probability models* because the probability that an event will occur is a linear function of the independent variables when the outcome is defined by 2 discrete values (0,1). Therefore, the conditional expectation of the outcome is equal to the conditional probability that the event will occur given the values of the independent variables. That is, this implies that the regression coefficient measures the change in the probability that the event will occur when the corresponding independent variable changes, holding all the other independent variables constant. The LPM is estimated as an ordinary least squares (OLS) regression with the binary-dependent variable usually represented dichotomously and the independent variables defined as discrete and/or continuous included on the right-hand side of the regression equation.

Hypothesis testing with the LPM is the same as in linear regression analysis of continuous variables, discussed elsewhere in this book, however, the fact that the LPM errors are heteroskedastic and nonnormal requires that bootstrapping or other robust standard error corrections are necessary. Further, the predicted probabilities resulting from an LPM can result in estimates less than 0 or greater than 1, violating a basic axiom of probability theory. Researchers often ignore this problem by assuming that negative predicted probabilities are equal to 0 and those greater than 1 are equal to 1. This may be a reasonable assumption under certain circumstances (for example, if most of the sample outcomes reside in the middle and not clustered at one or the other extreme), but cannot be applied generally.

Another drawback of the LPM is that it assumes that the marginal or incremental effect of an independent variable is constant throughout the probability range. This implies that the change in predicted probability is the same irrespective of the initial value of the independent variable. This may or may not be a valid assumption depending on the study question. For example, the effect of the independent variable may be only weakly related to the outcome probabilities near the extremes. Alternatively, as is often the case in clinical trials, where a participant starts at baseline may be highly predictive of how much of an outcome may be observed at follow-up. Therefore, one might expect the outcome probability to be related to the independent variables in a nonlinear manner.

Despite the limitations, the LPM remains an attractive approach, as it is easy to compute, the regression coefficients are easy to interpret, and it predicts well for values of the independent variables that are close to their sample means and outcomes that are not heavily concentrated at one extreme or the other.

## Nonlinear Models

In light of the highly prescribed circumstances under which the LPM is considered accurate and acceptable, one may choose a nonlinear function probability model for the outcomes, say $G(\cdot)$, with the restriction that $0 \leq G(z) \leq 1$ for all possible values of $z$. Since continuous cumulative distribution functions (CDFs) of random variables have this property by definition, they become obvious candidates. The 2 common CDFs are the standard logistic distribution, which gives the logit model, and standard normal distribution, which gives the probit model.

Let $Z = \beta_0 + \beta_1 X_{1i} + \beta_2 X_{2i} + \cdots + \beta_k X_{ki}$, then the logit or probit model takes the form $P(Y = 1|X's) = G(Z)$, where $G(\cdot)$ is the cumulative distributing function, $X_i$s are the independent variables and $\beta$s are the coefficients to be estimated. The outcome is $P(Y = 0|X's) = 1 - P(Y = 1|X's)$, since the probability sums up to 1. It follows that 1) as $Z$ ranges from $-\infty$ to $+\infty$, the cumulative distribution function range between 0 and 1, and 2) $P(Y = 1|X's)$ is nonlinearly related to independent variables.[1,2,3]

Since $Z$ is also nonlinear in the coefficients, the standard least-square methods are no longer valid. The maximum likelihood estimation (MLE) is used to estimate the coefficients and their asymptotic standard errors.[2] Standard statistical packages such as SAS and STATA report both of these estimates and standard errors of estimated coefficients. The asymptotic t-tests and confidence intervals can be evaluated just as with the least-square estimators.

In contrast to the LPM, the magnitude of each individual coefficient is *not* interpreted as the marginal effects of the independent variables. In fact, the effect of small changes in continuous independent variables on predicted probability depends on the values of *all* independent variables and estimated coefficients. Additionally, change in predicted probability depends on the initial value of the independent variables. In light of these implications, the change in probability is computed for independent variables at selected values of interest. Sample means of the independent variables are often used to obtain the effect of 1 unit change in the independent variables. If the aim of an analysis is to evaluate changes in the partial effects at different values of the independent variable, the minimum and maximum are also calculated and/or the lower and upper quartiles are estimated.

## Examples

The interpretation of the regression coefficients can best be illustrated with an example. This example analyzes the factors that influence the likelihood that a patient with Type 2 diabetes is prescribed metformin. The analysis includes demographic variables (age and gender), type of insurance (health maintenance organization, preferred provider organization, point of service plan, or other) and observable risk factors for myocardial infarction and heart failure as independent variables. The results are presented in Table 2. Suppose the primary variable of interest is age. The coefficient of age in the LPM is the marginal effect of age on the probability of receiving metformin. Therefore, for every *1 year* increase in age, the probability of being prescribed metformin *decreases* by 0.008 percentage point.

Continuing with this example using a nonlinear model approach, the coefficient (and associated p-values) of logit and probit models are presented in last 4 columns of Table 2. Let $\bar{Z} = \hat{\beta}_0 + \hat{\beta}_1 \bar{X}_1 + \hat{\beta}_2 \bar{X}_2 + \cdots + \hat{\beta}_k \bar{X}_k$ denote the value Z of at sample means of X's. Then, the value for logit $\bar{Z}_{Logit}$ is 0.3489 and for the probit models the value for $\bar{Z}_{Probit}$ is 0.2166 (from Table 2). Therefore, the effect of changing age by 1 year ($\Delta X_{age} = 1$) on the probability of being prescribed metformin can be calculated as follows:

$$\Delta \hat{P}(Y = 1 | X's)_{Logit} \approx \hat{\beta}_{age} \Delta X_{age} * g(\bar{Z}) = 0.0085$$

$$\Delta \hat{P}(Y = 1 | X's)_{Probit} \approx \hat{\beta}_{age} \Delta X_{age} * g(\bar{Z}) = 0.0085$$

Repeating these calculations for different values of $X_{age}$, while keeping all the other variables constant at their sample means, different values of predicted probabilities and marginal effects can be calculated. *Unlike the LPM*, both the predicted probabilities as well as marginal effects have a nonlinear relationship with age.

## Odds Ratio and Risk Ratio

When the independent variable of interest is binary, the results are presented in terms of odds ratio or in terms of risk ratio, which are also known as relative risks. The odds ratio is the ratio of odds (likelihood) of the event occurring; whereas the risk ratio is the ratio of probabilities of the event occurring in 2 different groups. Suppose the independent variable of interest is race (white or nonwhite). Then,

$$\text{Odds ratio} = \frac{\text{Odds for nonwhites}}{\text{Odds for whites}} = \frac{\frac{P_{N-W}}{1 - P_{N-W}}}{\frac{P_W}{1 - P_W}}$$

and,

$$\text{Relative risk} = \frac{\text{Probability of the event for nonwhites}}{\text{Probability of the event for whites}} = \frac{P_{N-W}}{P_W}$$

Researchers must exercise caution while calculating and interpreting these ratios.[4,5] Schulman and colleagues' study evaluated how often doctors recommend cardiac catheterization for hypothetical patients with chest pain and found that 84.7% of blacks and 90.6% of whites were referred for catheterization.[4] Therefore, the odds-ratio was equal to 0.574 and relative risk was equal to 0.934. Hence, the odds ratio implies that the blacks had approximately 40% lower *odds* of cardiac catheterization recommendation relative to the *odds* for whites. Similarly, the relative risk shows that the blacks had approximately 7% lower *probability* of referral for cardiac catheterization relative to the whites.

The misinterpretation of odds ratios as the relative risks is common. In the above case, if odds ratios are (*wrongly*) interpreted as relative risks (as they were in the media[6,7,8]), then it would mean that black patients had approximately 40% lower *probability* of referral than white patients. This misinterpretation of odds ratio overstates the magnitude of actual differences and implies discrimination. It is, therefore important to understand when to use odds ratio and when to use relative risk. Both the odds ratio and relative risk are calculated from the probabilities (or risk), as above.

In addition, if the odds ratio is less than 1, then the relative risk is also less than 1 and vice-versa, however their magnitudes may differ substantially. When the probability of an outcome in 2 groups being compared is less than 20%, the odds ratio approximates relative risk.[9,10] As a numerical example, suppose the probability of nonwhites contracting certain disease is 13%, that for whites it is 18%, then the odds ratio for nonwhite relative to white is equal to 0.68, and relative risk for nonwhite relative to whites is 0.72. This calculation shows that the value of odds ratio and risk ratio are close to each other. If however the probability of an outcome in either group is larger, then the magnitude of difference between odds ratio and relative risk increases, as was the case in the original example.

## Example

Going back to the earlier example, suppose now the variable of interest is gender. To calculate the odds ratio and the relative risk, the predicted probability of being prescribed metformin (while keeping all the other variables at their sample means) needs to be calculated separately for men and women. Using the information in Table 2, $\bar{Z}$ for men is $\bar{Z}_{Logit}^{Men}$ = 0.1589 and similarly, $\bar{Z}$ for women is $\bar{Z}_{Logit}^{Women}$ = 0.5654. Therefore, $P(Y = metformin|Men) = 0.5394$ and $P(Y = metformin|Women) = 0.6377$. Hence, the odds ratio (for men relative to women) is equal to 0.6660 and relative risk (for men relative to women) is 0.8462.

## 2. Categorical Outcomes

The binary outcomes discussed are a special case of categorical outcomes in which there are only 2 possible outcomes. Categorical outcomes in general can have an arbitrary number of possible outcome values. For example, a patient may be able to choose among any number of health care plans depending on the types of health or disease management programs that they are offered. Categorical variables are defined by the fact that they do not have any quantitative component. That is, the discrete ranking value assigned to a category does not imply value (for example, *greater* or *smaller*) or magnitude of some feature or trait relative to any other category. A health care provider might prescribe a patient with Type 2 diabetes metformin, thiazolidinediones, or sulfonylureas. In this example, each drug/class is a category to which the patients could be assigned but none of these categories can be referred to as *greater* or *smaller* than another, that is the value ordering of each category is irrelevant. Therefore, although the analysis of categorical variables is described above, using the ordinary least-square design is problematic.

## Multinomial Logit

Following on earlier examples, for a patient who may be prescribed any of the 3 antidiabetic drugs/classes, one approach is to define this variable as 1 if the drug is metformin; 2 if the drug/class is thiazolidinediones, and 3 if the drug/class is sulfonylureas. The appropriate modeling approach using these categorical variables is to designate one category as the *reference category*, calculate the log-odds for all the other categories relative to the designated reference category, and then allow the log-odds to be a function of the linear predictors. The choice of the reference category is arbitrary but is required for the estimation of the unknown parameters. Sometimes the first category, last category, or the category with the highest frequency is chosen and assigned as the reference category. Other times the research question guides the choice of the reference category. For example, if a health and disease management experiment is considering 2 treatment groups and 1 control group, the control group may be chosen as the reference category.

In our example, the metformin group is chosen as the reference category with thiazolidinediones and sulfonylureas as the categories for which log-odds are modeled. As in the case of logit and probit models discussed for the binary outcome case, MLE is generally used to obtain the estimates and asymptotic standard errors. Standard statistical packages (for example, SAS, STATA) provide the multinomial logistic procedure as well as other multinomial-estimation techniques (for example, multinomial probit, random parameters logit, or heterogeneous extreme value models).

## Interpreting Estimates

In multinomial logistic regression, the constraint that all probabilities sum to 1 means that one estimates one less regression equation than the number of categories. In the above example of prescriptions for antidiabetic drug, the metformin group is the reference category. Therefore, one relationship compares assignment of thiazolidinediones to that of metformin users and the second compares sulfonylureas users to metformin users. Hence, the interpretation of the odds ratio is the change in likelihood of being assigned to one drug/category (say, thiazolidinediones) relative to the reference category as it relates to one unit change in the independent (continuous) variable. As in the case of logistic regression for binary outcomes, estimated coefficients may be used to estimate the predicted probability of being assigned to any category as a function of the explanatory variables.

## Example

The earlier example is modified to allow for categorical variables. The variable of interest is the probability of being prescribed either metformin, or thiazolidinediones, or sulfonylureas, with the metformin group as the reference category. Table 3 provides the estimated coefficients and corresponding p-values. The predicted probability is estimated when all of the variables are held constant at their mean values. Therefore, let $\overline{Z}_m = \hat{\beta}_0^m + \hat{\beta}_1^m \overline{X}_1 + \hat{\beta}_2^m \overline{X}_2 + \cdots + \hat{\beta}_k^m \overline{X}_k$, for m = 2 (thiazolidinediones) and 3 (sulfonylureas). Then for thiazolidinediones, $\overline{Z}_{TZD}$ = -0.8941; and for sulfonylureas $\overline{Z}_{Sulf}$ = -1.2418 (Table 3). Therefore, $P(Y = Met|X') = 0.5890$; $P(Y = TZD|X') = 0.2409$ and $P(Y = sulf|X') = 0.1701$. By repeating these calculations for different values of $X_{age}$, while keeping all the other variables constant at their sample means, different values of predicted probabilities for all 3 categories can be calculated.

## 3. Conclusion

This chapter briefly describes the techniques used to analyze discrete outcomes. For binary outcomes, 2 regression techniques are discussed, along with their advantages and disadvantages. A unified example is presented to facilitate the comparison of different models. While presenting the results from the nonlinear regressions, it is important to remember that the estimated probabilities as well as the marginal effects of independent variables depend on all the independent variables, which is in contrast to the linear probability model. Multinomial categorical outcome estimation models are also discussed. In such cases, the LPM regression model is problematic and one must consider a logit- or probit-estimation approach.

## References:

1. Gujarati DN. *Basic Econometrics*. 3rd ed. New York, NY: McGraw-Hill; 1995.
2. Wooldridge JM. *Econometric Analysis of Cross Section and Panel Data*. Cambridge, MA: MIT Press; 2002.
3. Agresti, A. *Categorical Data Analysis*. 2nd ed. New York, NY: John Wiley; 2002.
4. Schulman KA, Berlin JA, Harless W, et al. The effect of race and sex on physicians' recommendations for cardiac catheterization. *N Engl J Med*. 1999;340:618-626.
5. Schwartz LM, Woloshin S, Welch HG. Misunderstandings about the effects of race and sex on physicians' referrals for cardiac catheterization. *N Engl J Med*. 1999;341(4):279-283; discussion 286-287.
6. Study suggests race, sex influence physicians' care. *The Wall Street Journal*. February 26, 1999:B6.
7. Doctor bias may affect heart care, study finds. *The New York Times*. February 25, 1999:A23.
8. Heart study points to race, sex bias. *Los Angeles Times*. February 25, 1999:12.
9. Zhang J, Yu KF. What's the relative risk? A method of correcting the odds ratio in cohort studies of common outcomes. *JAMA*. 1998;280:1690-1691.
10. Davies HT, Crombie IK, Tavakoli M. When can odds ratios mislead? *BMJ*. 1998;316:989-991.

## Part 5: Statistical Approaches and Methods

**TABLE 1:** Examples of Discrete Outcomes

| | Independent Variables | Dependent Variables |
|---|---|---|
| Binary variables | Gender (1 if male; 0 if female), | Hospitalization related to heart failure (1 if yes; 0 if no) |
| | Race (1 if white; 0 if nonwhite) | Insurance coverage (1 if yes; 0 if no) |
| | | Doctor visit (1 if yes; 0 if no) |
| Categorical variables | Region (1 if northeast; 2 if southeast; 3 if northwest; 4 if southwest) | Type 2 antidiabetes drug (1 if metformin; 2 if thiazolidinediones; 3 if sulfonylureas) |
| | Race (1 if Hispanic; 2 if Asian/Pacific; 3 if black; 4 if white; 5 if other or mixed | |

**TABLE 2:** Binary Outcome: Coefficients of All 3 Regressions

| | Mean | LPM | | Logit | | Probit | |
|---|---|---|---|---|---|---|---|
| | | Coeff | p-value | Coeff | p-value | Coeff | p-value |
| Constant | – | 1.0175 | <.0001 | 2.2127 | <.0001 | 1.3671 | <.0001 |
| Age | 56.5652 | -0.0082 | <.0001 | -0.0351 | <.0001 | -0.0217 | <.0001 |
| Male | 0.5326 | -0.0943 | <.0001 | -0.4065 | <.0001 | -0.2516 | <.0001 |
| HMO plan | 0.3425 | 0.0828 | 0.0006 | 0.3393 | 0.0010 | 0.2120 | 0.0009 |
| PPO plan | 0.4515 | 0.0905 | <.0001 | 0.3722 | 0.0002 | 0.2321 | 0.0002 |
| POS plan | 0.1057 | 0.0969 | 0.0006 | 0.4008 | 0.0010 | 0.2506 | 0.0008 |
| Heart failure risk | 0.2170 | 0.0133 | 0.3605 | 0.0593 | 0.3453 | 0.0368 | 0.3423 |
| MI risk | 0.3040 | 0.0064 | 0.6292 | 0.0253 | 0.6570 | 0.0155 | 0.6587 |
| Hypertension | 0.4975 | -0.0038 | 0.7547 | -0.0182 | 0.7309 | -0.0114 | 0.7275 |
| N | 6697 | | | | | | |

HMO=health maintenance organization, PPO=preferred provider organization, POS=point-of-service plan, MI=myocardial infarction

**TABLE 3:** Multinomial Outcomes: Coefficients and their P-Values

|  | Mean | Thiazolidinediones | | Sulfonylureas | |
|---|---|---|---|---|---|
|  |  | Coeff | p-value | Coeff | p-value |
| Intercept |  | -3.1906 | <.0001 | -2.4865 | <.0001 |
| Age | 56.56518 | 0.0429 | <.0001 | 0.0236 | <.0001 |
| Male | 0.532627 | 0.464 | <.0001 | 0.3262 | <.0001 |
| HMO plan | 0.342541 | -0.3036 | 0.0093 | -0.3677 | 0.0083 |
| PPO plan | 0.451546 | -0.429 | 0.0001 | -0.2681 | 0.0429 |
| POS plan | 0.105719 | -0.3916 | 0.0049 | -0.4036 | 0.0142 |
| Risk factors for heart failure | 0.216963 | -0.0637 | 0.3884 | -0.0559 | 0.5093 |
| Risk factors for MI | 0.304017 | -0.1263 | 0.0654 | 0.1187 | 0.1167 |
| History of hypertension | 0.497536 | 0.0284 | 0.6496 | 0.00336 | 0.9623 |
| N | 6697 |  |  |  |  |

HMO=health maintenance organization, PPO=preferred provider organization, POS=point-of-service plan, MI=myocardial infarction

CHAPTER 35

# Statistical Methods for Randomized Controlled Trials: Continuous Outcomes

Pedro Plans-Rubió, MD, PhD, MSc

Research in health and disease management and in pharmacoeconomics often involves continuous outcomes, such as measures of blood cholesterol or blood pressure. Continuous outcomes are amenable to statistical techniques of analysis based on the mean and standard deviation, and the adjustment of the effect of study variables on continuous outcomes is based on multiple linear regression analysis.

A continuous outcome is measured using a scale on which for any 2 continuous measurements, it is always possible to find one measurement in between. Blood cholesterol, blood pressure, glucose levels, weight, and blood cell count are a few examples, among many, of continuous outcomes. The types of data collected in research studies include categorical data (nominal or ordinal) and numerical data (counts and continuous outcomes). Categorical information can be grouped into categories and the corresponding values are binary (for example, yes/no).

Continuous outcomes must meet 2 conditions. First, each unit of change on the measurement scale must have an equal quantifiable value that supports standard arithmetic operators such as addition, subtraction, multiplication, and division. For this reason, continuous outcomes can be defined as interval variables. Second, values of continuous variables are measured in specific units when 0 represents the total absence of that unit and negative values reflect the negative of the unit (when appropriate).

## 1. Statistical Analysis for Continuous Outcomes

The comparison of continuous outcomes associated with 2 treatment strategies or in 2 groups of patients is done by carrying out a t-test or other statistical analysis using the mean and standard deviation of the groups being compared. Because continuous identically distributed random variables support the central limit theorem, mean values for continuous outcomes are by definition normally distributed. In this situation, the t-test provides a consistent measurement of the statistical significance of the efficacy of one treatment or program relative to another. It is possible to evaluate, for example, the efficacy of a new drug to reduce blood pressure by comparing the mean diastolic blood pressure reduction achieved in one group of 20 persons treated with the new drug and a group of 20 persons treated with the best available existing antihypertensive drug. Table 1 presents the results of a t-test, showing that a reduction of 10 mmHg achieved with the new drug is statistically significant, with a p-value < 0.001, than a reduction of 4.85 mmHg achieved with the comparator drug.

## 2. Pearson Correlation Coefficient

The association between continuous outcomes and patient characteristics defined by continuous variables, such as age and body mass index, can be assessed by calculating the Pearson correlation coefficient, denoted as "r." This coefficient shows how strong the relation is between 2 continuous variables. The values of the Pearson correlation coefficient ranges from -1 to 1, with a positive sign showing the 2 variables move together, and a negative sign if they move in opposition. The square of the correlation coefficient represents the fraction of the variation in one variable that may be explained by the other variable.[1] If r = 0.5, then 25% of the variation in the first variable is explained by movements in the same direction by the second variable. If r = -0.4, then 16% of the variation in the first variable is explained by movements in the opposite direction by the second variable. The Pearson correlation coefficient, however, does not give information on the impact of different values for patient characteristics on the outcomes.

## 3. Simple Linear Regression Models

Linear regression models can be used to assess the impact of patient characteristics on outcomes. Linear models can be simple or complex, depending on the number of independent variables included in the linear equation. A simple linear regression model can assess, for example, the impact of patient age or the impact of a new drug on blood pressure. To assess the impact of a new drug on blood pressure, diastolic blood pressure reduction (DBR) can be measured in a group of 20 patients treated with the new drug and 20 patients treated with the existing drug, and the simple linear regression equation is: DBR = a + b T. Where DBR is the variable diastolic blood pressure reduction (mmHg), T is the variable treatment with the new drug (1 = yes, 0 = no), b is the regression coefficient of the variable T and is the constant. The resulting equation derived from the data presented in Table 1 is: DBR = 4.85 + 5.15 T. The regression coefficient of the variable treatment with the new drug (T) is statistically significant, with p<0.001. This result shows that the impact on the diastolic blood pressure reduction of receiving the new treatment is significant, with a mean diastolic blood pressure reduction of 10 mmHg (4.85 + 5.15).

## 4. Multiple Linear Regression Models

When the 2 groups that are being compared, such as those included in the previous example, are not balanced across all patient characteristics, the regression coefficient of T (the variable treatment with the new drug) should be adjusted for the effect of the other independent variables. For example, the diastolic blood pressure reduction could depend not only on the new drug, but also on differences in the age, gender, body mass index, physical exercise and dietary habits between

## Part 5: Statistical Approaches and Methods

patients treated and not treated with the new drug.

Multiple linear regression models can be developed to adjust the regression coefficients of different independent study variables. Regression coefficients for the independent variables can be interpreted as weights that indicate how much each independent variable contributes to the observed outcomes, although they cannot be compared directly due to differences in units of measurement. Standardized regression coefficients solve this, making it possible to compare the weight of different independent variables on outcomes. Multiple regression coefficients for different study variables show the strength of each independent variable in accounting for the outcome, while taking into account the effect of all the other independent variables.

The goodness of fit of a multiple regression model is measured with the $R^2$ statistic, that is the square of the multiple correlation coefficient.[1,2] Therefore multiple correlation coefficient measures how strong the relation is between multiple independent variables and continuous outcomes. The significance of the $R^2$ statistic is assessed using the F statistic with degrees of freedom = N-p-1 (N = number of observations, p = number of independent variables). The hypothesis that $R^2$ is 0 is equivalent to the hypothesis that all regression coefficients are equal to 0. $R^2$ represents the proportion of the total variance in outcomes that is explained by the set of independent variables in the model. The adjusted $R^2$ represents a chance-corrected value for $R^2$.

If the patient groups considered in the previous example lost weight, this weight reduction may have an independent effect on the outcomes that should be taken into account. The new multiple regression model demonstrating the impact of both treatment with a new drug (T) and weight reduction (WR) is: BPR = $a + b_1 T + b_2$ WR. In this equation, $b_1$ denotes the multiple regression coefficient for variable T, and $b_2$ is the multiple regression coefficient for variable WR. A statistically significant multiple regression coefficient for variable T indicates that the new drug is associated with a significant diastolic blood pressure reduction, taking into account the effect of weight reduction.

If the regression coefficient of a variable changes when other independent variables are included in the multiple regression equation, a multiple regression model is necessary to determine the independent impact of this variable on the outcome. By contrast, when the regression coefficient does not change with other variables in the equation, the multiple regression model is not necessary.

Table 2 presents a multiple regression model to assess the impact of several independent variables on cholesterol levels in a sample of 312 patients. The multiple regression model includes the following variables: cholesterol-lowering therapy (yes/no), age (years), gender (male/female), HDL-cholesterol levels (mmol/l), triglyceride levels (mmol/l), systolic blood pressure (mmHg), diastolic blood pressure (mmHg), diet rich in cholesterol (yes/no), diabetes (yes/no), and smoking (yes/no). The model is associated with a multiple correlation coefficient of $R^2$=0.426, with p<0.001. The multiple regression analysis shows that patients treated with cholesterol-lowering therapies have lower-cholesterol levels, after taking into account the effect of other independent variables.

## 5. Building the Multiple Regression Model

Multiple regression models can be built with several independent variables which can be selected using a statistical program, which selects variables based on statistical criteria. Alternatively, they can be selected by the investigator, based on other criteria, such as the epidemiology of a condition and/or the clinical importance of the factors. Statistical programs, however, obtain the model with the lowest number of variables associated with the best goodness of fit.

Multicollinearity occurs in multiple regression models when 2 or more independent variables are so closely related to one another that the regression model cannot assess the independent contribution of each variable. To determine the degree to which these independent variables are correlated it is necessary to develop a correlation coefficient matrix. The correlation matrix shows the strength of correlation between the dependent variable and each independent variable and the intercorrelations between each of the independent variables.

Multicollinearity is detected by estimating the multiple correlation coefficients considering each independent variable as a dependent variable. A high-correlation coefficient resulting from comparing 2 variables indicates that the value of one is a linear function of the other variable and highly correlated. Since one independent variable could be correlated with several independent variables. One method to decide which variables to exclude from the model is to measure the proportion of its variability that cannot be explained by other independent variables in the model (the tolerance) and exclude the variables with low values.[3] Tolerance values ranges from 0 to 1, and it is generally considered that variables must have values higher than 0.25 to be included in a model.[4]

Statistical programs select variables using one of the following methods: forward selection, backward elimination, and stepwise regression. The forward selection method builds the model beginning with the variable with the highest correlation coefficient associated with the dependent variable adding each independent variable by strength of correlation in turn until the $R^2$ change is no longer statistically significant. Variables are included in the model taking into account the probability associated with the statistic F (p-to-enter) and/or F values (F-to-enter). The F test is used to assess the hypothesis that the change in $R^2$ is 0, which is equivalent to assessing the hypothesis that the regression coefficient of the entered variable is 0. The F value of the change in $R^2$ is the square of the t value of the regression coefficient. When the F statistic is statistically significant, the hypothesis that the change in $R^2$ is 0 is rejected, and the null hypothesis that the correlation coefficient is 0 is also rejected. In the software SPSS, for example, the program enters variables, by default, when p of the F statistic is $\leq 0.05$ or the F statistic is $\geq 3.84$.[2]

The backward selection method builds the model by entering all variables and removing variables by taking into account the minimum value of F required for each variable to remain in the model and the maximum probability associated with F to be removed. The SPSS program, in example, removes variables by default when p is >0.10 or the F statistic is <2.71.[2]

The stepwise procedure is a combination of forward and backward methods. The first variable is selected based on the forward method, and the second variable is selected based on the highest partial correlation and if it passes the specified entry criteria, it is also included in the model. The key difference between the forward method and the stepwise is that variables in the latter are examined for both entry and removal, taking into account a p-to-enter lower than p-to-remove or F-to-enter greater than F-to-remove.[2] The stepwise method finishes when no more variables meet entry and removal criteria.

## References

1. Neter J, Kutner NH, Nachtsheim CJ, Wasserman W. *Applied Linear Statistical Models*. 4th ed. Boston, MA: McGraw-Hill; 1996.
2. Norusis NJ. IBM SPSS Statistics 19.0: *Statistical Procedures Companion*. Upper Saddle River, NJ: Prentice Hall; 2012.
3. Kleimbaum DG, Kupper LL, Muller KE. *Applied Regression Analysis and the Multivariable Methods*. Belmont, CA: Duxbury Press; 1988.
4. Krzarowski W. *Principles of Multivariate Analysis*. Oxford, UK: Oxford University Press; 2000.

**TABLE 1.** Comparison of the Mean Diastolic Blood Pressure Reduction (mmHg) Achieved with a New Drug (treatment 1) and with the Existing Drug (treatment 2) Using the T-test

| | Treatment | N | Mean | Standard Deviation | Standard Error of Mean |
|---|---|---|---|---|---|
| Diastolic blood pressure (mm Hg) | 1 | 20 | 10.00 | 3.340 | 0.747 |
| | 2 | 20 | 4.85 | 2.254 | 0.504 |

| | Treatment | F | Sig. | t | df | Sig. (bilateral) | Difference of Means | Standard Error of Difference | 95% CI Superior | 95% CI Inferior |
|---|---|---|---|---|---|---|---|---|---|---|
| Diastolic blood pressure | Equal variances assumed | 1.124 | 0.296 | 5.715 | 38 | 0.000 | 5.150 | 0.901 | 3.326 | 6.974 |
| | Not equal variances assumed | | | 5.715 | 33.333 | 0.000 | 5.150 | 0.901 | 3.317 | 6.983 |

## Part 5: Statistical Approaches and Methods

**TABLE 2.** Multiple Regression Model Example

| Model | Regression Coefficients | | Standardized Coefficients | | p value |
|---|---|---|---|---|---|
| | B | Standard Error | Beta | Standard Error | |
| cholesterol-lowering therapy | -0.378 | 0.181 | -0.093 | -2.089 | 0.038 |
| age (years) | 0.019 | 0.004 | 0.276 | 4.495 | 0.000 |
| gender | 0.037 | 0.119 | 0.015 | 0.309 | 0.757 |
| BMI (Kg/m$^2$) | 0.017 | 0.015 | 0.059 | 1.132 | 0.258 |
| HDL-C (mmol/l) | 0.842 | 0.166 | 0.253 | 5.076 | 0.000 |
| TG (mmol/l) | 0.921 | 0.107 | 0.445 | 8.639 | 0.000 |
| SBP (mmHg) | 0.008 | 0.003 | 0.148 | 2.255 | 0.025 |
| DBP (mmHg) | -0.001 | 0.004 | -0.017 | -0.307 | 0.759 |
| diet rich in cholesterol | 0.137 | 0.115 | 0.055 | 1.190 | 0.235 |
| diabetes | 0.591 | 0.294 | 0.091 | 2.014 | 0.045 |
| smoking | -0.170 | 0.122 | -0.066 | -1.400 | 0.162 |
| (constant) | 0.484 | 0.870 | | 0.557 | 0.578 |

**Note:** This regression model was constructed to examine the relationship of cholesterol levels in 312 patients as a function of the following independent variables: cholesterol-lowering therapy (yes/no), age (years), gender (male/female), body mass index (BMI), HDL-cholesterol level (HDL-C), trygliceride levels (TG), systolic blood pressure (SBP), diastolic blood pressure (DBP), diet rich in cholesterol (yes/no), diabetes (yes/no) and smoking (yes/no).

CHAPTER 36

# Statistical Methods for Randomized Controlled Trials: Survival Analysis

Chenghui Li, PhD; and Qayyim Said, PhD

When evaluating the effectiveness of a health and disease management (HDM) program, researchers are often interested in determining whether or not the program successfully reduces the risk of certain medical or clinical outcomes such as hospitalization or mortality. One challenge in analyzing the data is that patients may move in and out of the program during the evaluation period as a result of changes in eligibility, insurance coverage, or loss to follow-up.[1]

If a patient never experiences an event before dropping out of the research population, his or her time to the event is regarded as *censored*. Another circumstance in which patient data are considered censored is when a patient completes the program over the entire evaluation period but never experiences the event of interest. Survival analysis is a statistical technique specifically designed to estimate time to occurrence of an event with censoring. In addition, it allows for comparisons among cohorts and can examine multiple explanatory variables to assist in determining specific patient or program characteristics that are associated with outcomes.[1] Information obtained from survival analyses can be used to evaluate and improve upon the design and effectiveness of HDM programs.[1]

This chapter provides an introduction to the basic concepts of survival analysis and a nontechnical summary of the 2 most commonly used techniques in survival analysis. The chapter also includes examples of how survival analysis has been applied to the evaluation of HDM programs.

## 1. Survival Function and Hazard Rate

One of the key concepts of survival analysis is the *survival function*, which represents the likelihood or probability that one will "survive" (or, an event will occur) beyond a specified time t. Time t is usually measured from the beginning of an evaluation period and through the end with measurements often taken in various increments such as weeks, months, or years, depending on the expected progression of the condition being studied. Although the name suggests mortality as the outcome measure of interest, the survival function is often used, and is suitable for, evaluating other time-dependent outcomes of interest. When other clinical and medical events are considered, "survival" denotes the absence of the outcome event of interest during the study period (for example, time to hospitalization or time to disease symptoms).

A related concept is the *hazard function*, which defines the *risk* or *rate* of an event. For example, imagine a person who has survived to time t for whom we want to know the risk that he or she will experience the outcome event in the next "moment" or period. The instantaneous risk that an outcome will occur at the next point in time t, given that one has not yet experienced the event, is the *hazard rate*. Individuals who experienced an outcome or were censored before or at time t, are no longer considered *at risk* for the outcome in the next period. Thus, the hazard is conditional on a person having "survived" or not experienced an event prior to or at time *t and also still being in the observation sample (uncensored)* thereafter. The hazard is regarded as a *rate* rather than a *probability* because it can be greater than 1.[2] For repeatable events, such as fractures or falls, the hazard rate can be interpreted as the *number of events per person per interval of time*.[2]

For instance, suppose the hazard rate of experiencing a fall for a patient enrolled in an HDM program is 0.1 per patient year, one can expect a patient to fall, on average, 0.1 times over a 12-month period if no censoring occurs during that time. This also assumes that the hazard rate remains constant over that period. If the same program enrolls 500 patients, 5 falls are expected over a 12-month period among all patients remaining in the program uncensored and assuming the hazard rate remains constant. This interpretation of the hazard rate as the expected number of events over a 1 unit-interval of time only applies to repeatable events and is not suitable for nonrepeatable events such as death. For those events, Allison suggests that researchers interpret the reciprocal of the hazard rate as the average length of time until an event occurs, assuming the hazard rate stays constant over the interval of time.[2]

For example, if the hazard rate for death is 0.1 per year for a 65-year-old man with diabetes and heart disease, then one can expect him to live, on average, for 10 years assuming the hazard rate remains unchanged over the next 10 years. This interpretation is also useful for repeatable events. Both interpretations, however, provide us intuitively the meaning of the estimated hazard rates. In reality, the hazard rate may vary over time. Our expectation of the survival will have to be adjusted accordingly over time. It is important to understand that the survival function and the hazard function are complementary ways of describing risk of a person experiencing an event over time. Given one, the other can be derived.

## 2. Survival Analysis Techniques

The 2 most widely used techniques for performing survival analysis are the Kaplan-Meier method and the Cox proportional hazards regression model.

### Kaplan-Meier Method

The Kaplan-Meier method is used to estimate the probability that a patient will survive each observational period conditional on the knowledge that he/she did not die in the previous period.[1] At each point in time, the Kaplan-Meier method estimates the *cumulative survival probability* as the product of all the conditional probabilities of surviving each observed period up to and including the current observation period. The mathematical form of the cumulative survival function denoted as S(t) is given by the following expression:

$$S(t) = P_1 * P_2 * \ldots * P_t$$

In the above expression, $P_1$ is the proportion of patients who survived the first period, $P_2$ is the proportion of patients who survived the second period, always conditional on having survived the preceding period, and so on. In general, the proportion of patients having survived up to period *i* is given by:

$$P_i = \frac{N_i - D_i}{N_i}$$

Where $N_i$ is the total number of patients *at risk* at the beginning of time *i*. At risk means that a patient has not experienced an event nor censored prior to time *i*. If a patient is censored at time *i* without experiencing an event, he/she will still be counted in $N_i$, but will be excluded from the at-risk set of the next time period, $N_{i+1}$. $D_i$ is the number of subjects who experienced an event at time *i*.

The Kaplan-Meier estimates of the survival probabilities are often presented as a survival curve that plots the estimated cumulative probability of survival or its complement, mortality (that is, 1 less the cumulative survival probability), as a step function of time. When comparing 2 groups, the difference in the estimated survival function between the treatment groups can be tested using the log-rank test, which is a large-sample nonparametric chi-square test that provides an overall comparison of the Kaplan-Meier curves under consideration.[3]

If the resulting p-value for the log-rank test is less than the specified significance level, usually 0.05, then it indicates statistically significant differences in overall survival across comparison groups. Several variations of the log-rank test such as the Wilcoxon, Tarone-Ware, Peto, and Flemington-Harrington tests are appropriate when specific criteria are met by the data.[3] They differ from the log-rank test in terms of the weights applied to observations at different time points and may be more applicable than the log-rank test when greater or fewer events occur during earlier or later parts of the study.[3]

Figure 1 provides an example of Kaplan-Meier curves from Rich et al (1995).[4] Rich and colleagues conducted a randomized control trial to examine the effect of nurse-directed multidisciplinary interventions on the rates of readmission within 90 days after hospital discharge for elderly patients with congestive heart failure (CHF). In this example, "survival" refers to *not being readmitted to hospital*. Figure 1 depicts the Kaplan-Meier curves for the probabilities of survival or not being readmitted to the hospital over the 90-day period of follow-up for both the control and treatment groups. Data on patients who died within the 90 days without being readmitted were considered as censored at the time of death. The authors found a statistically significant difference in the 90-day readmission rates between the nurse-directed multidisciplinary intervention group and the control group (p=0.035) indicating that the intervention significantly reduced the 90-day readmission rate among elderly patients with CHF.

## The Cox Proportional Hazards Model

Although the Kaplan-Meier method provides an estimate of the survival function, it does not take into account various patient or program characteristics that may impact the risk of experiencing an event over time. To assess the effect of various patient or program characteristics on the outcomes of a program, one can use the Cox proportional hazards model.

The Cox proportional hazards model is the most widely used method for analyzing survival data. A key assumption of Cox proportional hazards model is that of *proportional* hazards. In other words, if the risk of an event in one group at a particular time is twice that found in the other group when holding all other factors equal, then the hazard ratio will be the same regardless of the baseline hazard. For this reason, Cox proportional hazards models are considered nonparametric, since they do not require an assumption about the form of the baseline hazard function. The proportional hazards assumption requires that the hazards change proportionally as risk factors change. A detailed discussion regarding this assumption and the interpretation of the estimated hazard ratios can be found in Chapter 3 of Kleinbaum and Klein.[3]

The assumption of proportional hazards may not be applicable to the data under investigation and therefore should be tested before choosing the Cox proportional hazards regression model. A direct test is a log-log plot, which plots the log of the survival function against each covariate; if the log of the survival function is approximately parallel across different categories of covariates, it is a good indication that the proportionality assumption holds. In a Cox proportional hazards model without time dependence, an indirect test of the proportionality of the hazards is to include the product of a covariate and time t as an additional covariate and rerun the regression model. In this case the covariates are assumed to be independent of time in order to maintain the proportional hazards assumption. Thus, if the coefficient of the product term is significant, then it is an indication that the time-invariant proportional hazards assumption may not hold. In such a case, the Cox model can be extended to include time-variant (or time-dependent) variables.[2,3]

Thus far, the discussion has focused on time to the first event. However, in some cases, repeated events such as exacerbations of patients with chronic obstructive pulmonary disease may be of interest. The Cox proportional hazards models can be extended to model repeated events, including competing risks. Competing risks occur when there are at least 2 possible ways that a person can fail (for example, experience an event), but only one such failure type actually occurs in a given period.

For instance, patients may be at risk of dying from a stroke or cancer, but they cannot die from both. Discussions of these extensions are beyond the scope of this chapter.

## 3. Application to Disease Management

Survival analysis can be applied in several areas to evaluate and/or improve an HDM program as suggested by Linden and colleagues: "validation of risk stratification methods, tailoring of interventions to specific characteristics, understanding the timing between intervention, clinical and utilization impact, and ultimately, determining the degree of program intervention impact on utilization measures."[1] The following studies provide several practical applications of survival analysis in these areas.

The effects of the previously mentioned nurse-directed multidisciplinary interventions on rates of readmission amongst patients with CHF following hospital discharge is one such example.[4] A Cox proportional hazards model was used to determine whether the intervention itself was an independent predictor of readmission after adjusting for other potentially relevant covariates. The study determined that a nurse-directed multidisciplinary intervention improves quality of life and reduces hospital use and medical costs for elderly patients with CHF.[4]

A second study applied survival analysis to examine the long-term survival in elderly patients hospitalized for heart failure.[5] In this example, 2 models were used; the Kaplan-Meier survival curves were constructed to assess the probability of survival during the follow-up period and the Cox proportional hazards model was developed to identify independent predictors of long-term survival.[5] In a study of patients with diabetes mellitus, Young and colleagues used a Cox proportional hazards regression model to compare the predictability of mortality and hospitalization using the Diabetes Complications Severity Index and a simple count of complications; the former was found to perform slightly better than the latter.[6]

Several other studies have also been published using survival analysis to estimate the impact of HDM programs. A study of the use of telemanagement in an outpatient DM program for elderly patients with heart failure applied survival analysis to examine the impact of this program.[7] A randomized controlled trial to examine the effect of DM programs on mortality, health care utilization and costs among patients with heart failure examined outcomes amongst patients who participated in a HDM program and those who did not.[8] Patients who took part in the disease management program had fewer deaths compared with usual care, but no reduction in hospitalizations or cost-savings were found for the HDM programs.[8] Finally, survival analysis was used to compare the 2-year outcome between elderly patients with heart failure who enrolled in a combined hospital-based and home-based HDM program and those in usual care; the hybrid HDM programs was found to improve outcomes and was cost-effective over a long-term follow-up.[9]

Part 5: Statistical Approaches and Methods

## 4. Summary

This section provides a brief description of available survival analysis techniques that can be used for the evaluation of HDM programs. Survival analyses are particularly useful when data are censored and the risk of an event changes over time. The Kaplan-Meier method is used to estimate a survival curve from observed data. The log-rank test and related measures can be employed to compare survival curves across different treatment groups. Further, Cox proportional hazards models enable one to incorporate the effects of explanatory variables that may impact probability of survival providing the proportional hazards assumption is met. In the case where this is violated, relevant time-varying covariates should be considered.

## References

1. Linden A, Adams JL, Roberts N. Evaluating disease management program effectiveness: an introduction to survival analysis. *Dis Manag.* 2004;7(4):180-190.
2. Allison PD. *Survival Analysis Using SAS: A Practical Guide.* Cary, NC: SAS Institute Inc.; 1995.
3. Kleinbaum DG and Klein M. *Survival Analysis: A Self-Learning Text.* 2nd ed. New York, NY: Springer Science and Business Media; 2005.
4. Rich MW, Beckham V, Wittenberg C, et al. A multidisciplinary intervention to prevent the readmission of elderly patients with congestive heart failure. *New Engl J Med.* 1995;333(18): 1190-1195.
5. Huynh BC, Rovner A, Rich MW. Long-term survival in elderly patients hospitalized for heart failure: 14 year follow-up from a prospective randomized trial. *Arch Intern Med.* 2006;166: 1892-1898.
6. Young BA, Lin E, Von Korff M, et al. Diabetes Complications Severity Index and risk of mortality, hospitalization, and healthcare utilization. *Am J Manag Care.* 2008;14(1):15-24.
7. Gambetta M, Dunn P, Nelson D, et al. Impact of the implementation of telemanagement on a disease management program in an elderly heart failure cohort. *Prog Cardiovasc Nurs.* 2007; 22:196-200.
8. Galbreath AD, Krasuski RA, Smith B, et al. Long-term healthcare and cost outcomes of disease management in a large, randomized, community-based population with heart failure. *Circulation.* 2004;110:3518-3526.
9. Sindaco DD, Pulignano G, Minardi G, et al. Two-year outcome of a prospective, controlled study of a disease management programme for elderly patients with heart failure. *J Cardiovasc Med.* 2007;8(5):324-329.

**Figure 1:** Kaplan-Meier Curves for the Probability of Not Being Readmitted to the Hospital During the 90-Day Period of Follow-up[4]

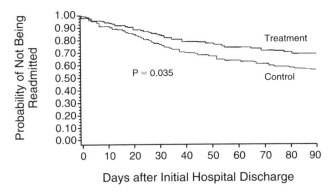

CHAPTER 37

# Statistical Methods for Randomized Controlled Trials: Confounders

Hans Petersen, MS

Lengthy and expensive randomized controlled trials (RCTs) for new drugs and other types of health care programs are routinely performed around the world to establish the safety and efficacy of these interventions. Central to the validity of these trials is the ability to satisfy the empirical condition that the intervention and control groups are similar in all aspects except for the treatment or program exposure. However, much of the evidence cited for the effectiveness of interventions is based on retrospective population database studies rather than RCTs. Though these studies also aspire to assign a causal inference between an intervention and the risk of disease, they do so without the stringent control over group assignment found in an RCT. Such studies are by their nature subject to bias and confounding. Indeed the validity of these studies is often questioned based on their potential for bias due to uncontrolled confounding factors.[1-4]

Confounding is a pernicious category of bias that must be controlled if valid causal inferences are to be made. Since study subjects in retrospective studies, by definition, have not been randomly assigned to an intervention, groups being compared may be unbalanced on important covariates and indeed may differ categorically by comorbidity burden or other measures. This may result in a biased estimate of the impact of a treatment or intervention. The bias induced from uncontrolled, unobserved or unobservable variables can be large relative to that found in an RCT. However, for various practical and ethical reasons, retrospective database studies sometimes may represent the best or only option to study certain diseases and interventions. In these instances researchers must attempt to control for potential sources of bias and confounding associated with observable variables.

A confounder is defined as an independent variable having a strong association both with the intervention exposure and with the outcome of interest (for example, the risk of the disease). In particular, a confounder must be directly associated with the treatment or intervention of interest and must also be an independent risk factor for the disease or outcome of interest. This relationship between the intervention, the potential confounding factor and the disease under investigation is the signature of the confounder. It distorts (over- or underestimates) the measure of association between exposure to the intervention and the health status or outcomes for the study subjects. The presence of a confounder results in the mixing of effects: the effects of the intervention of interest are mingled with the effects of other extraneous factors. In retrospective studies, several types of confounding may be present including confounding by indication for intervention exposure, confounding by other cofactors (for example, concomitant medication) and confounding by modifications of treatment effect.

# 1. Classic Examples of Confounder's Relationship with Exposure and Effect

An example of the confounder's relationship with exposure and effect could be coffee drinking in a study of the association between smoking and lung cancer. While coffee drinking is not known to cause lung cancer, it might appear to be in such a study because coffee drinking is strongly associated with smoking, a known cause of lung cancer. In this case the confounder, coffee drinking, is associated with the exposure (smoking), thus giving the appearance that it might also be associated with the outcome lung cancer. Another example of this relationship might be bowling in a study of coal mining and cancer. Again, while bowling is not known to cause cancer, it is a popular pastime among coal miners, and hence erroneously giving the appearance that it could be associated with cancer, a known risk from coal mining.

## Confounding by Indication

An example of a confounder by indication is an intervention given to treat an unrelated condition, which causes as a side effect the condition or outcome of interest, thereby mistakenly leading to the choice to treat with the comparator drug under study. Another example of a confounder by indication is a disease or condition in which the risk increase or decrease results from treatment with the drug of interest or from the disease or condition of interest. In either case, whether the confounder is an exposure or a condition, it must be recognized and data surrounding its presence must be captured so that it can be controlled for statistically.

## Confounding by Concomitant Medication

In the case of confounding by concomitant medication, it may appear that effect modification occurs due to other medication(s) in addition to the intervention of interest. For example, outcomes may mistakenly appear to be improved in the presence of the additional drug(s). Another explanation for this observation is that some patients are particularly compliant with their medications, including the treatment of interest. Such compliant patients are typically more conscious of their health care than the average patient. This health self-awareness will often lead to health-conscious behaviors, some of which may modify the outcome (disease) of interest. This form of confounding is sometimes referred to as the *healthy user effect*.

## Confounding by Effect Modification

Confounding by effect modification can result in several ways. Drug-drug interaction, for example, may result when a patient receives treatments for conditions in addition to the one of interest. The effects of combining these drugs may cause a shift in the outcomes related to the disease of interest; that is, to worsen or to improve. In both cases, the true effect of the intervention of interest is distorted. Another common example of effect modification is the impact of varying age groups. Older patients may respond differently to an intervention than younger patients, for example. Stratification of analyses by age group is often used as a way to control for such differences statistically. Effect modification may also be a result of variation in effect due to dosing differences. That is, the strength and frequency of dosing of a drug can have dramatic effects on the outcome of interest. These data must be captured and included as categorical and/or continuous variables describing exposure to control for these potential effects.

## 2. Finding and Controlling for Confounders

The published scientific literature is often the best place to start a search to identify known confounders. This, however, may not be sufficient. Important observations can sometimes take months or years to reach the public forum. It is often useful to consult with peers to determine if new confounders have been identified for the drug or disease of interest. Background variables commonly show up as confounders and, when possible, should be captured and controlled for in statistical models. These include variables such as age, socioeconomic status and education attainment. It is also important to note that unanticipated results discovered during analysis should not be discounted, but pursued.

Depending on the situation, confounders can be controlled for either at the study design stage, during analysis or both. Methods to control for confounders at the design stage include restricting and/or matching the patients sampled. Analytic methods can be used to control for confounding by using stratification and statistical modeling. The statistical modeling techniques include multivariate regression, propensity score methods, instrumental variables methods and Heckman selection bias methods.

## Sample Restriction

Restriction involves specifying the inclusion criteria such that subjects who are exposed to a confounding variable are excluded from the study. This method has the advantages of offering control over the effects of the confounder, being the least expensive approach in terms of time and effort, and simplifying the subsequent analysis. Disadvantages of this approach are that it does nothing to control for residual confounding, and it is impractical in situations where multiple confounders are present, as not all of these can feasibly be excluded. Moreover this approach can significantly reduce the sample size. This is of particular concern when adequate statistical power will be sacrificed if measures are taken that reduce the sample size.

## Matching

Matching involves grouping exposed and unexposed individuals together based on the presence of like confounders. Age and sex are common background confounders used in matching schemes. Employing this technique becomes more challenging as the number of matching factors increases. If the sample size is large, propensity score matching can be a useful approach to adjusting for confounding variables.

## Stratification

Stratification is a technique applied to a study sample prior to analysis. It can be used to assess if confounding exists or to reduce or eliminate the effects of confounding. The data are grouped into separate strata defined by grouping values of the confounding variable into *strata*. The impacts of the variable on outcomes are then evaluated within each stratum. Stratification permits the researcher to evaluate whether or not there is sufficient distribution of the confounder among the strata to make adjustment feasible. The technique is limited by the number of potential confounders. As this number increases so does the number of strata, and as the number of strata increases, the available subjects per stratum decrease.

## Statistical Modeling

Statistical modeling techniques such as regression represent powerful methods for controlling for multiple confounders. These techniques can require several iterations and assumed knowledge of the underlying distributions. Incorrect assumptions invariably lead to erroneous conclusions. It is often difficult to assure the best combination of covariates and the proper balance between them in complicated models. Inadequate sample size can also limit the ability of a mathematical model to fit multiple confounders.

## 3. Conclusion

Because confounding factors can distort the true relationship between a treatment and the risk of disease, it is critical that they be considered during the design stage of the study. Potential confounders must be identified and sufficient data to allow for their control during analysis must be captured in advance (*a priori*). Failure to do so will result in the irremovable distortion of effects estimates induced by the confounding factor(s).

## Part 5: Statistical Approaches and Methods

# References

1. Groenwold RHH, Hoes AW, Nichol KL, et al. Quantifying the potential role of unmeasured confounders: the example of influenza vaccination. *Int J Epidemiol*. 2008;37:1422-1429.
2. Berard A, Nakhai-Pour HR, Kulaga S. Impact of missing data on potential confounders in perinatal pharmacoepidemiologic studies using administrative databases. *Value Health*. 2009;12:A392.
3. Frankenstein L, Zugck C, Nelles M, et al. The obesity paradox in stable chronic heart failure does not persist after matching for indicators of disease severity and confounders. *Eur J Heart Fail*. 2009;11:1189-1194.
4. Sharif A. Predictors of new-onset diabetes after transplantation: the overlooked confounders. *Am J Transplant*. 2009;9:2858.

CHAPTER 38
# Statistical Methods for Randomized Controlled Trials: Missing Data in Outcomes Research Studies
Roger Luo, PhD

Missing data are a common phenomenon in clinical trials and retrospective database studies. Due to disease progression, the data missing in clinical trials pose a challenge to researchers and analysts. In recent years, clinical trials have increasingly included quality-of-life (QOL) measures to define patient-reported end points. Incompleteness of QOL data is an even more frequent phenomenon. In some therapeutic areas, such as cancer, special task forces have convened to consider how best to address the challenges of missing data.[1] For example, the National Cancer Institute of Canada (NCIC) Clinical Trials Group (CTG) QOL Committee was established in 1986. One of its achievements is a formal provision of guidelines to ensure completion of HRQOL data within the protocol requirements.[2]

There are many different philosophies and techniques to managing missing data.[3] Industry-sponsored, prospective, randomized, double-blind trials are traditionally conducted for regulatory approval of a new intervention. To meet government requirements of transparency, techniques for handling missing data tend to be simple and straightforward when analyzing clinical trial data. Such techniques are prespecified in study protocols with little room for deviation from the prespecified method in the phase of data management and analyses. For trials that are not intended for regulatory filing purposes, there is greater freedom in applying various techniques to handle missing data.[4] This section provides an overview and summary of those techniques.

## 1. Missing Mechanism

Nonresponse is a common challenge in survey research, clinical trials, and retrospective database studies. Nonresponse happens when respondents skip questions or entries and occurs with both explanatory variables and dependent variables. Traditional techniques to handle missing data can be grouped into 2 categories: deletion and imputation methods. Ignoring missing data by selecting to analyze only the available data can lead to biased conclusions. Techniques to impute values for missing variables become valuable in this case. However, before applying any imputation method, one must identify and understand the mechanisms of missing data.

Part 5: Statistical Approaches and Methods

There are 3 mechanisms of missing data:

1. **Missing completely at random (MCAR)**. An observation is said to be missing completely at random if the probability of missing is independent of all previous, current and future assessments. For this reason, we can assume that complete cases are effectively a random subsample of the full sample, and then discarding data in incomplete cases should not bias estimates. For empirical studies, a technique to assess the validity of this assumption is to compare the distribution of responses on a variable for the complete cases to the distribution on the same variable for the incomplete cases. If distributions differ, MCAR is not a valid assumption.

2. **Missing at random (MAR)**. Data are missing at random if the probability of missing a variable does not depend on missing values, but can be caused by exogenous conditions other than variables that have missing values. In this case it is often possible to make imputations for the missing values based on observable characteristics of the subjects.

3. **Missing not at random (MNAR)**. The missing not at random data mechanism may depend on the unobserved values. Within the framework of maximum likelihood or Bayesian inference, this mechanism is often termed *nonignorable*. This mechanism often seems plausible in QOL studies; for example, subjects who have worse QOL due to increased toxicity, disease progression, or death, may be more likely to complete survey instruments.

For MCAR, statistical inference based on the remaining available data is still unbiased although it may be inefficient if there are many missing values. For MAR and MNAR, we are not able to use data from patients when values of a variable are missing. This will potentially reduce final sample size. The subject deletion method is problematic because it depends on MCAR and could introduce bias when this assumption does not hold. Therefore, the available methods to impute missing values to make incomplete records useful become important.

# 2. Imputation Methods

## Mean Imputation

The mean imputation method replaces missing values with the mean of observed values. For example, in a patient survey study, we can use the mean of a QOL score to replace the missing QOL values for nonresponders. This technique is straightforward to implement but has some undesirable properties. First, because the sample size is reduced by nonresponse, standard variance formulas will underestimate the true variance. Second, estimates of quantities that are not linear in the data, such as the variance of the dependent variable or the correlation between a pair of variables, cannot be estimated consistently using standard complete-data methods on the complete data. Third, imputing means distorts the empirical distribution of the sampled values.

## Hot Deck Imputation

The hot deck imputation method uses values from similar responders to replace missing value of nonresponders. For example to estimate missing QOL values, a full sample is used to conduct a backward selection linear regression of QOL score on independent variables. This generates a list of significant independent variables associated with QOL. Patients are the stratified based on the values of those independent variables. In each stratum, there are patients with QOL scores and those without. Missing QOL values are replaced by the mean QOL estimated from responders' QOL scores in the same stratum. This technique is also simple to implement. However, it works only if the percentage of missing data is low so that each stratum has matching responders with nonmissing values.

## Cold Deck Imputation

Cold deck imputation replaces a missing value of an item with a value from an external source. For example, in a patient survey, if other studies suggested that patients with severe illness would have a mean QOL score of 3.7, moderate 5.5, and mild 7.9, then we can group patients into severe, moderate, and mild based on their disease conditions and assign the external QOL score to each of the nonresponder. In situations when the proportion of missing data is too great to use hot deck imputation, cold deck imputation can be useful. However, the external values chosen to replace the missing data points must be relevant to the study at hand. The difficulty is that when data are missing, one does not know whether or not the replacement value is relevant. In practice, one needs to conduct a literature search to define this value and support its validity.

## Regression Imputation

Regression imputation is a commonly used method for imputation of missing values. In this method the full sample is separated into responders and nonresponders. A linear regression model is conducted on the responder subgroup to establish a regression relationship of independent variables and QOL scores. The resulting regression is applied to the nonresponder subgroup and missing QOL scores are filled with the predicted QOL scores, thereby allowing subjects with missing observations to contribute to the analysis. The benefit of this technique is that the replacement value differs from individual to individual based on variables determined to be significant predictors of QOL. Theoretically, this technique provides a more relevant imputation for the individual missing datum. Although this technique still requires the rate of missing data to be low, this requirement is not as stringent as when hot deck imputation is employed.

## Stochastic Regression Imputation

Stochastic regression imputation is one step beyond regression imputation in the way that it replaces missing values. Imputation by stochastic regression uses a regression-predicted value plus a residual, drawn to reflect the uncertainty in the predicted value. With normal linear regression models, the residual will be normal with zero as its mean and a variance equal to the residual variance in the regression. In our example of the subject QOL variable, the linear regression estimated value will be added to a randomly drawn regression residual value and the combined value will replace the missing QOL score. This technique is considered the ideal approach to imputing missing values under MAR.

## Composite Methods

Composite methods are a way of utilizing several techniques together to generate estimated values to fill in missing information. For example, to combine the hot deck procedure and the stochastic regression imputation: a) first, patients are grouped into strata using the same grouping procedures as in hot deck imputation, b) next, stochastic regression is applied to impute within each stratum to replace missing patient QOL scores. Composite methods afford the opportunity to overcome limitations of one method to arrive at an educated guess of a missing value in almost any condition.

## Multiple Imputation Methods

Imputation of one value would greatly underestimate variance of the entire sample. One way to correct this problem is through multiple imputations in which we generate multiple estimates for one missing value. Multiple estimates are also a way to restore the variance of the original sample.

## 3. Summary

Missing data are a common challenge across study designs and types. In this section, we reviewed 3 mechanisms for handling missing data. Ignoring missing data and only analyzing the responder subsample is the least desirable as it may lead to biased results. Seven common techniques for imputing missing data are discussed and related to health economics and outcomes research examples. We conclude that in situations of missing data, one needs to understand the mechanism of data loss in a given sample and select the corresponding imputation technique appropriately.

# References

1. Ganz PA, Gotay CC. Use of patient-reported outcomes in phase III cancer treatment trials: lessons learned and future directions. *J Clin Oncol*. 2007;25(32):5063-5069.
2. Osoba D, Bezjak A, Brundage M, Pater J; National Cancer Institute of Canada Clinical Trials Group. Evaluating health-related quality of life in cancer clinical trials: the National Cancer Institute of Canada Clinical Trials Group experience. *Value Health*. 2007;10(suppl 2):S138-S145.
3. Enders CK. A Primer on the use of modern missing-data methods in psychosomatic medicine research. *Psychosom Med*. 2006;68(3):427-436.
4. Little R, Rubin DB. *Statistical Analysis with Missing Data*. Hoboken, NJ: John Wiley & Sons Inc.; 1987.

CHAPTER 39

# Statistical Methods for Randomized Controlled Trials: Sample Selection Bias Issues

Joanna Campbell, PhD

A primary outcome of interest in health and disease management (HDM) research is the effect of a particular treatment or intervention (for example, medication, device, or program) on outcomes, such as symptom resolution, occurrence of adverse events, and disease progression. Examples of research questions include: What is the effect of once-a-day proton-pump inhibitor (PPI) dosing on GERD symptoms? What is the effect of implantable insulin pumps on HbA1c levels? What are the effects of smoking cessation programs on quit rates?

This section presents the ways in which the nonrandom selection of a study sample can alter the perceived effect of an intervention on the outcomes of interest. Methods for identifying and addressing sample selection bias are also discussed.

## 1. Sample Selection

The ideal way to answer the question "What is the effect of an intervention on an outcome in a specific population?" is to construct a representative sample of the research population of interest, randomly assign patients within the sample to intervention and control groups, and compare the intervention and control groups on the mean outcome of interest. In practice, such a controlled experimental study design may not be practical or feasible requiring one to consider other types of study designs. Estimating a *true* treatment effect can be problematic when the study population is *not* a random sample of the research population thereby under- or overrepresenting certain characteristics of the population. This is often the case with observational studies and analyses of secondary data. As a whole, the bias resulting from a nonrandom sample used to infer a treatment effect are referred to as *sample selection bias*. There are several types of sample selection phenomena.

### Sample Selection Defined by Observed Explanatory Variables

This type of sample selection occurs when the study sample represents only a subset of the general population, eg, a sample may only include men, adults younger than 65 years of age, or patients at high risk. Drawing conclusions about a treatment effect estimated in a given subpopulation to the general population—*generalizing*—may not be valid. For instance, published studies have demonstrated that coronary angiograms are associated with different levels of effectiveness in predicting coronary risk in women compared with men, suggesting that research carried out primarily on men would have overestimated the effectiveness of angiograms in the general population creating a bias.[1]

## Sample Selection Defined by Outcomes

If a study population is limited to patients who are defined by a specific characteristic that is directly associated with the outcome or response variable (eg, change in systolic blood pressure [SBP]), generalizing the effects to patients who do not fit the narrow criteria for a given characteristic may not be valid. For instance, a study of the effects of an antihypertensive treatment may initially be conducted only in patients with extremely high SBP readings. Therefore, it is not appropriate to infer that the observed change in SBP attributable to the antihypertensive treatment (that is, the treatment effect) can or should apply if prescribed into patients with lower initial SBP measures.

## Incidental Sample Selection

Incidental selection refers to study samples that may be restricted through a secondary process. An example is an extension study of symptoms in patients with depression exposed to long-term antidepressant medication use. Often, patients continue in a study extension only if they have demonstrated a positive response to treatment in the preceding study phase. In this case, outcomes on subsequent depressive symptoms in patients who did not respond to treatment in the first phase are missing, yielding a *selected* study sample. Thus, generalizing the observed effectiveness of maintenance treatment in patients with an initial positive response to all patients who initiated antidepressant treatment is likely to overestimate the effectiveness.

## Ignorable Selection

In some instances, even though the study sample may not be representative of the general population, there is reason to believe that the average response to treatment does not vary systematically by the unobserved selection factors. A subtle variation of the ignorable selection phenomenon requires that if the treatment response systematically varies by the selection criteria, the selection process is entirely determined by variables that are already accounted for in the statistical model.[2]

Let us return to an earlier example—a study that is only conducted in men. The initial requirement for asserting *ignorable selection* would be satisfied if one could claim that gender had no effect on treatment response. The latter variation for asserting ignorable selection would be satisfied if it could be claimed that gender *only* affects response to the treatment of interest because women, on average, have lower levels of testosterone than men, and the model specification already includes a variable measuring testosterone levels.[3] Conceptually, this is similar to the concept of "missing completely at random"—where patients who have missing data are no more or less likely to respond to the intervention than patients with complete follow-up.

## 2. Identifying Sample Selection

To determine if there is selection bias, one must consider the processes used to generate the study sample. In other words, if there is reason to believe that the selection process has led to a sample that does not represent the intended population of interest, it is likely that analytic estimates derived from this sample will be subject to selection bias. For example, if the research question is "Does the intervention in question reduce disease progression *in advanced patients?*" then limiting the study sample to patients with advanced disease is appropriate. This limitation would *not* be appropriate if the research question was "Does the intervention in question reduce progression among *all* patients?"

Another potential source of selection bias arises when assignment of individuals to treatment groups is not random. This can occur even when the selection process itself yields the expected representative sample. In addition, there exist statistical tests to detect selection bias in a sample. These tests are generally associated with specific statistical methods used to compensate for sample selection bias such as the Heckman 2-step method and the truncated Tobit model. Conceptually, the *diagnostic* test considers the analytic results with and without the use of a statistical adjustment technique to determine if the 2 are statistically different. The details of these tests are explained in subsequent sections of this chapter.

## 3. Techniques for Addressing Sample Selection Bias

There are several methods that can be used to adjust for bias caused by sample selection. We briefly describe several commonly used methods in this section in the context of the sources of sample selection bias introduced earlier in this chapter. A list of additional resources is provided at the end of this chapter for readers interested in additional detail.

### Estimation of Treatment Effects in the Presence of Incidental Sample Selection

One of the most well-known methods for addressing incidental sample selection bias is the Heckman 2-step method.[4] A brief description is provided here, the reader is referred to Chapter 42 for a detailed explanation of this technique. The Heckman method statistically controls for differences between patients selected into the study population and those in the general population that are likely to influence the outcome of interest. The method employs 2 equations: a selection equation that uses data from both selected and nonselected participants, and a regression equation that uses data from the selected participants to predict outcomes.

The first equation produces a derived variable called *the inverse Mills ratio*, which is included in the second equation as a regression coefficient. The coefficient estimate associated with the intervention variable in the regression equation is an asymptotically unbiased estimate of the treatment effect in the general population when specific assumptions about the distributions can be met. In fact, the associated test for the presence of sample selection bias is a simple t-test of the coefficient estimate of the inverse Mills ratio in the outcomes equation provided the t-test is appropriately adjusted for heteroscedasticity (nonconstant variance in the error term).

The Heckman estimator is straightforward to implement and is a preprogrammed option in many statistical programs. In addition, the approach can be generalized to handle both continuous and discrete outcomes. Even so, there are several caveats to its use. Although not necessary, the estimates using this approach are more precisely estimated if there is at least one different explanatory variable in the selection equation that is not in the regression equation. (This is known as an *exclusion-restriction*.) Moreover, the results can be quite sensitive to the assumed normality of the error term in the treatment selection equation.[5]

## Estimation of Treatment Effects in the Presence of Sample Selection Defined by Outcomes

Consider the following hypothetical example. Patients with high blood pressure in a particular clinic are seen by 2 nurse-practitioners, one of whom practices *integrated care management* while the other provides *standard care*. Researchers at the clinic would like to study whether or not the integrated technique results in lower blood pressures, but realize that patients are only instructed to return to the clinic if the systolic blood pressure (SBP) remains above 150. Thus, the follow-up study population is restricted to patients with SBP greater than 150.

This is an example of a sample that is selected on the outcome variable; that is, there is no information, either on the outcome or explanatory variables, for patients with SBP less than 150. In effect, the outcome measure of interest is *truncated* at 150 and must be factored into the estimation procedure. Typically, estimation of treatment effects in a truncated sample is performed using a truncated Tobit model.[5] It important to note that the truncated Tobit model assumes a normal distribution. If the distribution of the error term is not normal or there is heteroscedasticity, the estimates from the Tobit model will not be consistent for the treatment effect in the general population.

## Estimation of Treatment Effects in the Presence of Sample Selection Defined by Observed Explanatory Variables

Consider the case of an analysis being performed on a study sample that is not representative of the general population as a result of oversampling of specific subpopulations, such as younger patients or ethnic minorities. In such an instance stratified analyses should be used for experimental data. For observational data, many statistical software packages have estimation routines that are designed to handle data from surveys with complex stratification designs using various weighting schemes. However, it should be noted that in the extreme case where data on significant subpopulations is completely unavailable, then statistical adjustments and stratification will have limited impact on increasing generalizability. An example is a study conducted only in men, *and* this is not an instance of ignorable selection. In this case, a frank and thoughtful discussion of the limitations of the data must be held.[6]

## 4. Nonrandom Treatment Assignment

A related class of bias involves nonrandom treatment assignment, referred to as *selection issues*. Nonrandom treatment assignment is not uncommon in treatment evaluation. Patients who elect to enroll in a study and agree to be randomized to receive an intervention or treatment may not be representative of the general patient population. Often these patients are more motivated than the typical patient; likewise, health care providers may direct patients toward programs where they are especially likely to benefit, or because they know that they have exhausted all other alternatives. If the variables that affect treatment assignment also impact the outcome of interest then naive comparisons of outcomes between patients who receive the treatment and patients who do not receive the treatment are biased. For instance, there is the hypothetical case in which sicker patients are both more likely to receive a particular treatment of interest and less likely to have positive disease outcomes. A simple comparison of outcomes for treated and nontreated patients will underestimate the true treatment effect in the *general population*.

Nonrandom treatment assignment can be motivated by observable (to the researcher) explanatory variables; for example, patients with COPD are more likely to receive smoking cessation therapy. Estimation of treatment effects when assignment is nonrandomly based on observable variables requires including all measures that affect the probability of receiving treatment in the outcome equation (that is, control function methods);[7] or matching methods such as propensity-score estimation.[8] Propensity score methods are discussed in detail in Chapter 40. Of note, treatment effects in the presence of nonrandom treatment assignment based on observable factors can also be estimated using the Heckman 2-step approach discussed earlier.

An example of this approach is Hay and colleagues study, *Cost Impact of Diagnostic Imaging for Lower Extremity Peripheral Vascular Occlusive Disease*.[9] In this study, the authors assess whether diagnostic imaging via contrast-enhanced magnetic resonance angiography (CE-MRA) lowers the costs associated with treating lower extremity peripheral vascular occlusive disease as compared to digital subtraction angiography (DSA). They note that a straightforward regression with treatment costs as the dependent variable, and a binary indicator for receipt of CE-MRA instead of DSA will result in a biased estimate of the impact of CE-MRA on treatment costs because more seriously ill patients are steered toward DSA rather than CE-MRA. Hay and colleagues use a modified Heckman method to correct for the nonrandom assignment of treatment with CE-MRA versus DSA.

## 5. Summary

Care must be taken in interpreting estimates of treatment effect when selection bias and nonrandom selection of the study sample are possible or suspected. This section described 3 ways in which nonrandom sample selection may bias estimation of treatment effects for a general population: selection on explanatory variables, in which the sample is not representative of the general population; selection on outcomes, in which the sample is restricted to observations within a specific range of outcomes; and incidental selection, in which the sample is generated by a secondary process.

Informal and statistical methods for detecting sample selection bias and determining its relevance to the study question are available. Methods for determining the presence of sample selection bias are directly linked to the statistical methods used for adjusting effects of bias, 2 of which are presented here: the Heckman 2-step method for addressing incidental selection, and the Truncated Tobit model for addressing selection on outcomes. Stratified analyses, or use of appropriate weighting schemes are recommended for analyses of samples selected on explanatory variables.

## Additional Reading

The reader is directed to the following useful references for additional information on this topic:

Cameron A, Trivedi P. Treatment evaluation. In: *Microeconometrics: Methods and Applications*. Cambridge, UK: Cambridge University Press; 2005:chap 25.

Wooldridge J. Censored data, sample selection, and attrition. In: *Econometric Analysis of Cross Section and Panel Data*. 2nd ed. Cambridge, MA: The MIT Press; 2010:chap 19.

Wooldridge J. Estimating average treatment effects. *Econometric Analysis of Cross Section and Panel Data*. 2nd ed. Cambridge, MA: The MIT Press; 2010:chap 21.

## References:

1. Shaw L, Merz CN, Pepine C, et. al. Insights from the NHLBI-sponsored Women's Ischemia Syndrome Evaluation (WISE) study: Part I: Gender differences in traditional and novel risk factors, symptom evaluation, and gender-optimized diagnostic strategies. *J Am Coll Cardiol.* 2006;47(3):S4-S20.
2. Manski CF. *Identification Problems in the Social Sciences.* Cambridge, MA: Harvard University Press; 1995:24.
3. Little R, Rubin D. Causal effects in clinical and epidemiological studies via potential outcomes: concepts and analytical approaches. *Annu Rev Public Health.* 2000;21:121-145.
4. Heckman JJ. Sample selection as a specification error. *Econometrica.* 1979;47:153-161.
5. Wooldridge J. Sample selection, attrition, and stratified sampling. In: *Econometric Analysis of Cross Section and Panel Data.* Cambridge, MA: The MIT Press; 2002:chap 17.
6. Cameron A, Trivedi P. Treatment effects and selection bias. In: *Microeconometrics: Methods and Applications.* Cambridge, MA: Cambridge University Press; 2005:chap 25.
7. Heckman JJ, Hotz V and J Walker. Choosing among alternative nonexperimental methods for evaluating the impact of social programs. *J Am Stat Assoc.* 1989;84:862-880.
8. Rubin D. Estimating causal effects from large data sets using propensity scores. *Ann Intern Med.* 1997;127(8):757-763.
9. Hay J, Lawler E, Yucel K, et al. Cost impact of diagnostic imaging for lower extremity peripheral vascular occlusive disease. *Value Health.* 2009;12(2):262-266.

CHAPTER 40

# Statistical Methods for Randomized Controlled Trials: Propensity Scores

Hans Petersen, MS; and Joel Hay, PhD

The propensity score is a useful statistical method that can be derived and employed during the analysis stage of a retrospective study.[1-8] It is used in a specialized analysis technique that has been developed to help control for bias and confounding. The propensity score is particularly useful in studies based on health care claims data making this technique particularly of interest to the Health and Disease Management (HDM) researcher. In essence this technique is a tool used to simulate the randomized controlled trial (RCT) setting when data may be subject to treatment selection bias. Specifically, the propensity score is the conditional probability, estimated using a logistic regression, of being assigned to a particular treatment based on a subset of individual patient-observed covariates (predictors).

When application of the technique is successful a researcher can expect the observed treatment effect to be an unbiased estimate of the true treatment effect. In the best case, application of the propensity score technique will render treatment assignment ignorable, as in an RCT. Success of the propensity score technique, however, depends heavily on the researcher's ability to identify and capture the necessary and sufficient covariates. To achieve this success, each of these covariates must be both observable and observed. A major benefit of the technique lies in encapsulation of multiple parameters, leading to a simplified analysis.

The propensity score method is most useful when there are no known unobservable explanatory factors that could be correlated with both treatment assignment and the outcomes of interest. This is referred to as the assumption of *strong ignorability*. When such an assumption is not plausible, alternative treatment selection bias methods, such as Heckman selection bias methods or instrumental variables methods may be more appropriate.

## The Propensity Score Method

For the HDM researcher or HDM program director, propensity score methods represent powerful tools for the investigation of treatment effectiveness. In practice, propensity score methods are relatively straightforward. For example, given the claims data for an enrolled population extracted to study the effectiveness of a particular drug or treatment, the first step is to collect as much pertinent information as possible. The initial goal of the analysis is to run a logistic regression using the collected variables to obtain a propensity score for treatment assignment. The propensity score can be specified as an output variable. The dependent variable is the treatment or *exposure*. This variable can be set to 1 if the patient has been treated and 0 otherwise (alternatively 1 can represent treatment A and 0 can represent treatment B). All other variables included in the propensity score model are the exogenous covariates (that is, variables that explain treatment selection but are not outcome variables of interest).

In practice, selection of the best set of covariates is as much an art based on knowledge and experience as it is a science. The logistic model yields a propensity score, defined as the predicted probability of receiving treatment. A benefit of working with claims data is that one can obtain the propensity score for both treated and untreated subjects. Thus each treated subject (case) can be matched to one or more untreated subjects (controls) based on the propensity score alone, or in combination with other variables. Hence, treated study subjects can be compared with untreated subjects having similar propensity for being treated. Given sufficient sample size and with proper controlling for confounders, the resulting comparison estimates the true effectiveness of the treatment.

## 1. Underlying Assumptions

Several underlying assumptions must hold true for the propensity score method to be successful. The first is that a similar propensity score within a subgroup of the cohort implies a similar covariate distribution. This assurance permits the assumption that treatment assignment is random, as in an RCT. Second, the assumption is that all exogenous covariates affecting either treatment assignment or the outcome have been included in the propensity score model and that treatment assignment depends solely on the measured covariates. The last assumption is that all subjects have a positive probability of receiving the treatment of interest. In most cases it will not be possible to assure all of these assumptions with complete certainty. For this reason, the study result remains an estimate of the true effect.

## 2. Uses of the Propensity Score

The propensity score is a versatile tool that can be used in the matching of cases and controls. Matching schemes employing the propensity score are greatly simplified since a large number of covariates can be reduced to a single number that retains their essential information. Matching is often indicated in studies having a high ratio of unexposed to exposed subjects. Popular matching schemes include nearest available, caliper, stratification, greedy, and Mahalanobis metric.[9-12]

The propensity score can also be used as a stratification variable for the grouping of similar cases. As the number of covariates increases in a model, so does the potential number of strata. Since the population size is fixed, increasing the number of strata reduces the available population for each stratum. Insufficiently populated strata limit the ability to estimate the effect of an exposure. Hence, an advantage of the propensity score is its ability to reduce the number of covariates thereby reducing the number of strata and increasing available subjects for each stratum.

Finally, the propensity score can be used as another variable for adjustment in a regression model. It may be used either as a continuous or categorical variable. It need not be used exclusively, but can be added in with other variables including those used to calculate the propensity score.

Researchers using datasets artificially manufactured to investigate their hypothesis have attempted to evaluate the conditions under which propensity score methods outperform traditional logistic regression models.[13] For mock-experimental datasets exhibiting fewer than 8 events per confounder, it has been demonstrated that propensity score methods yield less biased results than logistic regression. Conversely, for mock-experimental data sets with fewer than 7 events per confounder, traditional logistic regression yielded less biased results than propensity score regression.

## 3. Advantages and Limitations

Propensity score methods offer the potential for increased statistical efficiency (that is, unbiased results). In situations where a complex model is required to describe the probability of treatment, the propensity score offers a single composite variable that can be used alone or with other variables in final model. The propensity score is able to reveal areas in a stratified dataset with limited characteristic overlap between treated and untreated groups.

However, there is a considerable subjective component inherent to propensity score methods. In general, large sample sizes are necessary, and sufficient covariates for both the treatment and the outcome are required to maximize efficiency. As with logistic regression, adjustment is only possible for observed covariates. Neither should propensity score methods be used in a vacuum. Outside evidence always should be sought to support a causal association resulting from propensity score methods. The fact that an observed association is significant is not necessarily equivalent to defining whether or not it is clinically important. To be useful, findings should have the potential to translate into clinical practice, and not merely pique academic interest. As with any nonrandomized retrospective study, confounding by indication is possible. This is especially true in studies of rare outcomes. The results must reflect a true causal relationship to be useful.

A sensitivity analysis is often useful when employing these methods. One must look for the presence of exposure misclassification, outcome misclassification and confounder misclassification. In particular, one should be wary of *external adjustment*, a missing confounder.

## 4. Summary

Propensity score methods are a useful statistical tool for studying relatively rare outcomes in large populations and hence for guiding and supporting HDM programs. However, confounding by indication is common in studies of rare outcomes. Propensity score or logistic regression methods often represent the only alternative when randomization is not feasible for the study of a rare adverse event. As with any statistical method employed, it is only as good as the data captured to support it. Finally, sensitivity analysis is useful for gauging incomplete adjustment and examining other criteria for causality is a useful validity test.

# References

1. Hansen, BB. Propensity score matching to extract latent experiments from nonexperimental data: a case study. In: Dorans N, Sinharay S, eds. *Looking Back: Proceedings of a Conference in Honor of Paul W. Holland*. New York, NY: Springer Verlag; 2011:chap 9.
2. Rassen JA, Brookhart MA, Scheeweiss S. Applying propensity scores estimated in a full cohort to achieve balance in subgroup analyses. *Pharmacoepidemiol Drug Saf*. 2009;18:S15.
3. Shrier I. Propensity scores. *Stat Med*. 2009;28:1317-1318.
4. Alper AB, Campbell RC, Anker SD, et al. A propensity-matched study of low serum potassium and mortality in older adults with chronic heart failure. *Int J Cardiol*. 2009;137:1-8.
5. Austin PC, Lee DS. The concept of the marginally matched subject in propensity-score matched analyses. *Pharmacoepidemiol Drug Saf*. 2009;18:469-482.
6. Jo B, Stuart EA. On the use of propensity scores in principal causal effect estimation. *Stat Med*. 2009;28:2857-2875.
7. Wu CK, Luo JL, Wu XM, et al. A propensity score-based case-control study of renin-angiotensin system gene polymorphisms and diastolic heart failure. *Atherosclerosis*. 2009;205:497-502.
8. Karlin L, Arnulf B, Chevret S, et al. Use of the propensity score matching method to reduce recruitment bias in observational studies: application to the estimation of survival benefit of non-myeloablative allogeneic transplantation in patients with multiple myeloma relapsing after a first autologous transplantation. *Blood*. 2008;112:413-414.
9. Dyer M, Frieze A. Randomized greedy matching. Carnegie Mellon University Department of Mathematical Sciences. Paper 431. http://repository.cmu.edu/cgi/viewcontent.cgi?article=1430&context=math. Accessed April 24, 2013.
10. Lee WC, Wang LY. Reducing population stratification bias: stratum matching is better than exposure. *J Clin Epidemiol*. 2009;62:62-66.
11. Raynor WJ. Caliper pair-matching on a continuous variable in case-control studies. *Communications in Statistics-Theory and Methods*. 1983;12:1499-1509.
12. Rubin DB. Bias reduction using Mahalanobis-metric matching. *Biometrics*. 1980;36:293-298.
13. Cepeda MS, Boston R, Farrar JT, et al. Comparison of logistic regression versus propensity score when the number of events is low and there are multiple confounders. *Am J Epidemiol*. 2003;158:280-287.

CHAPTER 41

# Statistical Methods for Randomized Controlled Trials: Instrumental Variables Methods

Eberechukwu Onukwugha, PhD; and Emily S. Reese, MPH

The instrumental variables method is rooted in the statistical analysis of economic data, or econometrics. Researchers in the early part of the 20th century pioneered the method in an effort to identify supply and demand curves that were shifting over time or to estimate consumption functions using covariates that were measured with error.[1] In the latter half of the 20th century, the method found wider application in epidemiology and biostatistics. Regardless of the field of application, the instrumental variables approach is intended to address the issue of unobserved but relevant factors in analyses. This chapter uses 2 examples to illustrate the use of instrumental variables methods in outcomes research, with emphasis on disease management and health services utilization. Strengths and limitations of the method are discussed.

## 1. Medication Therapy Management Program Effects

Disease management program effects estimated using observational data are potentially biased if unobserved factors that determine program participation are correlated with the outcome of interest. For example, the program benefits associated with a medication therapy management (MTM) program for patients diagnosed with congestive heart failure (CHF) may include a reduced number of CHF-related hospitalizations over time. If individuals with more comorbidities are more likely to sign up for the MTM program, the estimated program benefit may be biased downward because individuals with multiple comorbid conditions are more likely to be hospitalized. Within the context of regression analysis, this bias can be addressed by implementing a proxy for the program participation indicator variable in a regression model of hospitalizations. The ideal instrumental variable:

    a. strongly predicts the likelihood of MTM participation; and

    b. is not statistically associated with the likelihood of a hospitalization conditional on program participation.

The instrumental variables method has been applied in various settings including studies of health services utilization. Instruments examined in the literature include the prescribing physician's preference for conventional or atypical antipsychotic medications;[2] the differential distances to catheterization, revascularization, and high-volume hospitals;[3] surgeons' preferred choice of antifibrinolytic agent;[4] travel distance and health insurance choice;[5] and more generally, persons sorting into programs based on unobservable factors.[6]

In the current example, a measure of the distance travelled by the patient serves as a potential instrument for the MTM program participation indicator in a model of hospitalizations. Patients who live farther away from the pharmacy providing the MTM service are less likely to participate compared to patients who live closer to a pharmacy that provides the MTM service. However, conditional on participation, the distance from the pharmacy is not expected to be correlated with the hospitalization events under consideration. Thus, the distance to the pharmacy provider might serve as a reasonable proxy for MTM participation in a model of hospitalizations.

In operationalizing the model, the following variables would be defined:

$$Y = \begin{cases} 1 & \text{hospitalizations related to CHF} \\ 0 & \text{no CHF hospitalizations} \end{cases}$$

$$X = \begin{cases} 1 & \text{MTM participation} \\ 0 & \text{no MTM participation} \end{cases}$$

$$Z = \begin{cases} 1 & \text{lives near pharmacy} \\ 0 & \text{does not live near pharmacy} \end{cases}$$

The model can be estimated in 2 steps[7]:

Step 1: $X = f(.., Z,...) \Rightarrow \hat{X}$

Step 2: $Y = f(\hat{X},...)$

In the first step, X is regressed on covariates, including the instrument, Z. The regression model is used to develop fitted values of X, denoted $\hat{X}$. The fitted values of X are included in Step 2 as a covariate in the model of hospitalizations with the following results:

1. The fitted value $\hat{X}$ is uncorrelated with the error term in the outcome (Y) equation because variation in X is now explained largely by Z.

2. The estimated program effect is not contaminated by factors that also are correlated with Y.

3. The fitted value has a causal interpretation in the hospitalization model, mimicking a situation in which assignment to an MTM program is based on a coin toss.

## 2. Health Services Utilization

The method of instrumental variables estimation is particularly useful in situations where a random experiment is not practical yet a causal interpretation is desired from the statistical analysis. Consider a situation in which researchers are interested in absenteeism in learning institutions and the patterns of health services utilization among educators. The research question is as follows: Are early education teachers more likely to visit physician's offices compared to their counterparts in secondary or graduate education?

The estimated correlation between office visits and early education teaching status may be overstated if unobserved factors are also associated with the likelihood of doctor visits. An unobserved factor might include the frequency of contact with young children. Early education teachers are more likely to come into close contact with young children and thus may have more frequent exposure to cold viruses, compared to their counterparts in secondary/graduate education. They may therefore be more likely to fall ill and visit the physician's office due to this reason and not as a result of their career choice in primary education.

Suppose that obtaining a bachelor's degree in early childhood education is highly correlated with teaching at a primary education level. Also, suppose that those with a bachelor's degree in early childhood education are no more likely than those without a bachelor's degree to visit a physician's office due to illness. An indicator for the possession of a bachelor's degree in early childhood education can serve as a reasonable instrument for early education teaching status in a model of physician visits. If the instrument coefficient is positive and statistically significant in the outcome equation, we can conclude, without the need for an experiment, that teaching at the primary level increases the likelihood of physician office visits.

The approach is illustrated graphically in Figures 1 and 2. Figure 1 describes the original situation in which we examine the association between X and Y (adjusted for other exogenous and potentially confounding factors).

**Figure 1.** Original Model

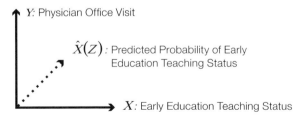

For the reasons described above, we believe that this estimated effect is subject to bias. Reconsidering Figure 1, imagine rotating the plane defined by X and $\hat{X}(Z)$ out towards you until $\hat{X}(Z)$ lies perpendicular to the Y-axis on the page. This leads us to consider Figure 2 in which we examine the (adjusted) association between and Y, where X isolates the effect of early education teaching status, allowing for a causal interpretation.

**Figure 2.** Adjusted for Unobserved Selection

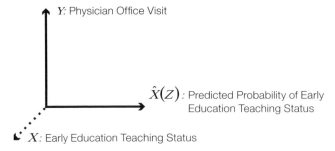

## 3. Strengths and Limitations

The theoretically elegant underpinnings of the instrumental variables approach often belie a challenging and potentially frustrating application. An important caveat with implications for empirical analysis relates to the properties of the instrumental variables estimator (IVE). The IVE offers large sample properties, unlike the ordinary least-squares estimator, which offers small sample properties.[7] The IVE's large sample property of consistency applies under a strict assumption of zero correlation between the instrument and the unmodeled component of the outcome equation; that is, the error term.[7]

This assumption is difficult to test formally and inconsistency of the IVE can arise if the assumption is not strictly satisfied.[7] The researcher desiring to employ the instrumental variables method should note other situations that can complicate the analysis and are likely to arise in empirical analysis: weak instruments, multiple endogenous variables, and interaction terms involving endogenous variables.

Weak instruments arise when the chosen instrument is weakly correlated with the endogenous variable, for example, the distance to the pharmacy is weakly correlated with the program participation decision or the possession of a bachelor's degree in early childhood education is weakly associated with working as a teacher in an elementary school. Weak instruments are of concern because they can significantly increase the bias associated with the effect of interest following the application of the instrumental variables method.[7,8,9] The bias does not necessarily decrease with larger samples sizes[8] therefore the use of claims data or hospital discharge data does not obviate the need to be concerned about weak instruments.

Methods for assessing the evidence for a weak instrument include using the partial $R^2$ or the F-statistic on the instruments.[8,9] The availability of more instruments than endogenous variables leads to an overidentified system of equations and allows the researcher to test instrument strength using the extra instruments.

However, in the presence of weak instruments, the benefits of the overidentified system have to be weighed against the potentially large bias in the estimated coefficients that may result from its use.[7]

Empirical analysis of program effects also should consider whether program effects are homogeneous or heterogeneous and whether the instrumental variables methods yield estimates of average program effects or local average program effects.[7,10,11] In addition, there may be subgroup differences that will require the inclusion of interaction terms in the first-stage model and/or the second-stage (outcome) model.[12] If the researcher chooses to model effect heterogeneity explicitly, it is possible to include interaction terms representing the product of the endogenous indicator variable and other exogenous covariates. The inclusion of these interacted terms in the outcome equation leads to multiple endogenous variables that will require their own instruments.[12]

## 4. Conclusion

Early work leading to the development of the instrumental variables method was concerned with the adverse impact of unobserved factors and that concern remains relevant today. With important caveats, the instrumental variables method facilitates testing for causal relationships between an endogenous variable such as disease management program participation and a clinical outcome in analyses using observational data. While they can be challenging to examine, these causal relationships are important to identify when conducting naturalistic studies to evaluate health outcomes associated with participation in health and disease management programs.

## References

1. Angrist JD, Krueger AB. Instrumental variables and the search for identification: from supply and demand to natural experiments. *J Econ Perspect*. 2001;15(4):69-85.
2. Wang PS, Scheeweiss S, Avorn J, et al. Risk of death in elderly users of conventional vs. atypical antipsychotic medications. *N Engl J Med*. 2005;353:2335.
3. Newhouse JP, McClellan M. Econometrics in outcomes research: the use of instrumental variables. *Annu Rev Public Health*. 1998;19:17.
4. Schneeweiss S, Seeger JD, Landon J, Walker AM. Aprotinin during coronary-artery bypass grafting and risk of death. *N Engl J Med*. 2008;358:771.
5. Lu M. The productivity of mental health care: an instrumental variable approach. *J Ment Health Policy Econ*. 1999;2:59.
6. Heckman J. Instrumental variables: a study of implicit behavioral assumptions used in making program evaluations. *J Human Res*. 1997;32:441.
7. Wooldridge JM. *Econometric Analysis of Cross Section and Panel Data*. Cambridge, MA: MIT Press; 2002.
8. Bound J, Jaegar DA, Baker RM. Problems with instrumental variables estimation when the correlation between the instruments and the endogenous explanatory variable is weak. *J Am Stat Assoc*. 1995;90:443-450.

Part 5: Statistical Approaches and Methods

9. Staiger D, Stock JH. Instrumental variables regression with weak instruments. *Econometrica*. 1997;65:557-586.
10. Imbens GW, Angrist JD. Identification and estimation of local average treatment effects. *Econometrica*. 1994;62(2):467-475.
11. Hogans JW, Lancaster T. Instrumental variables and inverse probability weighting for causal inference from longitudinal observational studies. *Stat Methods Med Res*. 2004;13:17-48.
12. Bond SJ, White IR, Walker AS. Instrumental variables and interactions in the causal analysis of a complex clinical trial. *Stat Med*. 2007;26:1473-1496.

# CHAPTER 42

# Statistical Methods for Randomized Controlled Trials: Heckman Selection Models

Eberechukwu Onukwugha, PhD

The sample selection model has been utilized in various settings to analyze program participation,[1] labor market participation,[2] and treatment effects.[3] A sample selection model is an econometric estimation approach used to overcome bias in situations where inference drawn by comparing groups based on a specified outcome may be obscured or distorted. The distortion is caused by unmeasured factors that are jointly associated with selection into the sample under study and with the outcome of interest. For example, suppose that only healthy women took part in a research study examining the relationship between postmenopausal estrogen use and heart disease. One might underestimate the risk of heart disease following estrogen use if the analysis does not account for the negative association between a defining characteristic of the sample under study (that is, *freedom from physical or mental illness*) and the outcome of interest (that is, heart disease). A proper analysis would need to explicitly include information about the selection process governing receipt of postmenopausal estrogen in the outcome equation. Thus, the sample selection problem is at its heart an omitted variables problem.[4]

The Heckman model builds on the strategy of identifying the omitted variable by first examining the selection process and then controlling for the risk of nonselection directly in the outcome equation. Specifically, the Heckman method applies a joint normal error term assumption to generate a first-stage estimator, and then uses the rules of truncated distributions to provide a second-stage correction factor that can be added to the outcome equation to correct for the underlying selection bias, assuming that all model assumptions hold. The following sections present a formal specification of the model, a discussion of strengths and limitations of the approach, and an empirical example of sample selection by considering the evidence for race disparities in specialist visits among men diagnosed with prostate cancer.

## 1. Model Specification

The sample selection model is specified as follows for an outcome of interest, y, and a selection process based on z:

1) $y = X\beta + \rho\sigma_1 \dfrac{\phi(-W\gamma)}{1-\Phi(-W\gamma)}$     2) $z = 1[W\gamma + \varepsilon_2 > 0]$

Equation [1] defines the outcome equation and equation [2] defines the selection equation. The second group of terms to the right of the equality sign in [1] includes 2 parameters and a quotient. The first parameter represents the correlation between equations [1] and [2], the second parameter represents the standard deviation of the error term (that is, $\varepsilon_1$) in a regression of y on X, and the third expression in this group represents the inverse Mills ratio. The expression on the right-hand side of [2] is an indicator function such that the variable 'z' is equal to 1 if the condition within the brackets is true and is equal to 0 otherwise.

The correlates, $X$, in the outcome equation do not have to be a strict subset of the correlates, $W$, in the selection equation in order to identify in [1].[5] If $X$ and $W$ are identical, the identification of depends on the nonlinearity of the inverse Mills ratio and, by extension, on the existence of sufficient variation in across the full sample.[5] Absent this variation in, the inverse Mills ratio is likely to be closely approximated by a linear function of $W$, which, in the case of $W = X$ and can lead to severe multicollinearity problems.[5] A correctly specified selection model likely will include variables that do not appear in the outcome equation so that the exact overlap of model covariates is not likely to be a concern in practice.

## 2. Estimation and Testing

Estimation of the sample selection model is accomplished either via maximum likelihood estimation of the joint process governing both the outcome and the truncation or using the Heckman model, aka the Heckit model.[5,6] The Heckman model[4] involves a 2-step estimation procedure:

1. Obtain the probit estimates of [2] using the full sample and then calculate the inverse Mills ratio for the selected sample.

2. Obtain the ordinary least-squares (OLS) estimates of [1] using the selected sample.

A test for selection bias is conducted using a t-test on the coefficient of the inverse Mills ratio in the outcome equation. The null hypothesis is that there is no selection bias and rejection of the null provides evidence for selection bias. The test for the statistical significance of the inverse Mills ratio is automatically calculated and reported by commonly used statistical packages.

Expansions of the model have largely focused on modifications to the outcome equation. These modifications have included the use of count variables and binary variables in the place of a strictly continuous outcome (5). The sample selection model in the case of 2 binary-dependent variables is known as the Heckprob model. Estimation of model parameters proceeds in a similar manner using maximum likelihood techniques. As with the Heckman model, thoughtful attention to the selection model results in a more convincing analysis of the outcome of interest in the case of incidental truncation.

## 3. Empirical Example: An Analysis Using SEER-Medicare Data

In the following, an empirical analysis of race/ethnic disparities in physician specialist visits is used to illustrate the effect of sample selection. The analysis utilizes data from the Surveillance, Epidemiology and End Results (SEER) cancer registries and linked Medicare claims data. The SEER-Medicare data provide treatment and physician visit information on 9,106 men aged 66 years or older and diagnosed with incident stage IV prostate cancer between 1994 and 2002.

The analysis examines the evidence for racial (for example, African American or Caucasian) disparities in sequential visits to specialists following an initial diagnosis of stage IV prostate cancer. For this analysis, a referral is defined as a visit to a medical oncologist/hematologist following a postdiagnosis visit to a urologist. Given that a referral can only be observed if there is a postdiagnosis urologist visit and determinants of observed urologist visits might also explain observed referrals, selection is a potential concern in this model. For example, in addition to educational and income levels, a patient's attitude to self-care, to multiple physician contacts, and towards proactive management of prostate cancer may affect whether or not they see a urologist after diagnosis and may also affect whether or not they see a medical oncologist/hematologist after the urologist visit.

The Heckprob model is specified as follows:

3) $\text{referral} = 1[X\gamma + \varepsilon_z > 0]$    4) $\text{urologist visit} = 1[W\gamma + \varepsilon_z > 0]$

The key covariate in the outcome model (Equation 3) is the indicator for African American race. Potential confounders include demographic, clinical (metastatic vs. nonmetastatic disease or M stage), and treatment-related measures.

The selection model (Equation 4) includes many of the same variables as the outcome model (Equation 3) with additional variables such as an indicator for patient residence in an urban location.

**TABLE 1.** Outcome Equation (Dependent Variable: Prob[referral=1])

| Independent Variables[1] | Model 1 (Probit) Full Sample | Model 2 (Heckman) Urologist Visit Sample | Model 3 (Heckman) Full Sample |
|---|---|---|---|
| Constant | -1.465** | -1.047** | -0.52** |
| African American | -0.154** | -0.117* | -0.068 |
| N | 9,106 | 6,764 | 9,106 |
| p-value on LR test for =0 | – | – | 0.0063 |
| Predicted Pr(referral=1) [95% CI] | 0.415 [0.412 – 0.42] | 0.462 [0.458 – 0.465] | 0.485 [0.482 – 0.488] |

\* $p < 0.05$, \*\* $p < 0.001$

[1] Other covariates include demographic, clinical, treatment, and physician visit measure.

Table 1 shows the results for the outcome equation based on various model specifications including a probit regression using the full sample (Model 1), a probit regression using the sample of patients with at least one urologist visit (Model 2), and a Heckprob regression using the full sample (Model 3). The results from the Heckprob model indicate that there is no difference between African Americans and Caucasians in terms of the likelihood of seeing a medical oncologist following a urologist visit while the results from an analysis using Model 1 or Model 2 show that African Americans are less likely to see a medical oncologist following a visit to a urologist postdiagnosis. Failing to account for sample selection regarding who sees an urologist leads to an underestimation (that is, 0.42 in Model 1 vs. 0.49 in Model 3) of the predicted probability of seeing a medical oncologist following a urologist visit.

## 4. Conclusion

To the extent that an implicit or explicit subgroup is used for estimating statistical model coefficients and drawing inference about program benefits or other comparisons, sample selection constitutes a potential source of bias in the case of nonrandom selection into the subgroup. The implications of this preselection for naturalistic studies of disease management program benefits cannot be ignored and the Heckman model provides an accessible method for reducing bias.

## References

1. Heckman J, Ichimura H, Smith J, Todd P. Characterizing selection bias using experimental data. *Econometrica*. 1998;66(5):1017-1098.
2. Heckman J, LaLonde R, Smith J. The economics and econometrics of active labor market programs. In: Ashenfelter O, Card D, eds. *Handbook of Labor Economics*. Vol. 3. New York, NY: Elsevier; 1999:1865-2097.
3. Imbens GW, Angrist JD. Identification and estimation of local average treatment effects. *Econometrica*. 1994;62(2):467-475.
4. Heckman JJ. Sample selection bias as a specification error. *Econometrica*. 1979;47(1):153-161.
5. Wooldridge JM. *Econometric Analysis of Cross Section and Panel Data*. Cambridge, MA: MIT Press; 2002.
6. Greene WH. *Econometric Analysis*. Upper Saddle River, NJ: Prentice Hall; 1997.

CHAPTER 43

# Statistical Methods for Randomized Controlled Trials: Bootstrap Method

Nalin Payakachat, BPharm, MSc, PhD

Evaluation of Health and Disease Management (HDM) programs requires reliable results to determine whether or not a program improves the health of a given population and if the program is worth the resources spent. Statistical ranges such as standard errors and confidence intervals are estimated to provide a sense of the reliability of statistical calculations. The classical approach to drawing statistical inference is defined by *a priori* assumptions of a parametric distribution (normal distribution) and requires a large sample size in order to provide accurate estimates. Bootstrap analysis is an alternative approach introduced by Efron in the late 1970s.[1] It is a nonparametric, computer-based method used to estimate statistical inferences without assuming a particular population distribution. The nonparametric bootstrap is *distribution free*, meaning that it does not require specific distribution functions. The term *bootstrap* refers to the use of an original dataset to generate new datasets that are called bootstrap samples. The bootstrap method estimates the sampling distribution through a large number of simulations and then constructs standard errors of the estimates.

This section introduces the general steps for carrying out the bootstrap method. Different types of bootstrap confidence intervals will also be overviewed. Examples of how this method may be applied to HDM program evaluations are provided, and limitations are discussed at the end of this section.

## 1. Bootstrap Procedures

The bootstrap method involves repeatedly resampling the data *with replacement* many times using sampling techniques such as the Monte-Carlo method to generate an empirical estimate of the entire sampling distribution.[2] As a rule, a sufficient number of sampling cycles must be run to ensure *stabilization* of the sample. One rule of thumb is to start with bootstrapping 1,000 cycles and check to see if the results have significant variability in the estimates. In general, the greater the number of sampling cycles, the better the stability of the results.

The first step in the bootstrap procedure is to construct an empirical probability distribution from the sample set $n$ by placing a $1/n$ probability at each point of the sample. Then, a subsample is randomly drawn *with replacement* from the sample set $n$. The generated bootstrap sample is called *a resample*. Each resample contains the same number of variables as the original sample, and it may include some of the original sample more than once and some may not be included at all. Parameters of interest are then calculated from this resample yielding a bootstrapped parameter value. The next step is to repeat the previous steps for $B$ times. The practical magnitude of $B$ depends on the statistics planned for the data. The larger the sample set $n$ is, the more accurate the bootstrap sampling distribution of these estimates will be. Typically, $B$ should be 50-200 to estimate the standard error of the parameter[2] and at least 1,000 to estimate confidence intervals.[3-5] Finally, a relative frequency histogram of the $B$ parameters is created by placing a probability of $1/B$ at each point of the estimated statistics. This distribution can be used to make inferences about the parameter. The conceptual justification of the bootstrap is if the sample set $n$ is a good approximation of the population of interest, the bootstrap method will provide a good approximation of the sampling distribution.

## 2. Bootstrap Confidence Intervals

There are 4 common approaches to calculate bootstrap confidence intervals including the normal approximation method, the percentile method, the bias-corrected and accelerated method, and the percentile-$t$ method.[2,4] The *normal approximation* method assumes that the sampling distribution of the statistic is *normal*, therefore ignoring the wealth of the bootstrap process. It may also mislead if used on a sampling distribution that is not normally distributed. The *percentile method* does not use an empirical sampling distribution. Rather, it calculates the $100(\alpha/2)$ and $100(1-\alpha/2)$ percentiles of the bootstrap distribution as the upper- and lower-confidence limits.

The *bias-corrected and accelerated method* is a modification of the percentile method that adjusts for the bias and skewness of the sampling distribution. This method is the most widely used in estimating a confidence interval using the bootstrap approach. The *percentile-t method* is a *double bootstrap* referring to sampling from a *resample*. This method is similar to the bias-corrected and accelerated method, which accounts for the skewness in the estimated sampling distribution and also transforms each bootstrap sample into a standardized $t^*$. The percentile-$t$ bootstrap confidence intervals are calculated using the $100(\alpha/2)$ and $100(1-\alpha/2)$ percentiles of $t^*$, which allows the estimation of the percentile-$t$ $100(1-\alpha)\%$ confidence interval.

## 3. Practical Applications

The bootstrap method can be applied in the evaluation of HDM programs to provide information regarding the variability of outcomes to inform decision making. There are several practical applications in HDM program evaluations using the bootstrap methods as demonstrated by the provided examples.

HDM programs typically consist of relatively small sample sizes and may have outliers (not normally distributed) that can violate the assumptions of the classical statistical inference approach. Under these circumstances, the bootstrap method provides an option to estimate outcomes and draw inferences. Linden and colleagues demonstrated the value of using the bootstrap methods for estimating the median cost decrease associated with a congestive heart failure (CHF) HDM program.[6] A pre-post model was employed to determine the population's average costs (per member, per month) attained in the program year when compared to the baseline year. These data were derived from a relatively small sample and were not normally distributed. The bootstrap procedure was performed using 1,000 samples derived from the cost differences of 94 randomly selected participants. Then, the median, standard errors, and 95% confidence intervals (the 2.5 and the 97.5 percentiles, the percentile method) were estimated. The bootstrap provided significantly lower-median difference and standard error when compared to the classical method. This discrepancy was explained by extreme outliers (skewed distribution) in the dataset demonstrating the importance of implementing the bootstrap method when data are skewed.

The bootstrap method is also widely used to solve the problem of estimating the standard error, bias and confidence intervals for the incremental cost-effectiveness ratios (ICERs) for HDM program evaluation. This procedure is similar to that described above except it includes 2 resampling steps for the intervention and control groups. Sample sets $n_i$ and $n_c$ represent the cost/effectiveness pairs from the intervention and control groups. Replications ($B$) of more than 2,000 cycles have been recommended to obtain stability in the bootstrap estimate of the variance of the ICER.[4,7] More details of this bootstrap procedure can be found elsewhere.[4,5] In economic evaluation of HDM programs, the population-based ICER is normally unobserved, which results in an unknown ICER sampling distribution.[4]

In such a case, parametric approaches may not be appropriate or must be used with caution. Smith and colleagues (2008) conducted a cost-effectiveness analysis of a telephonic HDM intervention in patients with heart failure from a health care system perspective.[8] The ICERs were computed to estimate the cost of increasing life expectancy through the use of the HDM intervention. Estimates of variability were calculated using nonparametric bootstrap method to provide confidence intervals given the unknown ICER distribution. Another study considered the cost-effectiveness of an HDM program compared to usual care in the elderly with major depression.[9] The bias-corrected and accelerated bootstrap method was employed to estimate confidence intervals for the mean cost differences as well as the ICERs of the HDM program.

The bootstrap method is useful when the sample distribution is unknown. If the sample is representative of the population, bootstrapping will provide a good approximation of the parameter's population distribution. Confidence in estimates from the bootstrap method grows with increased sample size as with other statistical methods.[2] A very small sample size (fewer than 20) can affect the accuracy of estimating statistical inferences in the bootstrap method. Extremely skewed distributions will also impact accuracy. When a sample size reaches 30 to 50 observations, and the sampling procedure is truly random, the bootstrap method is practical and beneficial applied in HDM research.

## 4. Conclusion

Accuracy of statistical estimates is crucial for HDM informed program evaluations. The bootstrap method can be employed to improve estimates and overcome limitations of classical statistical approaches. The ability to compute estimates for small sample size and data with non-normal distributions is beneficial for evaluating HDM programs. Finally, the bootstrap method is used to calculate uncertainty around the point estimate of the ICER in economic evaluation of the HDM program.

## References:

1. Efron B. Bootstrap methods: another look at the jackknife. *Ann Stat.* 1979;7:1-26.
2. Efron B, Tibshirani RJ. *An Introduction to the Bootstrap.* New York, NY: Chapman and Hall; 1993.
3. Mooney CZ, Duval RD. *Bootstrapping: A Nonparametric Approach to Statistic Inference.* Newbury Park, CA: SAGE Publications; 1993.
4. Briggs AH, Wonderling DE, Mooney CZ. Pulling cost-effectiveness analysis up by its bootstraps: a non-parametric approach to confidence interval estimation. *Health Econ.* 1997;6:327-340.
5. Campbell MK, Torgerson DJ. Bootstrapping: estimating confidence intervals for cost-effectiveness ratios. *Q J Med.* 1999;92:177-182.
6. Linden A, Adams JL, Roberts N. Evaluating disease management program effectiveness: an introduction to the bootstrap technique. *Dis Manage Health Outcomes.* 2005;13(3):159-167.
7. Chaudhary MA, Stearns SC. Estimating confidence intervals for cost-effectiveness ratios: an example from a randomized control trial. *Stat Med.* 1996;15:1447-1458.
8. Smith B, Hughes-Cromwick PF, Forkner E, Galbreath AD. Cost-effectiveness of telephonic disease management in heart failure. *Am J Manag Care.* 2008;14:106-115.
9. Bosmans J, de Bruijne M, van Hout H, et al. Cost-effectiveness of a disease management program for major depression in elderly primary care patients. *J Gen Intern Med.* 2006;21:1020-1026.

CHAPTER 44

# Statistical Methods for Randomized Controlled Trials: Model Validation

Nalin Payakachat, BPharm, MSc, PhD

Health and Disease Management (HDM) programs use a systematic, population-based approach to identify people who are at risk and who may benefit from a specific HDM intervention. Evaluating the population effects of these programs in terms of costs, clinical outcomes, and other outcomes is essential to inform decision making. Statistical analysis is crucial for measuring the value of HDM programs. Prediction models in HDM research programs attempt to identify characteristics of small segments of the population that are most likely to benefit from the programs. Accurate measurement of the population impact of a program is complicated by data availability, patient enrollment and drop out, confounding variables (such as insurance coverage changes), and, sometimes, lack of comparison or control groups. As a result, HDM research programs normally take place over short periods of time. These factors likely impact predictive validity of a program's evaluation. Model validation can be used in a predictive modeling process for evaluating HDM program effectiveness to ensure predictive ability and support policy decision makers for resources allocation.

The purpose of this chapter is to review model validation methods that are useful for evaluating predictive accuracy. The content discusses model validation approaches and related statistics used for a predictive model including explanatory power and cross-validation approaches in the context of their uses in HDM program evaluation. Examples of using the validation methods in HDM program evaluations are also provided.

## 1. Explanatory Power of a Predictive Model

When the outcome of a prediction model is a continuous variable such as costs, the predictive validity of the model is typically evaluated by measuring how close each estimated individual outcome is to the actual observed outcome. One of the most common measures is $R^2$. It is a single summary measure of predictive accuracy estimated as the fraction of the total variability in the response—also called the *explanatory power*—that can be accounted for by the model. $R^2$ values range from 0, indicating that the model explains none of the variation in the outcome, to 1, which indicates a perfect fit (that is, the model explains all of the variation).

Often, the validation of a model consists of nothing more than quoting the $R^2$ statistic from the model fit results. However, a high $R^2$ does not guarantee that the model fits the data well, and the $R^2$ statistic has little value in comparing models estimated using different methods of estimation. For example, the $R^2$ calculated from ordinary least squares is not comparable to the $R^2$ for the logistic method.

Another shortcoming of using $R^2$ is that it reflects the model accuracy across the whole range of the outcomes of interest. For example, an HDM program may have interest only in the high-cost end-users and no interest in the low-cost range. In this case, $R^2$ is not an appropriate to evaluate the model accuracy at the high-cost end because it cannot differentiate the high- and low-end ranges.[1] A further shortcoming is that data used in an HDM program is often not distributed normally. $R^2$ is sensitive to outliers and not robust if used to analyze a skewed data distribution. In this case, one must consider the *mean absolute prediction error* as the more appropriate estimate to reflect predictive accuracy because it takes into account the absolute value of the error, which is less sensitive to outliers.

Interpreting $R^2$ in the context of model prediction accuracy of HDM program evaluation must be done with caution. For example, the resulting $R^2$ of a predictive model using administrative claims data might be 0.20 (20%) but researchers need to clarify that this number does not mean that the model can correctly predict only 20%.[1] In the case of risk stratification in an HDM program, 20% is acceptable.

When researchers report goodness-of-fit, the $R^2$ statistic is often confused with adjusted $R^2$, but the 2 values should be interpreted differently. As such, researchers must interpret and report the $R^2$ statistic. Adjusted $R^2$ is a modification of $R^2$ that accounts for the number of explanatory terms in a model. Unlike $R^2$, the adjusted $R^2$ increases only if the new term improves the model more than would be expected by chance. Adjusted $R^2$ is particularly useful in a selection stage of model building, for example, stepwise regressions.

Buntin and colleagues quantified the differences between patients with chronic illnesses who enroll and those who do not enroll in HDM programs using 27,211 patients in a claims dataset.[2] One component of the analysis estimated the independent effects of demographic variables, insurance plan type, and prior utilization on enrollment in the program, and was used to assess the predictive power of the model. The Hosmer-Lemeshow test, which includes $R^2$, was employed to assess the model fit. However, the authors concluded that the models do not adequately predict enrollment, and the $R^2$ values were not high, which indicated that there are other unobservable variables associated with the outcomes (values not reported in the study results).

The receiver operating characteristic (ROC) curve is another estimate used to measure accuracy and can be used in a predictive model. It is calculated the area under the curve (AUC) from sensitivity versus 1-specificity across all prediction. Sensitivity is a fraction of all actual positives that are correctly predicted as such. Specificity is a fraction of negatives that are correctly predicted. These parameters are normally used for dichotomous outcome responses. A model that is able to distinguish 2 separate outcomes should have an AUC of at least 0.50 while a model with perfect discriminatory ability from the ROC curve yields an AUC of 1.0. More details of these calculations can be found in Hu and Linden.[3]

Tucker and Kramer applied the ROC curve approach to predict future high-risk members in terms of cost in 3 chronic diseases (diabetes, respiratory diseases, cardiac disease) in their organization.[4] Any member who was in the top 10% of the annual medical costs received a value of 1, and any member with medical costs below the top 10% received a value of 0. A hold-out method was used (see the internal validation process below) to create and test the prediction model. A total of 60,000 members were randomly selected from 2-years of member data (144,624 members) to develop the prediction model. The remaining members were used to test the prediction model. The ROC curve was employed to show the model's ability to predict those that were truly high-cost from those that were truly low-cost members. The AUC for the training and validation sets were 0.822 and 0.818 which are considered to have good discriminative ability for high-cost members.

## 2. Cross-validation

Explanatory power may not be a useful basis for assessing model performance, especially if researchers intend to use the model for further prediction. Another method for testing model performance is cross-validation. This method provides a better estimate of predictive accuracy than using goodness-of-fit measures. Internal cross-validation can be done using 3 methods. The simplest one is the hold-out method. Using this method, the data are separated into 2 sets: the *training* set and the *testing* set. The model's function is developed using the training set and used to predict the output values for the data in the testing set.

The second method is called the *k*-fold method in which data are divided into k subsets and the hold-out method is repeated k times. Each time one of the k subsets is used as the test set and the other *k-1* subsets are put together to form a training set. The average error across all *k* trials is computed. The advantage of the *k*-fold method is that it matters less how the data are divided. Every data point is in a test set exactly once and is in a training set *k-1* times. The variance of the resulting estimate is reduced as k is increased.

The last method is leave-one-out cross-validation: an extreme form of *k*-fold cross validation in which the number of subsets equals the number of data points in the original dataset. Thus, the model is fitted $n$ separate times on all the data except for one point and a prediction is made for that point. The average error is computed and used to evaluate the model, as previously described. Leave-one-out method is one of the methodologically strongest cross-validation methods, but widespread use is hindered by the necessary time consumption and computational expense.

External validation or out-of-sample validation uses a second dataset as a testing set for the model. This method provides researchers with more confidence for the obtained model and also implies external validity. In a study by Tu and colleagues 30-day and 1-year mortality following an acute myocardial infarction (AMI) were predicted using validated statistical models derived from hospital discharge administrative databases.[5] Logistic regression models using administrative databases on 52,616 patients in Ontario, Canada, were used to predict the outcomes. These models were subsequently validated using 2 external sets of AMI patients derived from administrative datasets from Manitoba, Canada, and California, US. The authors identified 11 variables in the Ontario AMI mortality prediction rules. The results showed that the model performed well in the 2 external datasets.

In another study, a prediction model was developed to predict what types of chest pain lead to early discharge in a population with a low prevalence of acute coronary syndrome (ACS).[6] The authors applied the $k$-fold procedure to validate the model and used the AUC of the ROC curve to present an overall measure of the discrimination abilities of the prediction model. The $k$-fold procedure was performed by randomly splitting the samples into 5 groups of approximately equal size. Approximately 80% of the samples were used as a training set. The model predicted by the training set was evaluated by calculating the area under the ROC curve as well as the specificity at 95% sensitivity among the remaining 20% patients in the validation set. This process was repeated 20 times, which implied 100 sets of validation sets. The prediction model had high discrimination (area under ROC of 0.81) showing that potential risk factors associated with ACS included age, hypertension, previous myocardial infarction, chest discomfort at presentation, and symptom duration.

## 3. Conclusion

Understanding model validation approaches and interpreting their related statistics are important to evaluate HDM program effectiveness. Predictive accuracy of a model used in HDM program evaluation plays an important role to support better resource allocation decisions.

### References:

1. Hu G, Root M. Accuracy of prediction models in the context of disease management. *Dis Manag*. 2005;8:42-47.
2. Buntin MB, Jain AK, Kattke S, Lurie N. Who gets disease management? *J Gen Intern Med*. 2009;24:649-655.
3. Linden A. Measuring diagnostic and predictive accuracy in disease management: an introduction to receiver operating characteristic (ROC) analysis. *J Eval Clin Pract*. 2005;12:132-139.
4. Tucker TL, Kramer TE. Predicting high cost members in a disease management setting. Available at: http://www.corsolutions.com/resources/papers/wp_predmodel.pdf. Accessed June 21, 2010.
5. Tu JV, Austin PC, Walld R, Roos L, Agras J, McDonald KM. Development and validation of the Ontario acute myocardial infarction mortality prediction rules. *J Am Coll Cardiol*. 2001;37:992-997.
6. Bjork J, Forberg J, Ohlsson M, Edenbrandt L, Ohlin H, Ekelund U. A simple statistical model for prediction of acute coronary syndrome in chest pain patients in the emergency department. *BMC Med Inform Decis Mak*. 2006;6:28.

CHAPTER 45

# Statistical Methods for Randomized Controlled Trials: Nonparametric Statistical Methods

Joel Hay, PhD

Classical statistical inference is built around estimating a parameter value (for example, the mean, variance, or a regression coefficient) given an assumed distribution for the random variable(s) associated with that parameter, and then determining how likely it is that the parameter's true value is either a specific value prespecified in a hypothesis test, or is greater than or equal (lesser than or equal) to some prespecified parameter value (for example, less than 0). The central limit theorem states that under relatively minimal assumptions regarding the random variables of interest, including independent and identical sampling of the observed sequence of random variable values, the estimated parameters will have normal distributions with calculable mean and standard errors, regardless of the underlying distributions of the random variables.[1] That is to say, under the central limit theorem, we do not have to make any parametric assumptions about the distributions of the underlying random variables, since the estimated parameters will still be normally distributed in many circumstances. This allows statistical inference and hypothesis testing to proceed under *nonparametric* distributional assumptions.

The central limit theorem provides a fundamental basis for statistical inference precisely because it does not require the analyst to determine the underlying distributions of the random variables before engaging in hypothesis testing or in estimating parameter confidence intervals. For example, a coin flip can only have 2 possible values (that is, heads or tails) and therefore cannot possibly be normally distributed. However, repeated fixed-size samples of coin flips will generate an average number of heads for each sample that does have a normal distribution centered on the true mean (for example, 50% for a fair coin) with a standard error that is an inverse function of the sample size.

If the analyst happens to know the true distributional functional form of the observed random variables, it is possible to improve the reliability and precision of the parameter estimates for any given sample. This insight forms the basis of maximum likelihood estimation, where given the assumed variable(s) distribution, one chooses the specific parameter values that maximize the joint probabilities of the observed variable values.[2] Maximum likelihood estimates have nice efficiency properties, such as the Cramér-Rao information inequality bound, which states that among all unbiased parameter estimates, the maximum likelihood estimator achieves the smallest possible variance.

If the distributional assumptions are correct then the maximum likelihood estimator will be precise, but if the distributional assumptions are incorrect, then the maximum likelihood estimator may not only be imprecise, but may also be biased and yield inaccurate statistical inferences. Often the statistical analyst is willing to take out some insurance against the possibility that the underlying random variable distributional assumptions are incorrect (or unknown) if that allows the parameter estimates to remain unbiased, with reasonable levels of precision and still allows accurate statistical hypothesis testing and confidence interval estimates.

When the analyst is unwilling to make any assumptions regarding the parametric distribution of the random variables, the resulting distribution-free statistical estimates are termed *nonparametric*. Generally the trade-off that is required for nonparametric estimation is that larger sample sizes are needed to generate the same level of precision that one can achieve with known parametric distributions. Nonparametric statistics are said to be *robust*. This means that their values and the resulting statistical inferences will not be unduly impacted by changes in the underlying random variable distributional assumptions.

## 1. Common Nonparametric Statistics

Although not typically thought of as such, one of the most frequently used nonparametric statistical analysis methods is ordinary least-squares (OLS) regression estimation. As long as the regression error terms are independent and identically distributed, and not correlated with the regressors, OLS maintains the property that it is the best linear unbiased estimator of the regression coefficients regardless of the error term distribution. Under the central limit theorem, statistical inferences can be carried out using known multivariate normal distributional assumptions for the regression coefficients, also regardless of the error term distribution. The OLS regression coefficient estimates are also maximum likelihood estimates if the analyst further assumes that the regression error terms are normally distributed, but they remain robust nonparametric estimates of the regression coefficients without assuming anything about the regression error term distribution.[3]

One of the most common approaches for developing nonparametric statistical estimation methods is simply to substitute a variable's rank-order values or sign values ( +/- ) for the observed values in a standard parametric statistical test. For example if one observed the following sequence of observations for a random variable {1,20000,3,0,5,200,9,1400} it would be difficult to maintain that the data came from a normally distributed variable or that statistical inferences based on assumed normality (or other distributional distributions) would be appropriate. If one substitutes the rank-order values for these values {2,8,3,1,4,6,5,7} then statistical inferences will preserve the value hierarchy without being sensitive to distributional assumptions. Based on this insight, some commonly used nonparametric tests have been developed to correspond to standard parametric tests.[4]

| Normal Theory-Based Test | Corresponding Nonparametric Test | Purpose of Test |
|---|---|---|
| t test for independent samples | Mann-Whitney U test; Wilcoxon rank-sum test | Compares 2 independent samples |
| Paired t test | Wilcoxon matched pairs signed-rank test | Examines a set of differences |
| Pearson correlation coefficient | Spearman rank correlation coefficient | Assesses the linear association between 2 variables |
| 1-way analysis of variance (F test) | Kruskal-Wallis analysis of variance by ranks | Compares 3 or more groups |
| 2-way analysis of variance | Friedman 2-way analysis of variance | Compares groups classified by 2 different factors |

Nonparametric Chi-square tests of contingency table data can also be used to determine whether or not variables are independent, regardless of their distributions. The Kolmogorov-Smirnov test can be used as a nonparametric test of equality of one-dimensional probability distributions used to compare 2 samples. The Kolmogorov-Smirnov statistic quantifies a distance between the empirical distribution functions of 2 samples without making any assumptions about their underlying functional form.

Another commonly used nonparametric estimation method is the proportional hazards model for estimating the impact of multivariate risk factors on survival probabilities (or other time to event probability models). Under weak assumptions, with this approach one can factor out the proportion of risk that is due to independent variables (for example, patient characteristics, Drug A, or Drug B) without making any assumptions about the distributional form of the underlying probabilities.[5,6]

One of the reasons for the popularity of instrumental variables methods to adjust for treatment selection bias and other types of endogeniety bias is that instrumental variables methods do not require specific distributional assumptions; although they do require specific assumptions about the correlations between the instruments and the other variables in the model.[7] This is a major advantage over Heckman selection bias methods and over some forms of propensity score methods.

Finally, bootstrapping methods are one of the most commonly used methods to generate nonparametric estimates of statistical sampling distributions. For many statistical models, parameter estimates can be straightforward, while the underlying distribution of those estimates may be either very difficult to compute or may follow complex or unknown distributions. In such cases, by re-estimating the parameters repeatedly from a sequence of randomly resampled series (with replacement) based on the original data one can develop an empirical distribution of the parameter values. This can be used to generate nonparametric confidence intervals for the estimated parameters or to undertake statistical hypothesis tests on the parameter values.

## 2. Disadvantages of Nonparametric Methods

Nonparametric statistical methods are characteristically opposite to Bayesian statistical methods. They attempt to minimize the distributional assumptions to achieve robust and reliable findings, while Bayesian methods require elaborate distributional assumptions in order to achieve estimator precision with minimal sample sizes. Since it is usually very difficult to validate distributional assumptions, nonparametric methods will maintain or increase their popularity relative to Bayesian methods as larger and more detailed electronic data become more feasibly analyzed.

As mentioned above, nonparametric statistics generally require larger sample sizes to achieve the same level of precision as parametric statistics. How big of a penalty this is depends on the particular situation. For example, a z-statistic only requires 63.7% of the sample size of a sign test if the underlying population is normally distributed. But this sample size penalty can be relatively small. For example, regardless of the underlying distribution, the Wilcoxon-Mann-Whitney test will never require more than 116% of the sample size necessary to achieve the same precision as the statistic based on the known distribution.[8]

Another key constraint of nonparametric statistics is that they often provide much less information on how changes in variables or parameters would impact findings, precisely because they are distribution free. For example, if the Kolmogorov-Smirnov statistic tells the analyst that 2 samples come from different distributions, it doesn't answer the question as to which distributions they come from or how different they actually are. A proportional hazards model can indicate how the relative risk of survival changes with a specific drug treatment, but it doesn't quantify that risk in absolute terms, since the underlying survival function remains nonparametric. Many of these issues can be dealt with using computer-intensive sensitivity analysis methods.

## 3. Conclusions

Nonparametric statistics provide useful and powerful methods to derive robust, precise and reliable parameter estimates without requiring restrictive assumptions on random variable distributions. Many well-known and widely used statistical methods are nonparametric, including OLS and instrumental variables regression methods. With the continuing advances in computational power, many statistical software packages such as STATA and SPSS have the ability to generate distribution free standard errors and parameter confidence intervals as a standard option for most statistical procedures. For many statisticians, the limitations of nonparametric statistics are a small price to pay for the confidence that the statistical results are robust and reliable, regardless of the underlying data distributions.

# References

1. Rice JA. *Mathematical Statistics and Data Analysis*. 3rd ed. Pacific Grove, CA: Duxbury Press; 2007.
2. Dhrymes P. *Econometrics: Statistical Foundations and Applications*. New York, NY: Springer-Verlag; 1974.
3. Angrist JD, Pischke JS. *Mostly Harmless Econometrics: An Empiricist's Companion*. New York, NY: Princeton University Press; 2009.
4. Hollander M, Wolfe DA. *Nonparametric Statistical Methods*. New York, NY: John Wiley & Sons Inc.; 1973.
5. Cox DR, Oakes D. *Analysis of Survival Data*. New York, NY: Chapman & Hall; 1984.
6. Yuan Y, Hay J, McCombs J. Mortality and hospitalization impacts of pharmacy consultation in ambulatory care. *Am J Manag Care*. 2003;9(1):101-112.
7. Greene W. *Econometric Analysis*. 6th ed. New York, NY: Prentice Hall; 2008.
8. Dallal GE. Nonparametric Statistics. http://www.jerrydallal.com/LHSP/npar.htm. Accessed April 29, 2013.

# Acronym Reference List

| ACRONYM | REFERENCE |
|---|---|
| ACA | Affordable Care Act of 2010 |
| ACE | angiotensin-converting enzyme |
| ACSUS | AIDS Cost and Services Utilization Survey |
| ADAS-Cog | Alzheimer's Disease Assessment Scale-Cognitive Subscale |
| ADL | activities of daily living |
| AHA | American Hospital Association |
| AHIMA | American Health Information Management Association |
| AHRQ | Agency for Healthcare Research and Quality |
| AMA | American Medical Association |
| AMIA | American Medical Informatics Association |
| APR-DRG | All Patient Refined Diagnosis Related Groups |
| APS-DRG | All Payer Severity-adjusted Diagnosis Related Groups |
| ARB | angiotensin II receptor blocker |
| ARRA | American Recovery and Reinvestment Act of 2009 |
| BASF | Beneficiary Annual Summary File (for Medicare enrollment and vital statistics) |
| BMI | body mass index |
| CAHPS | Consumer Assessment of Healthcare Providers and Systems |
| CAPI | computer-assisted personal interviewing |
| CASI | computer-assisted survey interviewing |
| CAT | computerized adaptive test |
| CCI | Chronic Condition Indicator |
| CCS | Clinical Classifications Software for ICD-9-CM or ICD-10 |
| CCW | Chronic Condition Data Warehouse |
| CDC | Centers for Disease Control and Prevention |
| CDS | clinical decision support |
| CER | comparative effectiveness research |
| CFA | confirmatory factor analysis |

*Acronym Reference List*

| ACRONYM | REFERENCE |
|---|---|
| CHD | coronary heart disease |
| CHF | congestive heart failure |
| CHMP | Committee for Human and Medicinal Products |
| CLAB | central line-associated bloodstream infection |
| CML | chronic myelogenous leukemia |
| CMS | Centers for Medicare & Medicaid Services |
| COPD | chronic obstructive pulmonary disease |
| COSTAR | Computer Stored Ambulatory Record System |
| CPI | Consumer Price Index |
| CPK | creatine phosphokinase |
| CPOE | computerized provider order entry |
| CPT | Current Procedural Terminology |
| CRC | category response curve |
| CTT | classical test theory |
| CVD | cardiovascular disease |
| DDI | drug-drug interaction |
| DEA | Drug Enforcement Administration |
| DIF | differential item functioning |
| DOD | U.S. Department of Defense |
| DQOL | **D**iabetes **Q**uality **of L**ife Measure |
| DRG | diagnosis-related group |
| DUE | drug-use evaluation |
| DUR | drug utilization review |
| ECOG | Eastern Cooperative Oncology Group |
| EDIS | emergency department information system |
| EFA | exploratory factor analysis |
| EHR | electronic health record |
| EHR-S | electronic health record system |
| EMA | European Medicines Agency |
| EMR | electronic medical record |
| EORTC | European Organisation for Research and Treatment of Cancer |

| ACRONYM | REFERENCE |
|---|---|
| EQ-5D | A standardized measure of health status developed by EuroQol |
| ER | emergency room |
| ES | effect size |
| FACT-L | Functional Assessment of Cancer Therapy-Lung |
| FIM | Functional Independence Measure |
| FS | functional status |
| FTE | full-time equivalent |
| GRC | global rating of change |
| GWAS | genome-wide association studies |
| HAI | health care-associated infection |
| HCPCS | Healthcare Common Procedure Coding System |
| HDM | health and disease management |
| HEDIS | Healthcare Effectiveness Data and Information Set |
| HELP | Help Evaluation through Logical Processing |
| HHS | U.S. Department of Health and Human Services |
| HIE | health insurance exchange |
| HIPAA | Health Insurance Portability and Accountability Act of 1996 |
| HIT | health information technology |
| HITAC | health information technology advisory committee |
| HITECH | Health Information Technology for Economic and Clinical Health Act of 2009 |
| HITRC | Health Information Technology Research Center |
| HMO | health maintenance organization |
| HOPPS | Hospital Outpatient Prospective Payment System |
| HOPPS PHP | Hospital Outpatient Prospective Payment System-Partial Hospitalization Program |
| HRQOL | health-related quality of life |
| IADL | instrumental activities of daily living |
| IC | Insurance Component |
| ICC | item characteristic curve |
| ICD-9 | International Classification of Disease, Ninth Revision |

*Acronym Reference List*

| ACRONYM | REFERENCE |
|---|---|
| ICD-9-CM | International Classification of Disease, Clinical Modification, Ninth Revision |
| IDS | integrated delivery system |
| IOM | Institute of Medicine |
| IQI | Inpatient Quality Indicators |
| IRB | institutional review board |
| IRT | item response theory |
| ISO | International Standard Organization |
| ISOQOL | **I**nternational **So**ciety for **Q**uality **o**f **L**ife Research |
| ISPOR | International Society for Pharmacoeconomics Outcome Research |
| JCAHO | Joint Commission for Accreditation of Health System Organizations |
| KBNI | Knowledge-Based Nursing Initiative |
| KID | Kids' Inpatient Database |
| LCL | lower control limit |
| LDS | limited data set |
| LPM | linear probability model |
| MAI | Medication Appropriateness Index |
| MAR | missing at random |
| MAX | Medicaid Analytic eXtract |
| MCAR | missing completely at random |
| MCID | minimally clinical important difference |
| MCO | managed care organization |
| MEDPAR | Medicare Provider and Analysis Review |
| MEPS | Medical Expenditure Panel Survey |
| MGMA | Medical Group Management Association |
| MHS | Military Health System |
| MID | minimal important difference |
| MNAR | missing not at random |
| MOS | Medical Outcomes Study |
| MPC | Medical Provider Component |

| ACRONYM | REFERENCE |
|---|---|
| MPIER | Medicare Physician Identification and Eligibility Registry |
| MPR | medication possession ratio |
| MS-DRG | Medicare Severity Diagnosis-Related Group |
| MTM | medication therapy management |
| MUE | medication use evaluation |
| NAHIT | National Alliance for Health Information Technology |
| NCBI | National Center for Biotechnology Information |
| NCHS | National Center for Health Statistics |
| NCQA | National Committee for Quality Assurance |
| NCVHS | National Committee on Vital and Health Statistics |
| NDC | National Drug Classification |
| NEDS | Nationwide Emergency Department Sample |
| NEHIS | National Employer Health Insurance Survey |
| NHANES | National Health and Nutrition Examination Survey |
| NHC | Nursing Home Component |
| NHDR | National Health Disparities Report |
| NHEA | National Health Expenditure Accounts |
| NHIS | National Health Interview Survey |
| NHLBI | National Heart, Lung, and Blood Institute (of the National Institutes of Health) |
| NHQR | National Health Quality Report |
| NIDDK | National Institute of Diabetes and Digestive and Kidney Diseases |
| NIH | National Institutes of Health |
| NIMH | National Institute of Mental Health |
| NIS | Nationwide Inpatient Sample |
| NMCES | National Medical Care Expenditure Survey |
| NNHS | National Nursing Home Survey |
| NPCD | National Patient Care Databases |
| NPI | National Provider Identifier |
| NRS | numeric rating scales |
| NSAID | nonsteroidal anti-inflammatory drug |

| ACRONYM | REFERENCE |
|---|---|
| NSCLC | non-small cell lung cancer |
| ONC | Office of the National Coordinator for Health Information Technology |
| OTC | over-the-counter |
| PCSQ | Pharmaceutical Care Satisfaction Questionnaire |
| PDE | prescription drug event |
| PDI | Pediatric Quality Indicators |
| PHR | personal health record |
| PPO | preferred provider organization |
| PQI | Prevention Quality Indicators |
| PRO | patient-reported outcome |
| PROMIS | Patient-Reported Outcomes Measurement Information System |
| PSI | Patient Safety Indicators |
| PSQ | Patient Satisfaction Questionnaire |
| PSU | primary sampling unit |
| QALY | quality-adjusted life years |
| QI | quality indicator |
| QIO | quality improvement organization |
| QOL | quality of life |
| QWB | Quality of Well-Being Scale |
| RBRVS | Resource-Based Relative Value Scale |
| RCI | Reliable Change Index |
| RCT | randomized controlled trial |
| rDUR | retrospective drug utilization review |
| REC | Regional Extension Center |
| ResDAC | Research Data Assistance Center |
| RHIO | Regional Health Information Organization |
| RIF | research identifiable file |
| RLS | restless leg syndrome |
| RMS | Regenstrief Medical Record System |
| ROC | receiver operating characteristic |

| ACRONYM | REFERENCE |
|---|---|
| RODS | Real-time Outbreak Detection System |
| RR | relative risk |
| SAF | standard analytical file |
| SASD | State Ambulatory Surgery Databases |
| SD | standard deviation |
| SEARCH | Study of the Effectiveness of Additional Reductions in Cholesterol and Homocysteine |
| SEDD | State Emergency Department Databases |
| SEER | Surveillance Epidemiology and End-Results |
| SEM | standard error of measurement |
| SF-36 | 36-item Short Form Health Survey |
| SHARe | **S**NP **H**ealth **A**ssociate **R**esource (genetic and clinical datasets) |
| SID | State Inpatient Databases |
| SIP | Sickness Impact Profile |
| SNP | single nucleotide polymorphisms |
| UCL | upper control limit |
| USHIK | US Health Information Knowledgebase |
| VA | US Department of Veterans Affairs |
| VAS | visual analogue scales |
| VCF | vertebral compression fracture |
| VistA | Veterans Health Information Systems and Technology Architecture |
| WHO | World Health Organization |
| WLQ | Work Limitations Questionnaire |
| WPAI | Work Productivity and Activity Impairment Questionnaire |

# Index

Locators followed by an "f" indicate figures; those followed by "t" indicate tables.

## A

AAA. *see* abdominal aortic aneurysm (AAA)
abdominal aortic aneurysm (AAA), 287
absenteeism (time lost from work), 188–189, 192–195
abstraction, medical record review, 76
abstraction tool, costs of developing, 76
ACA. *see* Affordable Care Act of 2010 (ACA)
ACE inhibitors, 60, 64
acquiescence response to PROs, 136
Acronym Reference List, 433–439
ACS. *see* acute coronary syndrome (ACS)
activities of daily living (ADL), 173
acute coronary syndrome (ACS), 426
ADAS-Cog. *see* Alzheimer's Disease Assessment Scale-Cognitive Subscale (ADAS-Cog)
ADHA. *see* Attention Deficit Hyperactivity Disorder (ADHD)
ADL. *see* activities of daily living (ADL)
administrative claims databases
    basic characteristics of, 6
    and benchmarking, 6, 13
    characteristics of claims datasets, 13–15
    derived from claims forms from providers, 15
    and evaluating effectiveness of HDM, 47
    for HDM program evaluation, 13
    limitations of, 24
    medical and pharmacy, 13, 16
    reliability and validity of, 28
    and use in billing and administration, 15
Affordable Care Act of 2010 (ACA), 48, 124
Agency for Healthcare Research and Quality (AHRQ)
    data available from, 7
    and gene-based technologies, 323
    and national medical expenditure surveys, 225
    and patient satisfaction, 208
    quality indicators, 117
Age-Related Eye Disease Study (AREDS), 329
age-related macular degeneration (AMD), 329
AHA. *see* American Hospital Association (AHA)
AHA Annual Survey Databases, 271
AHA Linkage Files, 271
AHIMA. *see* American Health Information Management Association (AHIMA)
AHRQ. *see* Agency for Healthcare Research and Quality (AHRQ)
AITC. *see* Austin Information Technology Center (AITC)
alleles, 324, 326
allergies, patient, 119
All Patient Refined Diagnosis Related Groups (APR-DRGs), 259
Alzheimer's Disease Assessment Scale-Cognitive Subscale (ADAS-Cog), 161
AMA. *see* American Medical Association (AMA)
Ambulatory Care Drug Database System, 245
ambulatory care-sensitive conditions, 267
ambulatory health care, 240
Ambulatory Sentinel Practice Network (ASPN), 246
AMD. *see* age-related macular degeneration (AMD)
American College of Cardiology, 151
American Health Information Management Association (AHIMA), 127
American Heart Association, 3
American Hospital Association (AHA), 257

*Index*

American Hospital Formulary Service number, 20
American Medical Association (AMA), 17, 241
American Medical Informatics Association (AMIA), 127
American Osteopathic Association, 241
American Productivity Audit and Work and Health Interview, 194
American Recovery and Reinvestment Act of 2009 (ARRA), 6, 79, 107, 124, 304
AMIA. *see* American Medical Informatics Association (AMIA)
Anatomical Therapeutic Chemical Classification System, 64
anchor-based approach
   and global rating of change (GRC), 162
   and Likert scale, 162
   and recognized end points, 161–162
anesthesia care, 119
Angina-Related Limitations at Work Questionnaire, 194
angiotensin II receptor blockers (ARBs), 60
Annual Survey of the AHA Annual Survey Database, 259, 264
antiepileptic drugs, 61
antipsychotic drugs, 64
antiretroviral drugs, 34
antithrombolytic therapy, 59–60
APR-DRGs. *see* All Patient Refined Diagnosis Related Groups (APR-DRGs)
ARBs. *see* angiotensin II receptor blockers (ARBs)
Area Resource File, 257, 259, 264
area under the curve (AUC), 424
AREDS. *see* Age-Related Eye Disease Study (AREDS)
ARRA. *see* American Recovery and Reinvestment Act of 2009 (ARRA)
Asheville Project, The, 199
ASPN. *see* Ambulatory Sentinel Practice Network (ASPN)
asthma quality-of-life questionnaire, 173–174
Attention Deficit Hyperactivity Disorder (ADHD)
   and genetic research, 327
   and Strengths and Difficulties Questionnaire (SDQ), 328
AUC. *see* area under the curve (AUC)
Austin Information Technology Center (AITC), 291
authorization requirements, 65

**B**

Back Pain Classification Scale, 134
backward elimination, method, 378
Barthel Index, 173, 326
baseline-pain levels, 137
baselines, 344
BASF. *see* Beneficiary Annual Summary File (BASF)
Bayesian adaptive trial study designs, 338
Bayesian inference, 394
Bayesian statistical methods, 430
BCDDP. *see* Breast Cancer Detection Demonstration Project (BCDDP)
Beck Depression Inventory, 134
Beneficiary Annual Summary File (BASF), 283
Beneficiary Identification and Records Locator Subsystem (BIRLS), 292
benzodiazepines, 62
beta-blockers, 48, 62, 64
bias-corrected and accelerated method, 420
billed, amount, 18–19
billing and claims denial, monitoring of, 119
binary-dependent variables, 416
Binary outcome: Coefficients of all 3 regressions, 372t
binary outcomes, 369
bioinformatics, 323
biological warfare agents, 91
biomarkers, 325
biomedical research, 360
Bioresearch Monitoring Information System (BMIS), 306
biostatistics, 409
bipolar disorder, 327
BIRLS. *see* Beneficiary Identification and Records Locator Subsystem (BIRLS)
block randomization scheme, 344

blood pressure reduction study, 379t
BMIS. *see* Bioresearch Monitoring Information System (BMIS)
body mass index assessment, 48
bootstrap
    analysis, 419
    confidence intervals, 419
    double, 420
    method, 419–420, 429
    procedure, 419
    sampling distribution, 419
bootstrap confidence intervals, 420
bootstrapped parameter, 420
bootstrapping, and error correction, 366
breast cancer, invasive, 341
Breast Cancer Detection Demonstration Project (BCDDP), 341
breast physical examination, 341
Brief Pain Inventory, 143
budget-neutrality, 5
Bureau of Labor Statistics, 41

**C**

CAHPS. *see* Consumer Assessment of Healthcare Providers and Systems (CAHPS)
caliper matching schemes, 406
cancer, 287–288
cancer sites, most common in elderly, 33
CAPI. *see* computer-assisted personal interviewing (CAPI)
cardiac catheterization study, 368–369
cardiovascular diseases (CVD), 32–33
cardiovascular risk factor levels, 341
care, convenience of, 210
Care Continuum Alliance, 3, 193, 197
case-control studies, 351
case-crossover study, 56
case-mix adjustments, 20
CASI. *see* computer-assisted survey interviewing (CASI)
CAT. *see* computerized adaptive tests (CAT)
cataracts, 329
categorical data (nominal or ordinal), 374
categorical measures, 365
categorical outcomes, 369

category response curves (CRCs), 164
CAT/IRT technology, 166
cause-effect relationship between HDM program and outcomes, 319
CCI. *see* Chronic Condition Indicator (CCI)
CCS. *see* Clinical Classifications Software (CCS)
CCW. *see* chronic condition data warehouse (CCW)
CDC. *see* Centers for Disease Control and Prevention (CDC)
CDC's Behavioral Risk Factor Surveillance System, 341
CDS. *see* clinical decision support (CDS)
CEA. *see* cost-effectiveness analyses (CEA)
CE-MRA. *see* contrast-enhanced magnetic resonance angiography (CE-MRA)
Census Bureau Research Data Center, 231
Center for Inherited Disease Research (CIDR), 328
Centers for Disease Control and Prevention (CDC)
    data available from, 7
    Division of Health Care Statistics., 239–240
    and listing of codes, 17
    and National Health Interview Survey (NHIS), 190–191
    and patient registries, 303
    and study of health and disease management, 223–224
Centers for Medicare & Medicaid Services (CMS)
    and comparing grades of health plans, 212
    and cost information, 270
    data available from, 7
    data obtained by, 224
    and documentation guidelines for medical records, 75
    and meaningful-use incentives, 108
    and Medicaid claims data, 23
    and quality improvement organization, 123
    reductions in health care costs, 4–5
    and severity-based DRG system, 20

## Index

central limit theorem, 374, 428
central line-associated bloodstream infections (CLABs), 118
CER. *see* comparative effectiveness research (CER)
Cerner Corporation, 263
CFA. *see* confirmatory factor analysis (CFA)
Charlson comorbidity index, 56
CHD. *see* coronary heart disease (CHD)
Checklist for Retrospective Database Studies—Report of the ISPOR Task Force on Retrospective Databases, 28
CHF. *see* congestive heart failure (CHF)
Children's Oncology Group, 326
Chi-square tests, 429
CHMP. *see* Committee for Human and Medicinal Products (CHMP)
chronic care management, 51
chronic condition data warehouse (CCW), 283
Chronic Condition Indicator (CCI), 269
chronic conditions
 defined, 269
 in the elderly, 282
chronic disease checklists, 244
chronic kidney disease (CKD), 356
chronic myelogenous leukemia (CML), 324
chronic obstructive pulmonary disease (COPD), 384, 402
CI. *see* confidence intervals (CI)
CIDR. *see* Center for Inherited Disease Research (CIDR)
CKD. *see* chronic kidney disease (CKD)
CLABs. *see* central line-associated bloodstream infections (CLABs)
claims
 and the coding/billing process, 40
 corrections/duplications of, 25
 duplicate, 40
 ineligible for reimbursement, 40
 zero dollar, 40
claims-based analyses, validity of, 33
claims databases
 identifying mortality, 29
 and miscoding, 41
 reviewing for consistency, 28–29
 reviewing for missing data, 28–29
 sources of, 22
classical test theory (CTT)
 and development of PRO instruments, 152
 item driven, 163
 and psychometric issues, 163
 scale driven, 163
Clinical Classifications Software (CCS), 265
clinical decision support (CDS), 99
clinical documentation, 74
clinical evidence, hierarchy of, 336
clinical trial data, 8
Clozaril National Registry (CNR), 302
CML. *see* chronic myelogenous leukemia (CML)
CMOP. *see* Consolidated Mail Outpatient Pharmacy (CMOP)
CMS. *see* Centers for Medicare and Medicaid Services (CMS)
CNR. *see* Clozaril National Registry (CNR)
coagulation and platelet function, 326
codes, use of, 15
codes of diagnosis, 16
coding errors, 25
Cohen's effect size (ES), 162
cohorts, defined, 350
cohort studies, 351–352
coinsurance amounts, 19
cold deck imputation method, 395
colorectal cancer screening, 48
commercial claims, 22
Committee for Human and Medicinal Products (CHMP), 142
Common uses of EHR data, 96t
comorbid conditions, 19–20
comorbidities, assessing, 56
comorbidity software programs, 265
comparative effectiveness research (CER), 298–299
compliance tracking, 84
complications, 19–20, 24
composite imputation methods, 396
computer-assisted personal interviewing (CAPI), 230

computer-assisted survey interviewing (CASI), 230
computerized adaptive tests (CAT), 166
Computerized Patient Record System (CPRS), 123, 291
computerized provider order entry (CPOE), 99
Computer Stored Ambulatory Record System (COSTAR), 122
conceptual framework and DURs, 58
concomitant medications and confounding factors, 389
condition-specific procedures, 31
confidence intervals, 419
confidence intervals (CI), 362
confidence limits, 362
confirmatory factor analysis (CFA), 158–159
confounding factors
    of concomitant medications, 389
    defined, 388
    and drug-drug interactions (DDIs), 390
    and effect modification, 390
    exposure and effect, 389
    by indication, 389
    known, 390
    and random allocation, 344
Congenital Defects registry, 303
congestive heart failure (CHF), 409
Congressional Budget Office, 126
Consolidated Mail Outpatient Pharmacy (CMOP), 293
Consolidated Standards Of Reporting Trials (CONSORT), 309
CONSORT. *see* Consolidated Standards Of Reporting Trials (CONSORT)
Consortium Data Access Committee, 329
Consumer Assessment of Healthcare Providers and Systems (CAHPS), 208
Consumer Price Index (CPI), 41
continuity of care, 210
continuous outcomes, 374–375
contrast-enhanced magnetic resonance angiography (CE-MRA), 402
control chart, components of, 116f
control group, 343
controlled experiment, 347

controlled substances, use of, 293
controlled trials, randomized. *see* randomized controlled trials (RCTs)
copayments, 19
COPD. *see* chronic obstructive pulmonary disease (COPD)
core data elements, 258
coronary heart disease (CHD), 59, 350
coronary heart disease risk, 341
correlation matrix, 377
COSTAR. *see* Computer Stored Ambulatory Record System (COSTAR)
cost attribution of illnesses, 39–40
cost-benefit of EHRs, 102
cost-containment strategies, 3
cost-effectiveness analyses (CEA), 294
cost-effectiveness analysis, 316
*Cost Impact of Diagnostic Imaging for Lower Extremity Peripheral Vascular Occlusive Disease*, 402
cost-of-illness
    assessing, 20
    studies, 38, 41
cost of or charge for a service, 18–19
costs, annual, 42
Cost-to-Charge Ratio (CCR) Files, 270
Council on Clinical Classifications, 17
counterfactual, establishment of, 5
Cox proportional hazards regression model, 382–384
Cox regression analysis, 355
CPI. *see* Consumer Price Index (CPI)
CPOE. *see* computerized provider order entry (CPOE)
CPRS. *see* Computerized Patient Record System (CPRS)
CPT. *see* Current Procedural Terminology (CPT)
Cramér–Rao information inequality, 427
CRCs. *see* category response curves (CRCs)
Cronbach's alpha, 156
cross-sectional studies, 365
cross-validation, 425
crosswalk, between systems, 93

*Index*

CTG. *see* National Cancer Institute of Canada (NCIC) Clinical Trials Group (CTG) QOL Committee
CTT. *see* classical test theory (CTT)
cumulative survival probability, 382–383
Current Population Survey, 190, 231–232
Current Procedural Terminology (CPT)
    category I codes: procedure or services, 17
    category II codes: performance measurement, 17
    category III codes: temporary, for new and emerging technologies, 17
    codes, 15–16
    factors for estimation, 19
    for outpatient procedures, 256, 292
    used to calculate expenditures, 19
CVD. *see* cardiovascular diseases (CVD)
cytogenetic testing, 324

**D**

Dartmouth COOP Functional Health Assessment Charts, 173
dashboards, 117
data, missing, 393–394
data mapping technologies, third-party, 96
Data Use Agreement (DUA), 259, 285
dates of service, 17–18
days' supply of medication dispensed, 16
DDIs. *see* drug-drug interactions (DDIs)
DDS. *see* VA Decision Support System (DSS)
death, cause of, 3
Decentralized Hospital Computer Program (DHCP), 123
decision-making support, clinical, 123
deductibles, 19
Defined Daily Doses, 64
Delphi Method, 144
demographics, basic, 29
demonstration projects
    defined, 340
    examples of, 341
Department of Health and Human Services (HHS), 112, 123, 225–226, 298
Department of Veterans Affairs (VA), 230
Department of Veterans Affairs (VA) Health Care System, 290
Determinants of outcomes and outcomes evaluated in demonstration projects, 342t
DHCP. *see* Decentralized Hospital Computer Program (DHCP)
diabetes, and renoprotective therapy, 60
Diabetes Complications Severity Index, 385
Diabetes Quality of Life (DQOL), 161, 173
diagnosis
    misleading, 31
    primary, 19
    uncertain, 31
    up-coding of, 32
diagnosis code, primary, 17
Diagnosis-Related Group (DRG)
    associated relative weight of, 19
    for identifying specific health care service use, 15
*Diagnostic and Statistical Manual of Mental Disorders*, 327
dialysis, chronic, 355
DIF. *see* differential item functioning (DIF)
differential item functioning (DIF), 165
digital subtraction angiography (DSA), 402
direct test, 384
disability, cause of, 3
discharge abstracts, 257
discharge diagnosis codes, 24
discrete outcomes, 365
disease
    chronic, 3
    prediction techniques, 51
    prevalence of, 305–306
    prevalence, irregularities in, 92
    registries, 28
    staging, 259
disease management, 3
Disease Management Association of America. *see* Care Continuum Alliance
disease progression, study of, 15
disease registries, 33–34
disease-specific instruments, 133–134, 175
disease state management (DSM), 211
distribution-based approach

and Cohen's effect size (ES), 161–162
and Reliable Change Index (RCI), 162
and standard deviation (SD), 162
and standard deviation error of measurement (SEM), 162
distribution-free statistical estimates, 428
documentation, incomplete, 25
documentation by exception rule, 76
DOD. *see* US Department of Defense (DOD)
dosing regimen and days supply, 21
double blind trial, 345–346
DQOL. *see* Diabetes Quality of Life (DQOL)
DRG. *see* Diagnosis-Related Group (DRG)
drug dictionary, 26
drug-disease contraindications, 62
drug-drug interactions (DDIs)
    as confounding factor, 390
    as contributing factor, 62
    and OTC medications, 62
drug regimens and patient adherence, 36
drug-use evaluation (DUE), 54
Drug Utilization, 66t
drug utilization information, 25
drug utilization reviews (DURs)
    defined, 53
    mandating of, 54
    scope of, 53–54
*drug visits*, 245
DSA. *see* digital subtraction angiography (DSA)
DSM. *see* disease state management (DSM)
DUA. *see* Data Use Agreement (DUA)
dual coverage, 35
dual eligibles, 24
DUE. *see* drug-use evaluation (DUE)
DURs. *see* drug utilization reviews (DURs)

**E**
Eastern Cooperative Oncology Group (ECOG), 160
EBM. *see* Evidence-Based Medicine (EBM)
ECHO measurements, 209, 211
ECOG. *see* Eastern Cooperative Oncology Group (ECOG)
econometrics, 409
ED. *see* emergency department (ED)

EDIS. *see* emergency department information systems (EDIS)
ED/Rx at discharge, 245
education programs, 64
EFA. *see* exploratory factor analysis (EFA)
Effectiveness of influenza vaccination to reduce mortality, 354t
EHR. *see* electronic health records (EHR)
EHR-S. *see* electronic health record systems (EHR-S)
electrocardiographic information, 325
electronic billing, 88
electronic clinical reminder system, 295
electronic data
    and disease management, 84
    and documentation and care coordination, 85
    in hospital emergency rooms, 89
    and improved quality of care, 89
    and interoperability, 84
    and issues of data protection, 84
    and issues of privacy, 84
    and reduction of cost, 89
    and research applications, 85
    and safety and disease surveillance, 85
    and tracking patient triage information, 89
electronic health records (EHR)
    barriers to adoption and use, 107
    benefits and limitations of, 98
    choosing the optimal system, 108
    closed, 85
    coding of symptoms, diagnoses, procedures, and treatments, 100
    comprehensive cost analysis, 126
    and considerations for providers, 95
    cost of, 7
    cost versus benefit, 102
    and data security, 125
    and declining compensation from Medicare, 112–113
    defined, 79–80
    direct subsidization of, 124
    and disease surveillance, 91
    ease of use, 109–110
    and economic barriers, 127

and errors, 95
establishment of, 7
and health research, 88
and identifying candidates for clinical trials, 90
increase in cost of care, 127
lack of standards and uniformity in, 308
limitations of, 6
meaningful-use incentives, 108–109
and the medical chart, 85
Medicare and Medicaid incentives for meaningful use of, 124
menu-driven fields, 101
methodological issues, 98
open, 86–92
patient access to, 86
patient portal, 86
and patient registries, 303
and patient safety, 90
potential of, 73
provider and staff training, 109–110
and real-time application, 115
replacing paper records, 76
and research applications, 92–95
specialized templates, 99
standardization, 101
standardization of data categories, 99
system interoperability, 101
system limitations, 107
technical assistance with, 124
and templates (electronic forms), 109
total costs of, 108
use in evaluations of HDM programs, 6
in the Veterans Health Administration (VHA), 294
electronic health record systems (EHR-S)
compatible software and hardware, 104
functional specifications of, 80–81
implementation of, 122
and integrated delivery systems (IDSs), 104
network, 80
and Regional Health Information Organizations (RHIOs), 104
electronic medical records (EMR), 79–80

Electronic Surveillance System for the Early Notification of Community-based Epidemics, 91–92
eligibility files, 21
EMA. see European Medicines Agency (EMA)
emergency care, availability of, 210
emergency department (ED), 240, 365
emergency department information systems (EDIS), 117
emotional role limitations, 190
empirical data, 360
employer-based health insurance, 229
employment status, 189
employment status, change in, 191
EMR. see electronic medical records (EMR)
Endicott Work Productivity Scale, 194
endogenous variables, 413
end-stage renal disease (ESRD)
and chronic dialysis, 355
and genetic research, 327
and Medicare, 281
enrollment data, 34
EORTC. see European Organisation for Research and Treatment of Cancer (EORTC)
epidemiologic database, 302
epidemiology, 255
episodes of care, 35
EQ-5D. see European Health Related Quality of Life (EuroQol)
ERIQA. see European Regulatory Issues on Quality of Life Assessment (ERIQA)
errors, random in PROs, 152–153
error term assumption, 415
ERT. see electronic health records (EHR)
ES. see Cohen's effect size (ES)
ESRD. see end-stage renal disease (ESRD)
ethical issues, 307
European Health Related Quality of Life (EuroQol), 190
European Medicines Agency (EMA), 141, 153, 301
European Organisation for Research and Treatment of Cancer (EORTC), 173
European Regulatory Issues on Quality of Life Assessment (ERIQA), 153

EuroQol. *see* European Health Related Quality of Life (EuroQol)
EuroQol instrument, 175
event files, individual, 231
Evidence-Based Medicine (EBM), 335
evolution of medicine, adjusting for, 94
Examples of discrete outcomes, 372t
experiments, 347
explanatory power, 423
exploratory factor analysis (EFA), 158–159
external validity, 28–29
extremity of response to PROs, 136

**F**

FACT-L. *see* Functional Assessment of Cancer Therapy-Lung (FACT-L)
factor analysis, 144, 158–159
FDA. *see* Food and Drug Administration (FDA)
feedback from patients, 120
fee-for-service plan, 22
FHS. *see* Framingham Heart Study (FHS)
FIM. *see* Functional Independence Measure (FIM)
financial return on investment and outcomes, 46
focus groups, 144
Food and Drug Administration (FDA)
 and active ingredients list, 64
 criteria for PRO instruments, 153
 and patient registries, 301
 PRO guidelines, 141
formularies, 57
formulary evaluation, 15
forward selection method, 377
Framingham Heart Study (FHS), 325, 350
Framingham SHARe, 325
free text entry and EHRs, 101
free text fields and EHRs, 101
FS. *see* functional status (FS)
FTE. *see* full-time equivalent (FTE)
full-time equivalent (FTE), 102
Functional Assessment of Cancer Therapy-Lung (FACT-L), 162
Functional Independence Measure (FIM), 173

functional limitation instruments that assess work outcomes, 201t
functional limitations in the workplace, 190
functional status (FS), 173

**G**

GAIN. *see* Genetic Association Information Network (GAIN)
ganglioneuroblastoma, 326
gene-based diagnostic and therapeutic technologies, 323–330
generic drugs
 and cost containment, 60
 defined, 60
 four main considerations of use, 60–61
 and legal requirements of state, 61
 and provider training, 64
Genetic Association Information Network (GAIN), 327
genetic information, 8
genetics
 alleles, 324
 and Attention Deficit Hyperactivity Disorder (ADHD), 327
 bcr-abl gene, 324
 and cancer, 326
 databases, 324
 and the DNA index, 326
 and eye disease, 329
 gene-based diagnostic and therapeutic technologies, 323–330
 genetics databases, 323–330
 genetic variants and disease, 323
 genomewide association studies (GWAS), 324–325
 and mental health, 327
 and the MYCN oncogene copy number, 326
 and Parkinson's Disease (PD), 328–329
 and polymorphisms of genes, 326
 research, 323–330
 and strokes, 326
 testing, 324
Genetics of Kidneys in Diabetes study, 327
genomewide association studies (GWAS), 324–325

*Index*

Genome-Wide Association Study of Neuroblastoma, 326
genotype frequencies, 327
genotype intensity data, 327
genotypic data, 329
GEP. *see* Good Epidemiological Practice (GEP)
GERD symptoms, 398
Glasgow Coma Scale, 118–119
Glasgow Outcome Scale, 326
global rating of change (GRC), 162
Good Epidemiological Practice (GEP), 309
Good Practices Working Group, 141
Google Health, 86
grace period, medication possession ratio, 38
GRADE. *see* Grading of Recommendations Assessment, Development, and Evaluation (GRADE)
Grading of Recommendations Assessment, Development, and Evaluation (GRADE), 309
GRC. *see* global rating of change (GRC)
greedy matching schemes, 406
grouper approach, 35
GWAS. *see* genomewide association studies (GWAS)

**H**

HAIs. *see* health care-associated infections (HAIs)
Hamilton Depression Rating Scale (HDRS), 319
Hawthorne effect, 344
hazard function, 382
hazard rates, 382
HCPCS. *see* Healthcare Common Procedure Coding System (HCPCS) codes
HCUP. *see* Healthcare Cost and Utilization Project (HCUP)
HCUP Cost-to-Charge Ratio (CCR) Files, 270
HDM. *see* health and disease management (HDM)
HDRS. *see* Hamilton Depression Rating Scale (HDRS)
Health and Disease Management (HDM)
  and avoiding preventable complications, 53
  and benchmarking, 53
  clinical and economic outcomes, 213
  and clinical outcomes, 381
  cost-benefit analysis of, 214
  and electronic health records (EHR), 84
  and electronic health record systems (EHR-S), 84
  and electronic medical records (EMR), 84
  evaluation of, 13
  and genetics databases, 8
  and health-related quality of life (HRQL), 172
  identifying medical conditions targeted for program, 38
  impact on health care costs, 47
  and improved patient care, 48
  and improvement in quality of care, 3
  and improving mortality rates, 53
  and incentives for providers, 48
  and limitation of claims, 49
  medical and pharmacy claims, 200
  and Medicare databases, 285–288
  meta-analysis of, 49
  and natural experiments, 347–348
  and nurse education, 360
  and patient registries, 298–309
  and patient-reported outcomes (PROs), 7
  and patient satisfaction, 213
  and people at risk, 423
  and pharmacoeconomics, 374
  programs for the chronically ill, 177
  reducing health care costs, 53
  and reducing morbidity, 53
  and reliable results, 419
  and the scope of claims databases, 28–42
  and survival analysis, 381
  and trigger event, 50
  and Veterans Health Administration (VHA), 294
  and work outcomes, 180
Health and Labor Questionnaire, 194
Health and Productivity Questionnaire, 194

Health and Work Performance
    Questionnaire, 200
Health and Work Questionnaire, 194
health care-associated infections (HAIs),
    232
Healthcare Common Procedure Coding
    System (HCPCS) codes, 32
Healthcare Cost and Utilization Project
    (HCUP)
    databases of, 257
    explained, 255
    HCUP database query system, 271
    HCUP database relationships, 278f
    HCUP databases, primary features of,
        279t–280t
    HCUP Fact Books, 269
    HCUP Facts and Figures, 269
    HCUP Statistical Briefs, 269
    and hospitalizations and readmissions,
        256
    longitudinal database on hospital care in
        US, 226
    and mortality information, 256
    and the potential for selection bias, 256
health care information technology (HIT),
    122
health care interventions, evaluations of, 4
health care plans, selection of, 207–208
health care quality
    clinical outcomes, 208–209
    components of, 209
    patient satisfaction as a measurement of,
        208
health care utilization measures, 48
Health Economics Research Center (HERC),
    293
health improvement interventions, 45
health index approach, 176
health index or health profile, 172, 175
health information exchanges, 104
Health Information Technology (HIT), 6
Health Information Technology for Economic
    and Clinical Health Act (HITECH), 4, 79,
    107
health insurance administrative claims data.
    see administrative claims databases

Health Insurance Cost, 228–229
health insurance eligibility, 21
Health Insurance Portability and
    Accountability Act of 1996 (HIPAA), 137,
    257, 291, 306
Health IT Research Center, 112
Health Maintenance Organizations (HMO),
    206, 319
health-related productivity loss, 188–189
Health-Related Productivity Questionnaire
    Diary, 194
health-related quality of life (HRQOL)
    clinically significant changes in, 174
    and functional status, 172
    and instruments used to assess, 141
    observable and nonobservable, 172
    and patient registries, 303
    and the progression health conditions,
        178
    and response shift, 178–179
    self-rated or proxy-rated, 180
    types of measurements to determine,
        176
Health Resources and Services
    Administration, 259
health services utilization patterns, 411
healthy user effect, 389
Heckit model. see Heckman model
Heckman estimator, 401
Heckman model, 416
Heckman selection bias methods, 390, 400
Heckprob model, 416
Heckprob regression, 418
HELP. see Help Evaluation through Logical
    Processing (HELP)
Help Evaluation through Logical Processing
    (HELP), 122
hematologist, 417
hepatitis C infection and antiviral treatment,
    60
HERC. see Health Economics Research Center
    (HERC)
heteroscedasticity, 400
HHS. see Department of Health and Human
    Services (HHS); US Department of Health
    and Human Services (HHS)

*Index*

HHS Interagency Work Group, 270
hierarchy of evidence in clinical trials, 307
high blood pressure, controlling, 48
HIPAA. *see* Health Insurance Portability and Accountability Act of 1996 (HIPAA)
HIT. *see* health care information technology (HIT); Health Information Technology (HIT)
HITECH. *see* Health Information Technology for Economic and Clinical Health Act (HITECH)
HIV-AIDS, 34
HIV and AIDS Costs and Use, 226
HMOs. *see* Health Maintenance Organizations (HMO)
hold-out method of validation, 425
homogeneity and internal consistency, 156
HOPPS. *see* Hospital Outpatient Prospective Payment System (HOPPS)
HOPPS–Partial Hospitalization Program (HOPPS PHP), 283
HOPPS PHP. *see* HOPPS–Partial Hospitalization Program (HOPPS PHP)
Hosmer-Lemeshow test, 424
Hospital Compare Website, 212
hospital discharge databases, 255, 271
hospitalization costs, computation of, 20
hospitalization episodes, 19
Hospital Outpatient Prospective Payment System (HOPPS), 283
hot deck imputation method, 395
HRQL instruments, 181t–182t
HRQOL. *see* health-related quality of life (HRQOL)
Human Genome Project, 323
hypothesis, 360
  statistical significance of, 361–362
  testing procedures, 361

**I**

IADL. *see* instrumental activities of daily living (IADL)
ICC. *see* Item Characteristic Curve (ICC)
ICD-9-CM. *see* Current Procedural Terminology (CPT)
ICD-9-CM codes, 231
ICD-9 codes. *see* Current Procedural Terminology (CPT)
ICERs. *see* incremental cost-effectiveness ratios (ICERs)
identifier mismatches, 29
IMAGE. *see* International Multi-Center ADHD Genetics (IMAGE)
implantable insulin pumps, 398
Important elements in a retrospective study design, 357t
imputation methods
  cold deck imputation method, 395
  composite imputation methods, 396
  hot deck imputation method, 395
  mean imputation method, 394–395
  multiple imputation methods, 396
  regression imputation method, 395
  stochastic regression imputation, 396
incidence of disease, 32
incidental selection, 399
incremental cost-effectiveness ratios (ICERs), 420
infections, hospital acquired, 24
inflation, effects of, 41, 47
influenza vaccine effectiveness, 352–353
information resources management (IRM), 291
inpatient claims, 19
Inpatient Quality Indicators (IQI), 266
Institute of Medicine (IOM), 77, 81, 123
Institutional Review Board (IRB), 291, 316
instrumental activities of daily living (IADL), 173
instrumental variables estimator (IVE), 412
instrumental variables method, strengths and limitations of, 409
insulin infusion protocol, 118
integrated care management, 401
integration of PHRs and EHRs, pros and cons, 86
integrity checks, 28
internal validity, 28–29
International Classification of Diseases, 15–16
International HapMap Project, 323

International Multi-Center ADHD Genetics (IMAGE), 328
International Neuroblastoma Pathology Classification, 326
International Neuroblastoma Staging System, 326
International Restless Legs Syndrome Study Group (IRLS), 148
International Society for Pharmacoeconomics and Outcomes Research (ISPOR), 141, 153, 298, 309
International Society for Quality of Life (ISOQOL), 141
International Standard Organization (ISO), 79
inter-rater reliability, 78
interviews, face-to-face, 144
inverse Mills ratio, 400, 416
IOM. see Institute of Medicine (IOM)
Iowa Priority Prescription Savings Program, 62
IQI. see Inpatient Quality Indicators (IQI)
IRB. see institutional review board (IRB); Institutional Review Board (IRB)
IRLS. see International Restless Legs Syndrome Study Group (IRLS)
IRM. see information resources management (IRM)
IRT. see item response theory (IRT)
ischemic stroke, 287
Ischemic Stroke Genetics Study (ISGS), 325
ISGS. see Ischemic Stroke Genetics Study (ISGS)
ISO. see International Standard Organization (ISO)
ISOQOL. see International Society for Quality of Life (ISOQOL)
ISPOR. see International Society for Pharmacoeconomics and Outcomes Research (ISPOR)
ISPOR PRO Task Force Reports, 141–142
ISPOR's PRO Good Research Practices Task Force, 148
Item Characteristic Curve (ICC), 164
item response theory (IRT)
   and category response curves (CRCs), 164
   and dichotomous items (yes/no), 164
   explained, 152
   and Item Characteristic Curve (ICC), 164
   and item difficulty, 164
   and item discrimination, 164
   linking (equating), 165
   and measurement precision, 164
IVE. see instrumental variables estimator (IVE)

**J**

JEHRI. see Joint Electronic Records Interoperability (JEHRI)
Joint Commission, The, 208
Joint Electronic Records Interoperability (JEHRI), 128
Joint Workforce Task Force, 127

**K**

Kaplan-Meier Curves, 387f
Kaplan-Meier method, 382–383
KBNI. see Knowledge-Based Nursing Initiative (KBNI)
KID. see Kids' Inpatient Database (KID)
Kids' Inpatient Database (KID), 258–260
KID Trends Files, 271
Knowledge-Based Nursing Initiative (KBNI), 119
knowledge translation, 323, 330
Kolmogorov-Smirnov test, 429–430

**L**

lack of clinical information, 24
LCL. see lower control limits (LCL)
LDS. see limited data set (LDS)
LDS data available from CMS, 283t–284t
Likert scale, 162, 175, 211
limited data set (LDS), 281
linear probability function, 366
linear probability model (LPM), 365
linear regression models, 375
linear regression models, multiple, 375–376
logistic method, 424
logistic regression, 405
log-log plot, 384

*Index*

log-rank test, 383
long-term care nursing units, 230
lower control limits (LCL), 115
LPM. *see* linear probability model (LPM)

**M**

Mahalanobis metric matching schemes, 406
MAI. *see* Medication Appropriateness Index (MAI)
major depressive disorder (MDD), 319
malpractice expenses, 19
mammography, 341
managed care organization, 22
managed care organizations (MCOs), 206
managed care plans and standards of practice, 50
MAR. *see* Missing at random (MAR)
matching schemes, 391, 406
mathematical model and multiple confounders, 391
MAX. *see* Medicaid Analytic eXtract (MAX) files
maximum likelihood estimation (MLE), 367, 427
MCAR. *see* Missing completely at random (MCAR)
MCID. *see* minimally clinical important difference (MCID)
MCOs. *see* managed care organizations (MCOs)
MDD. *see* major depressive disorder (MDD)
MDE. *see* Minimum Data Elements (MDE)
mean imputation method, 394
measurable variables and criterion validity, 159
measured covariates, 406
measurement error created by social desirability, 136
mechanisms of missing data, 394
Medicaid
    coverage provided, 23
    data, 24
    defined, 23
    and drug coverage, 23
    and federal government, 23
    and state governments, 23

Medicaid Analytic eXtract (MAX) files, 23
Medicaid claims data, 22
Medicaid-specific issues, 23–24
medical claims
    commonly used, 28
    discontinuous, 34
    purpose of, 20
medical conditions, direct and indirect costs of, 38–39
medical errors, reduction of, 122
Medical Expenditure Panel Survey (MEPS)
    Household Component (HC), 227–228
    Insurance Component (IC), 227–229
    limitations of, 235–236
    Medical Provider Component (MPC), 227, 229–230
    Nursing Home Component (NHC), 227, 230
    purpose of, 225
    strengths of data, 234–235
    usage of data, 232–234
Medical Group Management Association (MGMA), 102
medical home care, 125
medical liability, 75
Medical Outcomes Study (MOS), 133
Medical Outcomes Trust (MOT), 153
Medical Outcome Study 36-Item Short Form (SF-36), 190
Medical Record, The (TMR), 122
medical records
    abstracted, 255
    abstraction process, 78
    in ambulatory settings, 74
    cost of, 76
    and data quality, 77
    electronic, 73
    to evaluate clinical quality and effectiveness, 75
    functions of, 74
    in hospital settings, 74
    and illegible handwriting, 77
    levels of documentation, 77
    and multiple providers, 78
    other uses of, 74–75
    paper, 73, 76

and research, 76
medical surveillance, 84
Medicare
    Advantage Plans, 282
    claims, 33
    databases of, 281
    data quality and availability, 288–289
    eligible population, 282
    explanation of four part system, 281–282
    explained, 281
    and Health and Disease Management (HDM), 285–288
    limited datasets, 283
    Part D, 57
    and reduction of costs, 4–5
    research information packets, 285
    retrospective use of databases, 286–287
    types of data available, 282–285
Medicare and Medicaid beneficiaries, 23
Medicare and Medicaid patients, physicians refusal to see, 113
Medicare enrollment and vital statistics files, 283
Medicare Health Support (MHS), 286
Medicare Health Support Organizations (MHSOs), 286
Medicare Physician Identification and Eligibility Registry (MPIER), 283
Medicare Provider and Analysis Review (MEDPAR) file, 283, 287–289
Medicare Severity Diagnosis Related Groups (MS-DRG), 265
Medicare Severity DRG (MS-DRG) codes, 20
Medication Appropriateness Index (MAI), 58
medication possession ratio (MPR), 36–37, 365
medications
    adherence to, 365
        during hospitalization and lack of information, 25
    overutilization of, 59
    underutilization of, 59
medication therapy management (MTM), 211, 409–410
medication-use evaluation (MUE), 54
medication utilization analysis, 59–60

medicine, defensive, 75
Medline searches, 255
MEDPAR. see Medicare Provider and Analysis Review (MEDPAR) file
MEPS. see Medical Expenditure Panel Survey (MEPS)
MEPSnet, 231
MEPS online workbook, 232
meta-analyses of RCTs, 336
metropolitan statistical area (MSA), 244
MGMA. see Medical Group Management Association (MGMA)
MHS. see Medicare Health Support (MHS); Military Health System (MHS)
MHSOs. see Medicare Health Support Organizations (MHSOs)
microsatellite markers, 325
Microsoft Amalga Unified Intelligence System, 117
MID. see minimal important difference (MID)
Migraine Disability Assessment Questionnaire, 194
Migraine Work and Productivity Loss Questionnaire, 194
Military Health System (MHS), 348
minimal important difference (MID)
    and anchor-based approach, 161–162
    and distribution-based approach, 161–162
    explained, 160–161
    and responsiveness, 161
minimally clinical important difference (MCID), 174
Mini Mental Status Exam, 135
Minimum Data Elements (MDE), 340
missing at random (MAR), 394
missing completely at random (MCAR), 394
missing confounder, 407
missing not at random (MNAR), 394
MLE. see maximum likelihood estimation (MLE)
MNAR. see Missing not at random (MNAR)
model accuracy in outcomes, 424
model performance, 425
model specification, 399
model validation, 423

Index

molecular biology, 323
monetary incentive for research participants, 137–138
Monte-Carlo method, 419
mortality rates, high, 22
mortality study, 30
MOS. see Medical Outcomes Study (MOS)
MOT. see Medical Outcomes Trust (MOT)
MPIER. see Medicare Physician Identification and Eligibility Registry (MPIER)
MPR. see medication possession ratio (MPR)
MSA. see metropolitan statistical area (MSA)
MS-DRG. see Medicare Severity DRG (MS-DRG) codes
MTM. see medication therapy management (MTM)
MUE. see medication-use evaluation (MUE)
multicollinearity, 377
multinomial logit, 370
Multinomial outcomes: Coefficients and their p-values, 373t
multiple endogenous variables, 412
multiple imputation methods, 396
Multiple regression model example, 380t
multiple-sourced claims, 22
multistage probability design, 241
multivariable regression analyses, 55
multivariate regression, 366
myelodysplastic syndrome/myelodysplasia (MDS), 303
My HealtheVet, 86
myocardial infarction, 59, 325, 425

**N**

NAHIT. see National Alliance for Health Information Technology (NAHIT)
NAMCS. see National Ambulatory Medical Care Survey (NAMCS)
NAMCS and NHAMCS surveys
   access to, 244
   cross-sectional data, 245–247
   limitations of, 247–248
   privacy and confidentiality issues, 243
   and quality of care, 246
   strengths of, 247
   voluntary participation, 244

National Alliance for Health Information Technology (NAHIT), 80
National Ambulatory Medical Care Survey (NAMCS)
   explained, 239–240
   and systematic random samples, 241
National Cancer Institute of Canada (NCIC) Clinical Trials Group (CTG) QOL Committee, 393
National Cancer Institute's Surveillance Epidemiology and End-Results (SEER), 33
National Center for Biotechnology Information's (NCBI) database of Genotypes and Phenotypes (dbGaP), 325
National Center for Health Statistics (NCHS)
   databases of, 239
   and National Health Interview Survey (NHIS), 190
National Committee for Quality Assurance (NCQA), 48, 208
National Committee on Vital and Health Statistics (NCVHS), 298
National Death Index, 30
National Drug Classification (NDC)
   code recycling, 32
   codes, 15
   and information on drug dispensed, 20
National Employer Health Insurance Survey (NEHIS), 228
National Eye Institute, 329
National Health and Nutrition Examination Survey (NHANES), 242
National Healthcare Disparities Report (NHDR), 270
National Health Disparities Report (NHDR), 225
National Health Expenditure Accounts (NHEA), 230–231
National Health Interview Survey (NHIS), 190
National Health Provider Inventory, 230
National Health Quality Report (NHQR), 225–226, 270
National Heart, Lung, and Blood Institute (NHLBI), 324–325

National Hospital Ambulatory Medical Care Survey (NHAMCS)
  defined, 242
  estimates of medication use in hospital ambulatory care services, 241
National Hospital Discharge Survey (NHDS), 243, 263
National Institute of Diabetes and Digestive and Kidney Diseases (NIDDK), 327
National Institutes of Health (NIH), 6, 141, 163, 224
National Library of Medicine, 104
National Medical Care Expenditure Survey (NMCES), 226
National Nursing Home Survey (NNHS), 240
National Patient Care Databases (NPCD), 290, 291
National Provider Identifiers (NPIs), 18
National Survey of Ambulatory Surgery (NSAS), 242
Nationwide Emergency Department Sample (NEDS), 258–260
Nationwide Inpatient Sample (NIS), 258
natural experiments
  explained, 347
  and natural or manmade disasters, 347
  retrospective, 347–348
NCHS. see National Center for Health Statistics (NCHS)
NCHS surveys and data systems, 250t–251t
NCIC. see National Cancer Institute of Canada (NCIC) Clinical Trials Group (CTG) QOL Committee
NCQA. see National Committee for Quality Assurance (NCQA)
NCVHS. see National Committee on Vital and Health Statistics (NCVHS)
NDC. see National Drug Classification (NDC)
NDC code recycling, 26
nearest available matching schemes, 406
NECOSAD-II. see Netherlands Cooperative Study on the Adequacy of Dialysis-2 (NECOSAD-II)
NEDS. see Nationwide Emergency Department Sample (NEDS)

NEHIS. see National Employer Health Insurance Survey (NEHIS)
Netherlands Cooperative Study on the Adequacy of Dialysis-2 (NECOSAD-II), 355
neuroblastoma, 326
NHAMCS. see National Hospital Ambulatory Medical Care Survey (NHAMCS)
NHANES. see National Health and Nutrition Examination Survey (NHANES)
NHDR. see National Health Disparities Report (NHDR)
NHDS. see National Hospital Discharge Survey (NHDS)
NHEA. see National Health Expenditure Accounts (NHEA)
NHIS. see National Health Interview Survey (NHIS)
NHLBI. see National Heart, Lung, and Blood Institute (NHLBI)
NHQR. see National Health Quality Report (NHQR)
NIDDK. see National Institute of Diabetes and Digestive and Kidney Diseases (NIDDK)
NIH. see National Institutes of Health (NIH)
NIH Stroke Scale, 326
NIS. see Nationwide Inpatient Sample (NIS)
NIS Trends Supplemental files, 259, 271
nitroglycerin, 64
NMCES. see National Medical Care Expenditure Survey (NMCES)
NNHS. see National Nursing Home Survey (NNHS)
nonidentifiable data available from CMS, 284t–285t
nonidentifiable data files, 281
nonlinear function probability models, 367
nonparametric distributional assumptions, 427
nonparametric estimates, 428–429
nonrandom treatment assignment, 402
nonresponse in survey research, 393
nonsmall cell lung cancer (NSCLC), 306
nonsteroidal anti-inflammatory drugs (NSAIDs)

*Index*

and cardiovascular disease, 56
and colorectal cancer, 57
and gastrointestinal bleeding, 56
prescribing patterns of, 56
selective versus nonselective, 56
NPCD. *see* National Patient Care Databases (NPCD)
NPIs. *see* National Provider Identifiers (NPIs)
NRS. *see* numeric rating scales (NRS)
NSAIDs. *see* nonsteroidal anti-inflammatory drugs (NSAIDs)
NSAS. *see* National Survey of Ambulatory Surgery (NSAS)
NSCLC. *see* nonsmall cell lung cancer (NSCLC)
null hypothesis, 360
numerical data, 374
numeric rating scales (NRS), 143
Nursing Home Survey, 230

**O**

observable confounder, 336
observational analysis, 299
observational data, 8
observational studies, 76
observational study data, 319
observation sample, 382
odds ratios, 351, 368
Office of the National Coordinator for Health Information Technology (ONC), 107, 112, 123
Omnibus Budget Reconciliation Act, 54
ONC. *see* Office of the National Coordinator for Health Information Technology (ONC)
oncologist, 417
oncology, 324
OPAT. *see* Outpatient Parenteral Antimicrobial Therapy (OPAT)
OPC. *see* Outpatient Care File (OPC)
OPD. *see* outpatient department (OPD)
open blind trial, 345
opportunistic conditions, 34
ordinary least squares (OLS), 366, 428
OTC. *see* over the counter (OTC) medications
(OTC) medications, 25
outcome categories, 46

Outcome equations, 417t
Outcomes Movement, 172, 206
out-of-sample validation, 425
Outpatient Care File (OPC), 292
outpatient department (OPD), 240
outpatient files, 16
Outpatient Parenteral Antimicrobial Therapy (OPAT), 302
overdose, 63
over the counter (OTC) medications, 57
Oxford Handicap Scale, 326

**P**

paid, amount, 18–19
pain intensity and pain relief, 143
pain interference, assessment of, 143
pain severity, assessment of, 143
Pain Treatment Satisfaction Scale, 143
parameter of interest, 362
parameter value, 427
parametric distribution, 419
parametric statistical test, 428
Parkinson's disease (PD), 328–329
patient
 activities, monitoring of, 84
 age, 19
 cohort stratification, 51
 confidentiality provisions, 137
 demographic files, 16, 21
 discharge status (living or deceased), 19
 education, 3
 identification numbers, 16
 interview techniques, 59
 prescription drug usage, monitoring of, 126
 quality-of-life, 49
 registries, 8
patient-centered care, 3, 125, 207
patient diaries, 318–319
patient-focused approach, 209
patient interviews, 318–319
patient-observed covariates (predictors), 405
patient populations, identification of, 19
Patient Record Forms (PRFs), 242
patient registries

and administrative claims, 304
checklists for reporting results, 308
classifications of, 301–302
and clinical trials, 304
Clozaril National Registry (CNR), 302
combination registries, 309–310
Congenital Defects registry, 303
defined, 298
design and preparation of, 305–306
and development and conceptual
    applications of, 298
development of, 299–300
disease specific registries, 301–302
disease-specific registries, 303
and electronic health records (EHR),
    303–304
and ethical issues, 307
limitations and challenges of, 308
myelodysplastic syndrome/
    myelodysplasia (MDS) registry, 303
product-specific registries, 301–302
roles in health and disease management,
    298–309
SEER registry, 303
and sources of potential patients,
    301–302
and state governments, 303–304
and volunteer recruiting sites on the
    Internet, 303
patient-reported outcomes (PROs)
    administration methods, 141, 146–147
    and challenges of application, 151–152
    and clinical trials, 153
cognitive debriefing of instruments, 158
    and computerized adaptive tests (CAT),
        166
    defined, 133
    as defined by the FDA, 142
    design and development of instruments,
        141
    and differential item functioning (DIF),
        165
    and identification of unexpected
        problems, 151
    internal consistency of instruments, 156
    interpretability, assessment of, 160–161

inter-rater reliability assessments
    (interviewers), 157
item driven, 163
limitations of, 166
and long-term treatment outcomes, 134
measurement properties of, 151
methodologies for conducting, 135
and monitoring patients' disease
    progression, 151
overview, 5
and patient satisfaction, 207
and pharmaceutical companies, 151
pilot testing of instruments, 158
and psychometric merits of, 152
qualitative and quantitative outcomes,
    143
and randomized controlled trials (RCTs),
    316
and recall difficulties, 135
reliability of instruments, 156
and response rates, 134
and response sets, 136
responsiveness, assessment of, 160–161
scale driven, 163
scoring of, 147
stability of instruments, 157
test-retest reliability, 157
and translation into other languages,
    141, 148–149
uses for, 134
validated and nonvalidated instruments,
    141, 148
validity and reliability of, 153–157
validity of, 135
and the value of difficulty parameter, 164
Patient-Reported Outcomes Measurement
    Information System (PROMIS), 163
Patient Safety Indicators (PSI), 268
patient safety indicators (PSIs), 117
patient satisfaction
    and adherence to therapy and treatment
        regimens, 212
    clinical and nonclinical aspects of, 209
    historical perspective of, 206
    instruments to measure, 210

## Index

lack of standardization in measuring, 214
patient satisfaction instruments for different services in health care, 218t–219t
Patient Satisfaction Questionnaire (PSQ), 210–211
Patient Treatment File (PTF), 292
pay-for-performance measures, in HDM programs, 48
PBM. *see* Pharmacy Benefits Management (PBM)
PCSQ. *see* Pharmaceutical Care Satisfaction Questionnaire (PCSQ)
PD. *see* Parkinson's disease (PD)
PDE. *see* prescription drug event (PDE)
PDI. *see* Pediatric Quality Indicators (PDI)
Pearson correlation coefficient, 157, 375
Pediatric Quality Indicators (PDI), 267
peer-reviewed journal articles, 259, 261
percentile method, 420
percentile-t method, 420
periconceptional folate, 303
peripheral vascular disease, 59
peripheral vascular occlusive disease, extremitiy, 402
personal health records (PHR)
    and patient healthcare management, 86
    patient managed, 81
    unreliable and incomplete, 103–104
PGC. *see* Psychiatric GWAS Consortium (PGC)
Pharmaceutical Care Satisfaction Questionnaire (PCSQ), 211
pharmacoeconomics, 374
pharmacoepidemiology, 255
pharmacotherapy, 319
pharmacovigilance, 302
pharmacy benefits, 57
Pharmacy Benefits Management (PBM), 293
pharmacy claims, focus of, 20
pharmacy provider, 21
pharmacy services, 211
phenotyped case-control, 327
phenotypic data, 329
PHI. *see* protected health information (PHI)
Philadelphia chromosome, 324

PHR. *see* personal health records (PHR)
physical role limitations, 190
physician conduct, 210
physician identification numbers
    DEA numbers, 18
    license numbers, 18
physician orders, standardized, 64
physician services, 210
placebo group, 343
plasma phosphate and renal function loss, 356
population-based approaches, 256
population-based cancer registries, 303
population-based data sources, 223, 223f
population studies, 84
postmenopausal estrogen, 415
Potential Confounders to Consider for Retrospective DURs, 67t
PPI. *see* proton-pump inhibitor (PPI)
PPO. *see* preferred provider organization (PPO)
PQI. *see* Prevention Quality Indicators (PQI)
prediction models in HDM research programs, 423
predictive accuracy, 423
predictive validity, 160
preexisting conditions, 24
preferred provider organization (PPO), 22
Premier Health Care Alliance, 263
Premier Hospital database, 287
prescriber, 21
prescription databases, 54–55
prescription drug benefits, 57
prescription drug event (PDE), 283
prescription drug files, 20
prescription drugs, days' supply in claims data, 37
presenteeism (decreased on-the-job productivity), 188–189, 192–195, 199–200
prevalence of disease, 32
Prevention Quality Indicators (PQI), 267
PRFs. *see* Patient Record Forms (PRFs)
primary sampling units (PSUs), 240–241
principal theory, 360
private insurers, claims data from, 22

probability theory, 366
probit regression, 418
procedural coding, 4, 82, 100
Procedure Classes, 266
PRO domain, 156
productivity, lost, 3
productivity and work outcomes, 188–189, 196
productivity instruments, important questions, 197–198
productivity instruments that assess presenteeism and absenteeism, 202t
*Product of a Hospital, The*, 133
product safety, monitoring of, 8
PRO instruments, 7, 135–136, 141
PROMIS. *see* Patient-Reported Outcomes Measurement Information System (PROMIS)
propensity score, 406
propensity score analysis, 56
propensity score methods, 338, 402, 405–406
prophylactic enoxaparin, 64
proportional hazards, 384, 429
PRO response options, 145t
PROs. *see* patient-reported outcomes (PROs)
prospective observational study, 298
prospective studies
    analysis of results, 350–351
    defined, 350
    designing of, 350
    and odds ratios, 351
    versus retrospective studies, 355
Prospective versus retrospective study design, 356f
prostate cancer, stage IV, 417
protected health information (PHI), 304, 306
proteinuria, 327
proton-pump inhibitor (PPI), 398
provider activities, monitoring of, 84
provider number, 16
PSIs. *see* patient safety indicators (PSIs)
PSQ. *see* Patient Satisfaction Questionnaire (PSQ)
PSUs. *see* primary sampling units (PSUs)
Psychiatric GWAS Consortium (PGC), 327

psychiatry and associations between genetics and disease, 327
psychometric methods for PRO instrument development, 152
psychometric methods recommended for PRO instrument validation, 154t–155t
psychotropic medications, 59
PTF. *see* Patient Treatment File (PTF)
Public Health Service Act, 243

Q

QALYs. *see* quality-adjusted life years (QALYs)
QI. *see* Quality indicators (QIs)
QIO. *see* quality improvement organization (QIO)
QOL. *see* quality-of-life (QOL)
qualitative measures, 365
qualitative versus quantitative outcomes, 365
quality-adjusted life years (QALYs), 176
quality control checks, 244
Quality Enhancement by Strategic Teaming (QuEST), 319
quality improvement organization (QIO), 123
Quality indicators (QIs), 117
quality of care, 6
quality-of-care data, requiring physicians to report, 49
quality-of-life (QOL), 141, 143, 393
Quality of Well-Being Scale (QWB), 175, 190
quantitative comparative controlled experiments, 343
quantitative empirical analyses, 335
quasi-experiments, 347
query language, standard, 120
QuEST. *see* Quality Enhancement by Strategic Teaming (QuEST)
QWB, 190

R

racial disparities, 417
radioactive fallout, 347
Ramsey Sedation Scale, 118–119
RAND Health Insurance Experiment, 172
randomization, methods of, 344

*Index*

randomized controlled trials (RCTs), 4–5, 336
randomized controlled trials (RCTs)
   clinical maneuvers (interventions), 343
   comparative studies (comparison of two or more interventions), 343
   and confounding factors, 388–391
   confounding factors in, 344
   controls and placebos, 343
   defined, 343
   and discrete outcomes, 365
   and ethics, 346
   and experimental treatments, 344
   and the Hawthorne effect, 344
   inclusion and exclusion criteria, 345
   investigators, 343
   key features of, 343–344
   limitations of, 346
   participants or subjects (study populations), 343
   and perceptions of treatments, 345
   and pharmacotherapy versus surgical intervention, 345
   and random allocation, achieving, 344
   and risk-benefit ratio, 345
   types of trials in, 345
   use of data from, 315–319
rating scale, 56
RBRVS. *see* Resource-Based Relative Value Scale (RBRVS)
RCD. *see* Research Data Center (RDC)
RCI. *see* Reliable Change Index (RCI)
rDURs. *see* retrospective DURs (rDURs)
readjustment counseling centers (Vet Centers), 290
real-time analysis, 116, 119–120
real-time applications, 115–121
real-time data, 115–120
real-time data monitoring, 115
real-time EHR applications, 121
Real-time Outbreak Detection System (RODS), 91
recalibration, 128, 179
recall bias, 193, 318, 353
receiver operating characteristic (ROC), 160, 424

recombinant tissue plasminogen activator (rt-PA), 287
RECs. *see* Regional Extension Centers (RECs)
reference category, 370
Regenstrief Medical Record System (RMS), 122
Regional Extension Centers (RECs), 111, 124
Regional Health Information Organizations, 104
registry-based data collection, 308
registry data, advantages of using, 307
registry design, 305
registry development, 8, 224, 298–299
Registry of Patient Registries (RoPR), 309
regression analysis
   for binary outcomes, 365
   for categorical outcomes, 365
regression coefficients, 367, 376
regression discontinuity analysis, 5
regression error term distribution, 428
regression estimation, 135, 428
regression imputation method, 395
regression model, 348, 366, 376–377, 384–385
reimbursement by the insurance company, amount, 19
Relative risk (RR) and odds ratios (OR), 353t
Relative risk of disease in men and women treated with simvastatin, 353t
Reliable Change Index (RCI), 162
renal replacement therapy, 355
renal therapy, protective, 60
ResDAC. *see* Research Data Assistance Center (ResDAC)
Research Data Assistance Center (ResDAC), 23, 282
Research Data Center (RDC), 243
research identifiable files (RIFs), 281
research purposes, de-identifying for, 22
research recruitment for PROs, 137–138
residential units (RUs), 228
Resource-Based Relative Value Scale (RBRVS), 19
resources, utilization of, 47
resource utilizations, 318
respondent burden, 147, 156

response items, 164
response rate, 7, 64, 133–135, 138, 227–229
response sets, 135–136
response shift to PROs, 136
restricted randomization, 344
restriction, exclusion, 390, 400
retrospective case series, 158
retrospective cohort study, 55, 358
retrospective cost-effectiveness, 294
retrospective DURs (rDURs)
    and appropriate drug dosage, 63
    and appropriateness of drug therapy, 58
    and case-control studies, 55
    and case-crossover studies, 55
    and claims-based studies, 53, 54
    and comorbid conditions, 56
    defined, 53
    and drug-disease contraindications, 62
    and drug-drug interactions (DDIs), 62
    drug utilization issues, 61
    and the elderly, 58
    involving generic drugs, 61
    and Medicare Part D, 57
    methodological issues, 53–55
    and over the counter (OTC) medications, 57
    and patients' insurance coverage, 57
    and prescribing errors, 56
    and retrospective cohort studies, 55
    seven categories of, 58
    and specificity of drugs, 55
    and State Medicaid agencies, 58
    study designs, 55
    and therapeutic duplication, 63
retrospective patient recall, 305
retrospective studies
    data sources, 357
    designing of, 338
    explained, 355
    versus prospective studies, 355
    types of, 358
RIF data available from CMS, 283t
RIFs. see research identifiable files (RIFs)
risk adjustment for disease level, 51
risk factors, 31
risk ratios, 368

risk stratification, 424
risk stratification methods, 385
RMS. see Regenstrief Medical Record System (RMS)
ROC. see receiver operating characteristic (ROC)
RODS. see Real-time Outbreak Detection System (RODS)
RoPR. see Registry of Patient Registries (RoPR)
RTCs. see randomized controlled trials (RCTs)
rt-PA. see recombinant tissue plasminogen activator (rt-PA)
RUs. see residential units (RUs)

**S**

safety, monitoring of, 298
SAFs. see standard analytical files (SAFs)
sample selection methods, 338, 398–400
SAQ. see self-administered questionnaire (SAQ)
SASD. see State Ambulatory Surgery Databases (SASD)
schizoaffective disorder, 327
schizophrenia, 327
SD. see standard deviation (SD)
SDO. see Standard Developing Organization (SDO)
SDQ. see Strengths and Difficulties Questionnaire (SDQ)
SEARCH. see Study of the Effectiveness of Additional Reductions in Cholesterol and Homocysteine (SEARCH)
SEDD. see State Emergency Department Databases (SEDD)
SEER. see National Cancer Institute's Surveillance Epidemiology and End-Results (SEER)
SEER registry, 303
Selected registries from 1998 to 2008, 310t–311t
selection bias, 14, 294, 315, 398
selection issues, 402
self-administered questionnaire (SAQ), 228

*Index*

SEM. *see* standard deviation error of measurement (SEM)
sensitivity analysis, 407
sentiment analysis, 120
sentinel effect, the, 65
sentinel events or safety signals, 117
service date coding, 18
severity-adjusted codes, 20
SF-36 (Short Form 36) Health Status Questionnaire, 175–177
SGA. *see* subjective global assessment (SGA)
SHARe. *see* SNP Health Association Resource (SHARe)
short form health survey (SF-36), 133
Sickness Impact Profile, 175, 190
SID. *see* State Inpatient Databases (SID)
single blind trial, 345
single-sourced claims, 22
Slone Epidemiology Center at Boston University, 303
smoking cessation, 48, 138, 398, 402
SNP Health Association Resource (SHARe) databases, 224
  databases for genetic testing, 324
  and integrated genetics databases, 325
social desirability response to PROs, 136
Social Security Act, and Medicare, 281
Social Security Administration (SSA) death file, 292
socioeconomic status, low, 24
socioeconomic status of patients, 51
software programs, statistical, 232
Spearman-Brown adjustment, 156
specific conditions, and PROs, 134
stabilization of samples, 419
standard analytical files (SAFs), 283
standard care, 401
Standard Developing Organization (SDO), 80
standard deviation (SD), 162
standard deviation error of measurement (SEM), 162
standard errors, 419
standardized coding of data, lack of, 111
standard query language, 94
Stanford Presenteeism Scale, 194

State Ambulatory Surgery Databases (SASD), 258, 261–262
State Emergency Department Databases (SEDD), 258–260, 262
State Inpatient Databases (SID), 258, 261
statins, 59
statistical analysis, 423
statistical calculations, 419
statistical modeling techniques, 391
statistical process control, 115, 118
stem cell transplantation, 260
stepwise procedure, 378
stepwise regression, 377, 424
stickers in patient charts, 64
stochastic regression imputation, 396
strata, 344
stratification, 351, 391
stratification matching schemes, 406
stratified analyses, 390, 401
stratified randomization, 344
stratified sample, 258
Strengthening the Reporting of Observational Studies in Epidemiology (STROBE), 309
Strengths and Difficulties Questionnaire (SDQ), 328
STROBE. *see* Strengthening the Reporting of Observational Studies in Epidemiology (STROBE)
stroke, ischemic, 287, 326
strokes, 59
structural validity, 158
Study of the Effectiveness of Additional Reductions in Cholesterol and Homocysteine (SEARCH), 325
subjective global assessment (SGA), 355
Supplemental Files for Revisit Analyses, 271
support, social, 51
surgical procedures, 19
Surveillance Epidemiology and End Results (SEER), 287–288, 303, 341, 417
survey data, 28
survey design, 225, 228–230, 247
survival analysis, 381–383
survival curve, 383
survival function, 381

syndromic surveillance systems, 116

**T**
target populations, identifying
    based on medical condition, 30
    in chronic medical conditions, 45
    for health and disease management, 30
    using claims data, 45
teaching and illness figure, 412f
telehealth
    defined, 87
    programs, 127
telemedicine
    defined, 87
    group therapy sessions, 87
    and heart monitoring, 87
    over the Internet, 87
    to provide health care to rural areas, 87
    and remote monitoring devices, 87
    and sending reminders, 87
terminology and definitions (for chapter 14), 168t
test-retest reliability, timing of, 157
theory based test, 429t
therapeutic duplication
    defined, 63
    due to miscommunication, 63
    and OTC medications, 63
therapeutic index, narrow, 61
thrombosis, deep venous, 60
time horizon, 35
time t, 381
time-varying covariates, 385
TMR. *see* Medical Record, The (TMR)
Transparent Reporting of Evaluations with Nonrandomized Designs (TREND), 309
TREND. *see* Transparent Reporting of Evaluations with Nonrandomized Designs (TREND)
triple blind trial, 345–346
true score theory. *see* classical test theory (CTT)
Truncated Tobit model, 401, 403
Truven Health Analytics, 263
t-test, 416
tumor registries, 34

Type I and Type II errors in hypothesis testing, 364t

**U**
UCL. *see* upper control limits (UCL)
underdose, 63
undiagnosed conditions, 31
Uniform Billing Forms, 257
uninsured patients, 255
unique physician identification number (UPIN), 284
United States National Center for Health Statistics, 17
United States President's Council of Advisors on Science and Technology, 330
universal provider identification numbers (UPINs), 18
unmeasurable variables, 316
unmeasured factors, 415
up-coding to increase reimbursement, 25
UPIN. *see* unique physician identification number (UPIN)
UPINs. *see* universal provider identification numbers (UPINs)
upper control limits (UCL), 115
urologist, 417
uroselective alpha-blockers, 348
US Census Bureau, 190
US Department of Defense (DOD), 128
US Department of Health and Human Services (HHS). *see* Department of Health and Human Services (HHS)
US Department of Veterans Affairs (VA), 86, 123
US Health Information Knowledgebase (USHIK), 226
USHIK. *see* US Health Information Knowledgebase (USHIK)
utilization reviews, 75

**V**
VA. *see* Department of Veterans Affairs (VA)
vaccine effectiveness, 352
VA/Centers for Medicare and Medicaid Services (CMS) Data, 292–293
VA Decision Support System (DSS), 292

## Index

VA disability benefit, 290
VA Information Resource Center (VIReC), 290–291
validation assessments, 33
validation methods
    cross-validation, 425
    external validation, 425
    hold-out, 425
    k-fold method, 425
    out-of-sample validation, 425
    prediction model, 423
validity of patient-reported outcomes (PROs)
    concurrent validity, 160
    construct validity, 158
    content validity, 157–158
    convergent validity, 159
    criterion validity, 159
    discriminate validity, 159
    divergent validity, 159
    extreme groups validity, 160
    face validity, 157
    known groups validity, 160
    predictive validity, 160
    and reliability, 153–157
    structural validity, 158
*Value in Health*, 141, 148
VA Medical SAS Datasets, 292
VA outpatient pharmacy, 293
VA patient Medicare utilization data, 291
variable analysis, 5
variables
    background, 390
    behavioral health, 308
    binary-dependent, 416
    categorical, 369–370
    confounding, 390
    continuous, 365
    core set, 261
    demographic, 424
    dependent, 348, 360, 393
    endogenous, 413
    explanatory, 370, 393
    independent, 360
    instrumental, 338, 347
    missing, 307
    multiple explanatory, 381
    omitted, 415
    outcome, 401
    output, 405
    random, 374, 428
    response, 399
    selection methods of, 377
    stratification, 406
    time-dependent, 384
VAS. *see* visual analogue scales (VAS)
VCFs. *see* vertebral compression fractures (VCFs)
vertebral compression fractures (VCFs), 32
Veteran Integrated Service Networks (VISNs), 290
Veterans Health Administration (VHA)
    data available from, 7, 290
    data resources of, 291–292
    datasets for inpatient care, 292
    and death information, 292
    functions of, 290
    and Health and Disease Management (HDM), 294
    as an insurer, 290
    programs described, 224
    and standard medical benefits package, 290
    strengths and limitations of data, 295–296
    surveys to assess quality of life, 295
    and the VA formulary, 294
    Vital Status Files, 292
Veterans Health Information Systems and Technology Architecture (VistA), 86, 123, 291
VHA. *see* Veterans Health Administration (VHA)
videoconferencing and consultation capabilities, 87
VIReC. *see* VA Information Resource Center (VIReC)
Virginia Cancer Registry, 34
VISN data warehouses, 293
VISNs. *see* Veteran Integrated Service Networks (VISNs)

VistA. *see* Veterans Health Information Systems and Technology Architecture (VistA)
VISTA database, 294
visual analogue scales (VAS), 143
Vital Status File, 292, 294

**W**
waiver programs, 16
weighting procedures, 231
Wellcome Trust Case Control Consortium (WTCCC), 329
Well-Integrated Screening and Evaluation of Women Across the Nation (WISEWOMAN), 341
wellness programs, employer-based, 138
WHO. *see* World Health Organization (WHO)
Wilcoxon-Mann-Whitney test, 429
Wilson and Cleary model, 172–173
WISEWOMAN. *see* Well-Integrated Screening and Evaluation of Women Across the Nation (WISEWOMAN)
WLQ. *see* Work Limitations Questionnaire (WLQ)
work disability, 191
workforce productivity, 188
Work Limitations Questionnaire (WLQ), 194
work outcomes
 and productivity, 188–189
 terminology, 189
workplace productivity and illness, 188–189, 192
Work Productivity and Activity Impairment Questionnaire (WPAI), 194
Work Productivity and Activity Impairment Questionnaire–Allergy Specific, 194
Work Productivity and Activity Impairment Questionnaire-general health version (WPAI:GH), 194
Work Productivity and Activity Impairment Questionnaire-specific health problem version (WPAI:SHP), 194
Work Productivity Short Inventory, 194
work role-related outcomes, 189
World Health Organization (WHO), 17, 64, 172

WPAI. *see* Work Productivity and Activity Impairment Questionnaire (WPAI)
WPAI:GH. *see* Work Productivity and Activity Impairment Questionnaire-general health version (WPAI:GH)
WPAI:SHP. *see* Work Productivity and Activity Impairment Questionnaire-specific health problem version (WPAI:SHP)
WTCCC. *see* Wellcome Trust Case Control Consortium (WTCCC)

**Z**
zero dollar claim, 40